L) 39

MW01295080

Gambling Disorder

Andreas Heinz
Nina Romanczuk-Seiferth
Marc N. Potenza
Editors

Gambling Disorder

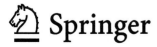 Springer

Editors
Andreas Heinz
Department of Psychiatry
and Psychotherapy
Charité – University Medicine Berlin
Berlin
Germany

Nina Romanczuk-Seiferth
Department of Psychiatry
and Psychotherapy
Charité – University Medicine Berlin
Berlin
Germany

Marc N. Potenza
Department of Psychiatry
Yale University
New Haven, CT
USA

ISBN 978-3-030-03058-2   ISBN 978-3-030-03060-5   (eBook)
https://doi.org/10.1007/978-3-030-03060-5

Library of Congress Control Number: 2018966544

© Springer Nature Switzerland AG 2019
This work is subject to copyright. All rights are reserved by the Publisher, whether the whole or part of the material is concerned, specifically the rights of translation, reprinting, reuse of illustrations, recitation, broadcasting, reproduction on microfilms or in any other physical way, and transmission or information storage and retrieval, electronic adaptation, computer software, or by similar or dissimilar methodology now known or hereafter developed.
The use of general descriptive names, registered names, trademarks, service marks, etc. in this publication does not imply, even in the absence of a specific statement, that such names are exempt from the relevant protective laws and regulations and therefore free for general use.
The publisher, the authors, and the editors are safe to assume that the advice and information in this book are believed to be true and accurate at the date of publication. Neither the publisher nor the authors or the editors give a warranty, express or implied, with respect to the material contained herein or for any errors or omissions that may have been made. The publisher remains neutral with regard to jurisdictional claims in published maps and institutional affiliations.

This Springer imprint is published by the registered company Springer Nature Switzerland AG
The registered company address is: Gewerbestrasse 11, 6330 Cham, Switzerland

Contents

What Is an Addiction?

Andreas Heinz and Anne Beck

1.1 Introduction

When should behavioural problems such as pathological gambling be considered to be an addiction?

If we want to define addictive disorders, we can look at current classification systems, neurobiological findings and the intuitions that structure both clinical and biological research. In this chapter, we will start with the classification systems and their underlying ideas, discuss the plausibility of neurobiological correlates and consistency of respective findings and finally compare some key theories about addiction that are currently guiding research.

In ICD-10 as well as DSM-IV, substance-related addictions are characterized by the development of tolerance to the effects of the drug of abuse, the manifestation of withdrawal symptoms upon detoxification, strong craving to consume the drug (this criterion was only recently introduced in DSM-5 and was not previously listed in DSM-IV) and reduced control of drug intake (in DSM-IV and DSM-5, this criterion is differentiated into the aspect of long-term high drug intake on the one hand and unsuccessful attempts to reduce it on the other hand). Further criteria describe harmful consequences of drug intake as well as a substantial increase in time spent to acquire and consume the drug of abuse at the expense of other activities [1–3]. In ICD-10 and DSM-IV, harmful drug use in the absence of further key aspects of substance dependence was classified as a separate category, while in DSM-5, harmful use, associated social problems and impairment of important obligations have been included together with the previously listed symptoms of

A. Heinz (✉) · A. Beck
Department of Psychiatry and Psychotherapy, Charité—Universitätsmedizin Berlin, Berlin, Germany
e-mail: andreas.heinz@charite.de; anne.beck@charite.de

© Springer Nature Switzerland AG 2019
A. Heinz et al. (eds.), *Gambling Disorder*, https://doi.org/10.1007/978-3-030-03060-5_1

addiction into a dimensional approach that classifies substance use disorders [2]. A rationale behind this decision was that in epidemiological studies, there is a continuous increase in drug-related problems rather than sharp boundaries distinguishing harmful use from addiction. On the other hand, it has been criticized that if DSM-5 criteria are applied, legal restrictions (e.g. due to alcohol being illegal in many countries) can turn the desire to consume a glass of wine in the evening into a substance use disorder if acquiring and consuming the illegal drug causes social problems and, for example, due to incarceration, impairs performance in accordance with important social obligations [4]. With respect to non-substance-related disorders, DSM-5 was the first classification system to include certain behavioural syndromes in the wider category of addiction [2]. More specifically, pathological gambling, which in DSM-IV was classified as a disorder of impulse control, is now included in this wider addiction category. Transferring the concepts of substance-related addiction into the area of behavioural syndromes, tolerance development can be compared to the observation of increasing amounts of money required to satisfy the gambler's desire to participate in the game, withdrawal symptoms can be represented by restlessness and dysphoria when gambling is interrupted, craving and a rather large amount of time dedicated to the addiction can be indicated by a gambler being preoccupied with his or her game, and loss of control can be reflected in unsuccessful attempts to control or even stop gambling. Further rather specific syndromes associated with pathological gambling are chasing losses, i.e. the attempt to regain larger amounts of money previously lost in the gamble by increasing stakes, the use of gambling as a maladaptive tool to cope with negative emotions as well as the reliance on others to provide enough money to continue gambling. In accordance with the dimensional approach of DSM-5, social problems and impaired role performance, which previously represented criteria for harmful addictive behaviour, are now also included as criteria used to classify gambling disorder as an addiction.

Current classification systems claim that all symptoms are to be treated equal and that the presence or absence of two or more symptoms fulfilling the criteria listed above suffices to diagnose an addiction [2]. However, it is immediately clear that with respect to neurobiological research, some of the symptoms listed above have rather clear-cut biological correlates, while others are so deeply embedded in social interactions and legislation that the search for neurobiological correlates appears to be not only hopeless but also misguided. A famous example is the now abolished criterion "repetitive problems with the law", which was reflected in "illegal acts associated with gambling" in the former classification of pathological gambling in DSM-IV. But even beyond such descriptions of problematic behaviour that clearly depend upon legislation, social problems and impairments in role performance depend very strongly on cultural and social settings as well as demands on the individual [4]. The same is true with respect to the time required to get and consume a drug of abuse or to participate in gambling: This criterion is strongly influenced by the availability of the desired acts, which is of course reduced when the substance is illegal or gambling is prohibited. Accordingly, neurobiological research has largely focussed on the development of tolerance, withdrawal symptoms associated with the sudden interruption of drug intake or gambling, craving for the addictive behaviour or drug of abuse as well as reduced control in dealing with drug intake or gambling [5–8].

1.2 Addiction Versus Dependence: Conceptual Changes

Traditionally, there has been a shift in focus when dealing with addictive disorders: Some decades ago, Edwards focussed on the "dependence" aspect of addictive behaviours, suggesting that tolerance development and withdrawal symptoms are at the core of drug-related problems [9]. Specifically, Edwards [9] suggested that all drugs of abuse cause biological alterations when chronically consumed, which result in withdrawal symptoms once their intake is stopped. In accordance with this hypothesis, Koob and Le Moal suggested that such neuroadaptive changes due to chronic drug intake result in establishing a new homeostasis, which depends on the continuation of drug consumption [5]. For example, alcohol stimulates GABAergic inhibition in the brain [10], and a long-term downregulation of GABA-A receptors has been observed in detoxified alcohol-dependent patients [10–12]. This down-regulation of GABA-A receptors apparently balances the inhibitory effects of alcohol on GABA-A receptors. However, once alcohol intake is suddenly stopped, for example, in severe alcohol dependence during night sleep, GABA-A receptors remain downregulated, while there is a lack of the inhibitory effect of the drug of abuse. The loss of homeostasis represents a dysbalance between excitation and inhibition and contributes to withdrawal symptoms such as seizures [13]. Furthermore, if such inhibitory drug effects interact with second messenger systems in core areas of the autonomic nervous system including the locus coeruleus, impaired inhibition of this brain area can contribute to vegetative withdrawal symptoms [14–16]. According to Edwards [9], such withdrawal symptoms regularly occur following chronic drug intake and are a hallmark of substance dependence [9]. Moreover, Edwards [9] suggested to focus on the dependence aspect of addictions, because the term "addict" itself can have stigmatizing effects. Today, we see a shift of the research focus away from questions of drug tolerance and dependence towards what is considered to be key aspects of addition, i.e. strong drug craving and loss of control [2]. This shift of focus enabled the American Psychiatric Association to classify pathological gambling as an addiction: Tolerance development and withdrawal symptoms are particularly strong if the consumed drug of abuse has inhibitory effects on certain brain areas including the autonomic nervous system. Gambling and other addictive behaviours, however, are usually not sedative and—unlike drugs of abuse—do not directly interfere with inhibitory and excitatory systems in the central nervous system [5, 17, 18]. While there can be dysphoria and restlessness in gamblers who are suddenly interrupted when participating in their game or when being confronted with gambling machines they are not allowed to use [19, 20], such withdrawal symptoms are usually rather mild and hard to distinguish from some aspects of craving for the behaviour. Therefore, both research on non-substance-related addictions including gambling and a current neurobiological focus on brain areas and neurotransmitter systems associated with motivation and executive control shifted research on substance dependence towards the "addiction" aspect, i.e. craving and control impairment.

1.3   Key Neurobiological Findings in Addiction Research

Indeed, neurobiological research on addiction has its most consistent findings with respect to the correlates of drug craving and a bias towards drug intake at the expense of other activities, which—when consciously not accepted and accompanied by claims that the person actually wants to do otherwise—often counts as an indicator of control impairment. Further aspects of control impairment include impulsive responding to small rewards that are immediately available instead of waiting for larger rewards and by impaired motor control when having to interrupt a motor tendency to respond to certain stimuli [21]. However, these different aspects of impulsivity often do not correlate at all with each other, questioning the concept of "impulsivity" as a coherent and useful construct in addiction research [22].

More consistent results have been acquired with respect to drug craving and aspects of loss of control associated with dopamine dysfunction in the ventral striatum and further brain areas associated with the so-called reward system [23, 24]. Indeed, all drugs of abuse release dopamine in the ventral striatum and thus reinforce drug consumption [25]. Unlike natural reinforcers, drugs of abuse continue to release dopamine upon re-exposure; thus the dopamine response to drugs fails to habituate. Moreover, dopamine release associated with drugs of abuse is usually much higher than dopamine release associated with natural reinforcers [25–29]. However, direct evidence for sensitized or increased dopamine release, as postulated by some addiction theories [30, 31], is hard to verify in humans, because even functional magnetic resonance imaging with its time frame of seconds is not able to track phasic dopamine release alterations appearing in the range of milliseconds [32]. However, recent research suggest that such short bursts of dopamine release indeed activate the ventral striatum as measured with optogenetic functional magnetic resonance imaging in awake rodents [33], thus suggesting that studies on cue-induced functional activation of the ventral striatum elicited by drug versus neutral or nondrug reward anticipatory cues indeed reflect alterations in dopaminergic signalling.

It is quite plausible that certain gambles and other addictive behaviours repetitively and unphysiologically strongly activate dopamine release in the ventral striatum, and in accordance with this hypothesis, indirect evidence for ventral striatal dysfunction in gambling has been reported [6, 34–37]. In this context, compensatory downregulation of dopamine receptors in the ventral striatum and blunting of functional activation of this brain area elicited by non-addictive reward-indicating cues has repeatedly been observed [6, 35, 38–40]. Such alterations in dopaminergic neurotransmission and the associated functional activation have often but not always been associated with the experience of subjective craving [41–43]. Craving, however, is a conscious process reported by the individual and requires a certain degree of self-reflection and openness towards one's own experiences as well as interpersonal trust for sharing it with an observer. More direct ways to assess drug craving are measures of implicit drug approach tendencies as observed with the alcohol approach-avoidance task (alcohol AAT [44, 45]), where it has been observed that, for example, alcohol-dependent patients tend to pull alcohol cues towards themselves and need more time when required to push them away compared with nondrug-related stimuli [44, 45].

While there is some evidence that alterations in the so-called reward system contribute to craving for drugs as well as non-substance-related addictions including gambling, there is less consistent neurobiological findings with respect to the clinical symptom of impaired control over drug intake or gambling. An aspect of loss of control that is directly related to reward system alterations in addiction is given by an unconscious bias of behaviour towards drug consumption or pathological gambling at the expense of other activities. Such behavioural biases may be due to the fact that drugs of abuse as well as behavioural addictions activate dopamine release in the ventral striatum more strongly than natural reinforcers [25], thus reinforcing drug consumption or pathological gambling more strongly. Furthermore, increased presynaptic dopamine release can lead to neuroadaptive alterations, e.g. in the availability of dopamine D2 receptors, as observed for chronic alcohol intake in rodents [46] as well as in human alcohol-dependent patients [41, 42, 47]. Downregulation of dopamine receptors may help to explain why natural reinforcers fail to activate the ventral striatum in addicted subjects [39, 40, 48]. However, why do drug-associated cues continue to activate the ventral striatum in many studies [40, 49, 50]? Animal experiments have shown that cues that predict reward are attributed with the same salience and motivational value as the reward itself, due to a shift of phasic dopamine release from reward reception to the surprising presentation of the conditioned cue that reliably predicts reward [32, 51]. Drug cues, which are associated with high drug reward, could thus cause increased ventral striatal activation due to such conditioning processes [52]. Beyond such conditioning processes, Robinson and Berridge [31] suggested that drugs "sensitize" dopamine release [31], with repeated drug use being associated with increased psychomotor stimulant properties of, e.g., cocaine and drug cues, which elicit increased dopamine release in individuals that tend to react strongly to reward-associated stimuli [53, 54]. If such experiments in animals can be transferred to humans, it is quite plausible that some but not all individuals are prone to strongly react to drug-associated cues. On the other hand, salience attribution per se should not be confounded with a strong approach bias towards the drug of abuse. In fact, Beck et al. [49] observed that functional activation of both the amygdala and the ventral striatum was increased in patients who prospectively remained abstinent rather than relapsed to alcohol use [49]. Increased amygdala activation, which was functionally connected to the centre of origin of dopaminergic neurons in the brainstem, may also help to attribute salience towards potentially negative stimuli such as alcohol pictures in patients who consciously decided to remain abstinent. Observing increased activation of the ventral striatum in prospective abstainers but not relapsers was surprising but may also be due to salience attribution rather than eliciting an approach bias by activation of this limbic part of the striatum [55].

The effects of Pavlovian conditioned stimuli on unrelated instrumental choice behaviour can be assessed using Pavlovian-to-instrumental-transfer tasks, in which such Pavlovian cues are presented as background stimuli while performing an unrelated choice. Applying such studies in humans, Garbusow et al. observed that appetitive cues tend to increase approach behaviour and aversive cues tend to decrease approach behaviour to a larger degree in detoxified alcohol-dependent patients compared to healthy controls [56], and assessment of the effects of alcohol cues in such settings is currently carried out. Such studies may help to shed more light on the effects of drug cues on approach behaviour and, in a larger theoretical framework, on reduced control of addictive behaviour due to an unconscious bias of instrumental choice towards drugs or pathological gambling.

1.4   Executive Control and Addictive Behaviour

Neurobiological correlates of reduced control of drug intake or addictive behaviour have also been associated with impaired executive control functions. In alcohol dependence, neurotoxic effects of alcohol intake can contribute to cortical atrophy, particularly in the prefrontal cortex, and thus impair executive functions such as working memory [57, 58]. Again, such neurotoxic drug effects are hard to observe in pathological gambling, where cortical functioning is rather unimpaired on a structural level. Also, studies in subjects at risk failed to reveal impaired frontocortical control functions and rather pointed to a bias of information processing towards drug-associated choices in association with ventral striatal activation [59]. Furthermore, some studies in alcohol-dependent patients suggest that bottom-up information processing from the ventral striatum to the prefrontal cortex rather than top-down control of motivational systems by the prefrontal cortex is impaired in alcohol dependence [60]. These observations are in line with current studies emphasizing the role of the ventral striatum in cortico-striatal-thalamic neurocircuits, which regulate complex behaviour [61, 62]. Altogether, impaired control is a key concept of addictive behaviour; however, whether there are clinically relevant alterations in non-substance-related addictions with respect to cortical control functions remains to be explored in more depth.

1.5   Addictions Versus Compulsions

So far, these considerations suggest that drug addiction is characterized by a bias of information processing particularly in the so-called reward system towards drug consumption and drug-associated cues. With respect to pathological gambling, there has also been observed reduced activation of the ventral striatum by non-gambling-related stimuli predicting financial reward (e.g. [6, 34]), while increased activation of various brain areas including the prefrontal cortex has been observed by drug-associated stimuli in pathological gambling (e.g. [63]). Do these neurobiological correlates suggest that addictions are specific types of compulsions, i.e.

which similarities and differences can be identified when comparing obsessive-compulsive (OCD) and addictive disorders?

It has long been shown that human choice behaviour largely depends upon information processing in fronto-striatal-thalamic neurocircuits [64]. With respect to drug addiction, Volkow and others have repeatedly observed that there is reduced glucose utilization in the frontal cortex in different substance-related addictions [65–67]. OCD, on the other hand, has been associated with increased glucose utilization in the frontal cortex and associative striatum [68–70]. More recent studies with functional magnetic resonance imaging revealed that different obsessive-compulsive behaviours such as washing or hording are associated with specific fronto-striatal-thalamic networks, which also include activation of further limbic brain areas such as the anterior insula [71]. Exposure to drug-related cues has also been associated with brain activation patterns inside and outside of fronto-striatal-thalamic networks [72]. However, the direction of the respective changes appears to be different between OCD and addiction, with increased long-term glucose utilization in the frontal cortex being observed in obsessive-compulsive disorders, while these brain areas are rather hypoactive in addiction except when momentarily activated by drug-associated cues [49, 73]. Clinically, we and others have observed that compulsions are rather permanently manifesting repetitive actions, which phenomenologically differ considerably from cue-induced drug craving and consumption [74, 75]. Therefore, while craving and drug consumption can be experienced as rather "compulsive" by patients, neurobiological similarities are limited and substantial differences are evident.

1.6   Summary and Outlook

Altogether, this review of neurobiological correlates of key symptoms of addiction suggests that tolerance development and withdrawal symptoms constitute core aspects of addiction [9]; however, such symptoms are usually rather mild in non-substance-related addictions due to the rather low sedative effects of such activities. Strong craving and a bias towards addictive behaviour, on the other hand, have repeatedly been associated with altered functional activation of neural circuits known to regulate choice behaviour, which strongly rely on ventral striatal activation embedded in circuits including the prefrontal cortex and thalamus as well as further limbic brain areas [76]. Such alterations can bias behaviour towards the drug of choice or the preferred addictive behaviour at the expense of other activities. However, we should be careful to rely on craving and reduced control as the only indicators of addictive behaviour: Every passion including dedicated research or romantic love can be characterized by strong craving and a certain focus of attention on this activity at the expense of others [77]. Therefore, it does not suffice to label some activities as helpful and others as harmful, because then social and legal tendencies, e.g. to ban a certain drug including alcohol from public consumption or to prohibit gambling, decide whether a certain behaviour is an addiction or not. Conceding this would mean that dominating morals and legislation and not medical criteria decide what behavioural syndromes constitute a clinically relevant mental malady. To avoid such confounds with changing morals, the diagnosis of a clinically relevant mental malady should, in our view, require that two of three criteria are fulfilled:

The first one is a decision on whether certain symptoms of a disorder are medically relevant, i.e. whether they can *generally* impair human life to a relevant degree (the disease criterion). This decision is not one based on natural science evidence but rather on plausibility and common sense. Not being able to roll your tongue is not a disease, because you do not need to roll your tongue to survive as a human being, while being unable to swallow is a symptom of a disease, because as humans we need to consume food to survive.

The second and third one depend upon the individual assessment of the consequences of these symptoms, i.e. do they harm the person by causing suffering (the illness criterion) or a severe limitation of social participation (the sickness criterion [77]).

With respect to key symptoms guiding the diagnosis of a disease, developing tolerance to a drug of abuse and showing withdrawal symptoms that can be lethal as in delirium tremens are clearly symptoms of a disease, because their manifestation can be life threatening. Other aspects of addictions such as strong craving and loss of control do not directly jeopardize human survival but can severely impair human life with others [77]. Assessing whether this is indeed the case, value judgements play a stronger role than when assessing withdrawal symptoms. Therefore, we have to be careful not to exclusively rely on symptoms such as craving and reduced control when diagnosing an addiction. Kant [78] has suggested that addictions are always characterized by a certain disinterest in another human being as an independent person with his or her own goals and way of life [78], and we suggest that beyond craving and loss of control, behavioural addictions are characterized by such a reduced interaction with other human beings. However, we warn that all these assessments strongly rely on contemporary value judgements and may be revised in the future in more tolerant or less liberal societies. Therefore, diagnosing an addiction in the absolute absence of tolerance development and withdrawal symptoms may not be recommendable and we indeed do not recommend to do so. We have suggested that other criteria to diagnose a medically relevant disease including harm to the person's health or role functioning or an increased amount of time necessary to acquire the drug of abuse or to gamble are of limited value: Physical harm, e.g. resulting from liver toxity of alcohol intake, can be objectified quite easily, while harmful effects on social interactions depend on legalization or punishment of drug consumption or gambling and also affect the time required to acquire or consume a drug of abuse or to find a place to gamble. Therefore, we feel that at the core of the medical diagnosis of a disease, a general impairment of mental functions relevant for human life needs to be diagnosed, and this diagnosis should rely on core aspects of addictions including tolerance development, withdrawal symptoms, craving and impaired control of the respective behaviour.

Furthermore, we suggest that diagnosing symptoms that indicate that a medical disease is present (the disease criterion) does not suffice to actually diagnose a clinically relevant mental malady. There are human beings who show clear indications of medically relevant dysfunctions including acoustic hallucinations, who neither suffer from them nor are impaired in their common performance of daily activities [79]. Therefore, beyond the medical disease aspect, the individual has to either suffer from these symptoms (the illness criterion) or be severely impaired in his or her social participation (the sickness criterion), particularly with respect to activities of daily living such as personal hygiene or food consumption etc. [77]. Beyond the assessment of generally relevant medical symptoms, any diagnosis of a clinically relevant disorder thus needs to also assess the personal consequences of such symptoms including individual suffering or the impairment to cope with activities of daily living [77]. We emphasize such a cautious approach to diagnosis in order to avoid that dictatorships or other ideological groups can start defining any unwanted behaviour as an addiction, for example, critical blogging in the Internet or, as was the case in ninetieth century, the attempts to escape from slavery as drapetomania [80, 81]. Behavioural addictions can have a profound negative impact on the life of the afflicted subjects; however, we have to make sure that diagnosing such an addiction is not abused to label socially unwanted behaviour, which is performed by individuals in spite of negative social pressure, as a mental malady. Therefore, the cautious approach of the American Psychiatric Association [2], which only classified gambling as an addictive disorder and abstained from labelling more behavioural syndromes including involvement in excessive sexual contacts or shopping, is quite warranted [2]. We hope that this book and its review of clinical as well as neurobiological findings on behavioural addictions will help to promote such a cautious and rational approach towards behavioural addictions.

References

1. American Psychiatric Association. Diagnostic and statistical manual of mental disorders. 4th ed., text rev. edn. Washington, DC; 2000.
2. American Psychiatric Association. Diagnostic and statistical manual of mental disorders (DSM-5). Washington, DC and London: American Psychiatric Publishing; 2013.
3. World Health Organization. ICD-10, international statistical classification of diseases and related health problems. 10th revision edn. Genf; 2013.
4. Heinz A, Friedel E. DSM-5: important changes in the field of addictive diseases. Nervenarzt. 2014;85(5):571–7.
5. Koob GF, Le Moal M. Drug abuse: hedonic homeostatic dysregulation. Science. 1997;278(5335):52–8.
6. Romanczuk-Seiferth N, Koehler S, Dreesen C, Wustenberg T, Heinz A. Pathological gambling and alcohol dependence: neural disturbances in reward and loss avoidance processing. Addict Biol. 2015;20(3):557–69.
7. Romanczuk-Seiferth N, van den Brink W, Goudriaan AE. From symptoms to neurobiology: pathological gambling in the light of the new classification in DSM-5. Neuropsychobiology. 2014;70(2):95–102.
8. Volkow ND, Fowler JS. Addiction, a disease of compulsion and drive: involvement of the orbitofrontal cortex. Cereb Cortex. 2000;10(3):318–25.
9. Edwards G. Withdrawal symptoms and alcohol dependence: fruitful mysteries. Br J Addict. 1990;85(4):447–61.

10. Krystal JH, Staley J, Mason G, Petrakis IL, Kaufman J, Harris RA, Gelernter J, Lappalainen J. Gamma-aminobutyric acid type A receptors and alcoholism: intoxication, dependence, vulnerability, and treatment. Arch Gen Psychiatry. 2006;63(9):957–68.
11. Clapp P, Bhave SV, Hoffman PL. How adaptation of the brain to alcohol leads to dependence: a pharmacological perspective. Alcohol Res Health. 2008;31(4):310–39.
12. De Witte P. Imbalance between neuroexcitatory and neuroinhibitory amino acids causes craving for ethanol. Addict Behav. 2004;29(7):1325–39.
13. Heinz A, Beck A, Wrase J, Mohr J, Obermayer K, Gallinat J, Puls I. Neurotransmitter systems in alcohol dependence. Pharmacopsychiatry. 2009;42(Suppl 1):S95–S101.
14. Akaoka H, Aston-Jones G. Opiate withdrawal-induced hyperactivity of locus coeruleus neurons is substantially mediated by augmented excitatory amino acid input. J Neurosci. 1991;11(12):3830–9.
15. Maldonado R, Stinus L, Gold LH, Koob GF. Role of different brain structures in the expression of the physical morphine withdrawal syndrome. J Pharmacol Exp Ther. 1992;261(2):669–77.
16. Rasmussen K, Beitner-Johnson DB, Krystal JH, Aghajanian GK, Nestler EJ. Opiate withdrawal and the rat locus coeruleus: behavioral, electrophysiological, and biochemical correlates. J Neurosci. 1990;10(7):2308–17.
17. Koob GF, Volkow ND. Neurocircuitry of addiction. Neuropsychopharmacology. 2010;35(1):217–38.
18. Tsai G, Gastfriend DR, Coyle JT. The glutamatergic basis of human alcoholism. Am J Psychiatry. 1995;152(3):332–40.
19. Chamberlain SR, Lochner C, Stein DJ, Goudriaan AE, van Holst RJ, Zohar J, Grant JE. Behavioural addiction—a rising tide? Eur Neuropsychopharmacol. 2016;26(5):841–55.
20. Grusser SM, Poppelreuter S, Heinz A, Albrecht U, Sass H. Behavioural addiction: an independent diagnostic category? Nervenarzt. 2007;78(9):997–1002.
21. De Wit H. Impulsivity as a determinant and consequence of drug use: a review of underlying processes. Addict Biol. 2009;14(1):22–31.
22. Rupp CI, Beck JK, Heinz A, Kemmler G, Manz S, Tempel K, Fleischhacker WW. Impulsivity and alcohol dependence treatment completion: is there a neurocognitive risk factor at treatment entry? Alcohol Clin Exp Res. 2016;40(1):152–60.
23. Breiter HC, Aharon I, Kahneman D, Dale A, Shizgal P. Functional imaging of neural responses to expectancy and experience of monetary gains and losses. Neuron. 2001;30(2):619–39.
24. Knutson B, Adams CM, Fong GW, Hommer D. Anticipation of increasing monetary reward selectively recruits nucleus accumbens. J Neurosci. 2001;21(16):RC159.
25. Di Chiara G, Bassareo V. Reward system and addiction: what dopamine does and doesn't do. Curr Opin Pharmacol. 2007;7(1):69–76.
26. Di Chiara G, Imperato A. Drugs abused by humans preferentially increase synaptic dopamine concentrations in the mesolimbic system of freely moving rats. Proc Natl Acad Sci U S A. 1988;85(14):5274–8.
27. Fuchs H, Nagel J, Hauber W. Effects of physiological and pharmacological stimuli on dopamine release in the rat globus pallidus. Neurochem Int. 2005;47(7):474–81.
28. Gessa GL, Muntoni F, Collu M, Vargiu L, Mereu G. Low doses of ethanol activate dopaminergic neurons in the ventral tegmental area. Brain Res. 1985;348(1):201–3.
29. Martel P, Fantino M. Influence of the amount of food ingested on mesolimbic dopaminergic system activity: a microdialysis study. Pharmacol Biochem Behav. 1996;55(2):297–302.
30. Flagel SB, Robinson TE, Clark JJ, Clinton SM, Watson SJ, Seeman P, Phillips PE, Akil H. An animal model of genetic vulnerability to behavioral disinhibition and responsiveness to reward-related cues: implications for addiction. Neuropsychopharmacology. 2010;35(2):388–400.
31. Robinson TE, Berridge KC. The neural basis of drug craving: an incentive-sensitization theory of addiction. Brain Res Brain Res Rev. 1993;18(3):247–91.
32. Schultz W, Dayan P, Montague PR. A neural substrate of prediction and reward. Science. 1997;275(5306):1593–9.
33. Ferenczi EA, Zalocusky KA, Liston C, Grosenick L, Warden MR, Amatya D, Katovich K, Mehta H, Patenaude B, Ramakrishnan C, Kalanithi P, Etkin A, Knutson B, Glover GH,

Deisseroth K. Prefrontal cortical regulation of brainwide circuit dynamics and reward-related behavior. Science. 2016;351(6268):aac9698.

34. Balodis IM, Kober H, Worhunsky PD, Stevens MC, Pearlson GD, Potenza MN. Diminished frontostriatal activity during processing of monetary rewards and losses in pathological gambling. Biol Psychiatry. 2012;71(8):749–57.
35. Balodis IM, Potenza MN. Imaging the gambling brain. Int Rev Neurobiol. 2016;129:111–24.
36. Quester S, Romanczuk-Seiferth N. Brain imaging in gambling disorder. Curr Addict Rep. 2015;2(3):220–9.
37. Reuter J, Raedler T, Rose M, Hand I, Glascher J, Buchel C. Pathological gambling is linked to reduced activation of the mesolimbic reward system. Nat Neurosci. 2005;8(2):147–8.
38. Beck A, Schlagenhauf F, Wüstenberg T, Hein J, Kienast T, Kahnt T, Schmack K, Hägele C, Knutson B, Heinz A, Wrase J. Ventral striatal activation during reward anticipation correlates with impulsivity in alcoholics. Biol Psychiatry. 2009;66(8):734–42.
39. Hagele C, Schlagenhauf F, Rapp M, Sterzer P, Beck A, Bermpohl F, Stoy M, Strohle A, Wittchen HU, Dolan RJ, Heinz A. Dimensional psychiatry: reward dysfunction and depressive mood across psychiatric disorders. Psychopharmacology. 2015;232(2):331–41.
40. Wrase J, Schlagenhauf F, Kienast T, Wustenberg T, Bermpohl F, Kahnt T, Beck A, Strohle A, Juckel G, Knutson B, Heinz A. Dysfunction of reward processing correlates with alcohol craving in detoxified alcoholics. NeuroImage. 2007;35(2):787–94.
41. Heinz A, Siessmeier T, Wrase J, Buchholz HG, Grunder G, Kumakura Y, Cumming P, Schreckenberger M, Smolka MN, Rosch F, Mann K, Bartenstein P. Correlation of alcohol craving with striatal dopamine synthesis capacity and D2/3 receptor availability: a combined [18F]DOPA and [18F]DMFP PET study in detoxified alcoholic patients. Am J Psychiatr. 2005;162(8):1515–20.
42. Heinz A, Siessmeier T, Wrase J, Hermann D, Klein S, Grusser SM, Flor H, Braus DF, Buchholz HG, Grunder G, Schreckenberger M, Smolka MN, Rosch F, Mann K, Bartenstein P. Correlation between dopamine D(2) receptors in the ventral striatum and central processing of alcohol cues and craving. Am J Psychiatry. 2004;161(10):1783–9.
43. Volkow ND, Wang GJ, Telang F, Fowler JS, Alexoff D, Logan J, Jayne M, Wong C, Tomasi D. Decreased dopamine brain reactivity in marijuana abusers is associated with negative emotionality and addiction severity. Proc Natl Acad Sci U S A. 2014;111(30):E3149–56.
44. Wiers CE, Stelzel C, Park SQ, Gawron CK, Ludwig VU, Gutwinski S, Heinz A, Lindenmeyer J, Wiers RW, Walter H, Bermpohl F. Neural correlates of alcohol-approach bias in alcohol addiction: the spirit is willing but the flesh is weak for spirits. Neuropsychopharmacology. 2014;39(3):688–97.
45. Wiers RW, Eberl C, Rinck M, Becker ES, Lindenmeyer J. Retraining automatic action tendencies changes alcoholic patients' approach bias for alcohol and improves treatment outcome. Psychol Sci. 2011;22(4):490–7.
46. Rommelspacher H, Raeder C, Kaulen P, Bruning G. Adaptive changes of dopamine-D2 receptors in rat brain following ethanol withdrawal: a quantitative autoradiographic investigation. Alcohol. 1992;9(5):355–62.
47. Volkow ND, Wang GJ, Fowler JS, Logan J, Hitzemann R, Ding YS, Pappas N, Shea C, Piscani K. Decreases in dopamine receptors but not in dopamine transporters in alcoholics. Alcohol Clin Exp Res. 1996;20(9):1594–8.
48. Garavan H, Pankiewicz J, Bloom A, Cho JK, Sperry L, Ross TJ, Salmeron BJ, Risinger R, Kelley D, Stein EA. Cue-induced cocaine craving: neuroanatomical specificity for drug users and drug stimuli. Am J Psychiatry. 2000;157(11):1789–98.
49. Beck A, Wustenberg T, Genauck A, Wrase J, Schlagenhauf F, Smolka MN, Mann K, Heinz A. Effect of brain structure, brain function, and brain connectivity on relapse in alcohol-dependent patients. Arch Gen Psychiatry. 2012;69(8):842–52.
50. Schacht JP, Anton RF, Myrick H. Functional neuroimaging studies of alcohol cue reactivity: a quantitative meta-analysis and systematic review. Addict Biol. 2013;18(1):121–33.
51. Schultz W. Dopamine reward prediction-error signalling: a two-component response. Nat Rev Neurosci. 2016;17(3):183–95.

52. Heinz A, Schlagenhauf F, Beck A, Wackerhagen C. Dimensional psychiatry: mental disorders as dysfunctions of basic learning mechanisms. J Neural Transm (Vienna). 2016;123(8):809–21.
53. Flagel SB, Akil H, Robinson TE. Individual differences in the attribution of incentive salience to reward-related cues: implications for addiction. Neuropharmacology. 2009;56(Suppl 1):139–48.
54. Flagel SB, Clark JJ, Robinson TE, Mayo L, Czuj A, Willuhn I, Akers CA, Clinton SM, Phillips PE, Akil H. A selective role for dopamine in stimulus-reward learning. Nature. 2011;469(7328):53–7.
55. Zink CF, Pagnoni G, Martin ME, Dhamala M, Berns GS. Human striatal response to salient nonrewarding stimuli. J Neurosci. 2003;23(22):8092–7.
56. Garbusow M, Schad DJ, Sebold M, Friedel E, Bernhardt N, Koch SP, Steinacher B, Kathmann N, Geurts DE, Sommer C, Muller DK, Nebe S, Paul S, Wittchen HU, Zimmermann US, Walter H, Smolka MN, Sterzer P, Rapp MA, Huys QJ, Schlagenhauf F, Heinz A. Pavlovian-to-instrumental transfer effects in the nucleus accumbens relate to relapse in alcohol dependence. Addict Biol. 2016;21(3):719–31.
57. Adams RA, Huys QJ, Roiser JP. Computational psychiatry: towards a mathematically informed understanding of mental illness. J Neurol Neurosurg Psychiatry. 2016;87(1):53–63.
58. Pfefferbaum A, Sullivan EV, Mathalon DH, Shear PK, Rosenbloom MJ, Lim KO. Longitudinal changes in magnetic resonance imaging brain volumes in abstinent and relapsed alcoholics. Alcohol Clin Exp Res. 1995;19(5):1177–91.
59. Stuke H, Gutwinski S, Wiers CE, Schmidt TT, Gropper S, Parnack J, Gawron C, Hindi Attar C, Spengler S, Walter H, Heinz A, Bermpohl F. To drink or not to drink: harmful drinking is associated with hyperactivation of reward areas rather than hypoactivation of control areas in men. J Psychiatry Neurosci. 2016;41(3):E24–36.
60. Park SQ, Kahnt T, Beck A, Cohen MX, Dolan RJ, Wrase J, Heinz A. Prefrontal cortex fails to learn from reward prediction errors in alcohol dependence. J Neurosci. 2010;30(22):7749–53.
61. Deserno L, Huys QJ, Boehme R, Buchert R, Heinze HJ, Grace AA, Dolan RJ, Heinz A, Schlagenhauf F. Ventral striatal dopamine reflects behavioral and neural signatures of model-based control during sequential decision making. Proc Natl Acad Sci U S A. 2015;112(5):1595–600.
62. Schlagenhauf F, Rapp MA, Huys QJ, Beck A, Wustenberg T, Deserno L, Buchholz HG, Kalbitzer J, Buchert R, Bauer M, Kienast T, Cumming P, Plotkin M, Kumakura Y, Grace AA, Dolan RJ, Heinz A. Ventral striatal prediction error signaling is associated with dopamine synthesis capacity and fluid intelligence. Hum Brain Mapp. 2013;34(6):1490–9.
63. Lorenz RC, Kruger JK, Neumann B, Schott BH, Kaufmann C, Heinz A, Wustenberg T. Cue reactivity and its inhibition in pathological computer game players. Addict Biol. 2013;18(1):134–46.
64. Alexander GE, DeLong MR, Strick PL. Parallel organization of functionally segregated circuits linking basal ganglia and cortex. Annu Rev Neurosci. 1986;9:357–81.
65. Adams KM, Gilman S, Koeppe RA, Kluin KJ, Brunberg JA, Dede D, Berent S, Kroll PD. Neuropsychological deficits are correlated with frontal hypometabolism in positron emission tomography studies of older alcoholic patients. Alcohol Clin Exp Res. 1993;17(2):205–10.
66. Volkow ND, Chang L, Wang GJ, Fowler JS, Ding YS, Sedler M, Logan J, Franceschi D, Gatley J, Hitzemann R, Gifford A, Wong C, Pappas N. Low level of brain dopamine D2 receptors in methamphetamine abusers: association with metabolism in the orbitofrontal cortex. Am J Psychiatry. 2001;158(12):2015–21.
67. Volkow ND, Wang GJ, Shokri Kojori E, Fowler JS, Benveniste H, Tomasi D. Alcohol decreases baseline brain glucose metabolism more in heavy drinkers than controls but has no effect on stimulation-induced metabolic increases. J Neurosci. 2015;35(7):3248–55.
68. Baxter LR Jr, Phelps ME, Mazziotta JC, Guze BH, Schwartz JM, Selin CE. Local cerebral glucose metabolic rates in obsessive-compulsive disorder. A comparison with rates in unipolar depression and in normal controls. Arch Gen Psychiatry. 1987;44(3):211–8.

69. Baxter LR Jr, Schwartz JM, Bergman KS, Szuba MP, Guze BH, Mazziotta JC, Alazraki A, Selin CE, Ferng HK, Munford P, et al. Caudate glucose metabolic rate changes with both drug and behavior therapy for obsessive-compulsive disorder. Arch Gen Psychiatry. 1992;49(9):681–9.
70. Schwartz JM, Stoessel PW, Baxter LR Jr, Martin KM, Phelps ME. Systematic changes in cerebral glucose metabolic rate after successful behavior modification treatment of obsessive-compulsive disorder. Arch Gen Psychiatry. 1996;53(2):109–13.
71. Mataix-Cols D, Wooderson S, Lawrence N, Brammer MJ, Speckens A, Phillips ML. Distinct neural correlates of washing, checking, and hoarding symptom dimensions in obsessive-compulsive disorder. Arch Gen Psychiatry. 2004;61(6):564–76.
72. Kuhn S, Gallinat J. Common biology of craving across legal and illegal drugs – a quantitative meta-analysis of cue-reactivity brain response. Eur J Neurosci. 2011;33(7):1318–26.
73. Goldstein RZ, Volkow ND. Dysfunction of the prefrontal cortex in addiction: neuroimaging findings and clinical implications. Nat Rev Neurosci. 2011;12(11):652–69.
74. Huys QJM, Beck A, Dayan P, Heinz A. Neurobiology and computational structure of decision making in addiction. In: al. Me, editor. Phenomenological neuropsychiatry: bridging the clinic and clinical neuroscience. Posted at the Zurich Open Repository and Archive, University of Zurich. 2013.
75. Schoofs N, Heinz A. Pathological gambling. Impulse control disorder, addiction or compulsion? Nervenarzt. 2013;84(5):629–34.
76. Heinz AJ, Beck A, Meyer-Lindenberg A, Sterzer P, Heinz A. Cognitive and neurobiological mechanisms of alcohol-related aggression. Nat Rev Neurosci. 2011;12(7):400–13.
77. Heinz A. Der Begriff der psychischen Krankheit. Berlin: Suhrkamp; 2014.
78. Kant I. Anthropologie in pragmatischer Hinsicht. Stuttgart: Reclam; 1983.
79. van Os J. "Schizophrenia" does not exist. BMJ. 2016;352:i375.
80. Beard DJ, Findlay JA. Drapetomania—a disease called freedom. FL: Broward Public Library Foundation; 2000.
81. Naragon MD. Communities in motion: drapetomania, work and the development of African American slave cultures. Slavery Abolition. 1994;15(3):63–87.

Gambling Disorder as a Clinical Phenomenon

Christopher J. Hunt and Alexander Blaszczynski

2.1 Games and Gambling in Antiquity

The exact origins of gambling have faded into obscurity but its presence dates to antiquity. Archaeological findings offer evidence of games of chance played as long back as approximately 4000 years BC. Murals and artefacts around this period indicate that board games such as the forerunners of draughts and backgammon and astragals (knucklebones) used as dice thrown to determine the number of steps to move playing pieces [1–3] were commonly accepted as leisure pursuits. The oldest known Eastern games of Wei-kin in China and Go in Japan emerged around 2300 years BC. These games relied on chance as the determinant of outcomes, but the exact point in time when players began to risk items of value either to enhance excitement in competition or for personal gain remains unknown. What is known is that reference to gambling can be found in ancient Egyptian mythical accounts of deities and demigods and in Mediterranean and Eastern culture folklores.

Indications are that many games laid the foundation for activities that subsequently met the definition of gambling, that is, an agreement between two or more participants to risk an item of value on the outcome of an event determined wholly or to some extent by chance for purposes of obtaining a gain/profit. Roulette, for example, has its origins in Grecian and Roman soldiers wagering on the turn of numbered chariot wheels; the throwing of dice and lots in appeal to religious divination represents the forerunner of modern dice games; legends about keno claim a history dating back to efforts to raise money to fund wars and build the Great Wall in ancient China; horse and chariot races later evolved into national wagering events; and simple early card games diverged into the multiple card game formats played today, such as poker, baccarat and blackjack. In contemporary times,

C. J. Hunt · A. Blaszczynski (✉)
Brain Mind Centre, School of Psychology, The University of Sydney,
Sydney, NSW, Australia
e-mail: christopher.hunt@sydney.edu.au; alex.blaszczynski@sydney.edu.au

© Springer Nature Switzerland AG 2019
A. Heinz et al. (eds.), *Gambling Disorder*, https://doi.org/10.1007/978-3-030-03060-5_2

technological and electronic advances have given rise to sophisticated electronic gambling devices mimicking traditional games, and the Internet offers global opportunities for virtually all forms of gambling.

Societal acceptance of gambling has fluctuated from extremes of widespread indulgence to attempted suppression for as long as gambling has been in existence. For example, Confucius (551–479 BC), whose philosophy formed the basis of much Chinese moral reasoning throughout subsequent centuries, reportedly referred to gambling as unproductive and as violating filial duty [4]. There is then evidence of legal proscriptions against gambling in China during the Warring States period (c. 476–221 BC) and during the Tang dynasty (c AD 618–907 [4]). Similar religious and legal restrictions on gambling in Europe were enacted in response to the social and economic impacts of excessive gambling: public disorder, creation of poverty and personal and familial distress, cheating and exploitation and as it was viewed as an activity contrary to Protestant work ethics or religious tenets [5, 6]. Accordingly, religious edicts prohibiting gambling and statutes banning certain activities, limiting losses or preventing recovery of gambling debts were enacted across many jurisdictions. By 1882, virtually every European province prohibited gambling [7] with the temperance movement in the latter part of that decade temporarily successful in tempering the consumption of alcohol and gambling in America. In the current era, the full circle has turned with gambling, although not universally adopted and accepted, becoming a multibillion dollar global industry, incorporating 24/7 convenient, anonymous and easy access to gaming and wagering products through multiple land-based options and via online devices (smartphones, tablets and laptops).

2.2   Gambling to Excess

Numerous anecdotal and case history accounts of individuals, including historical celebrities, falling prey to the lure of gambling have been chronicled over the ages [6]. Documented in these writings is the extent to which individuals wreaked havoc on their wealth, incurred debt leading to poverty and imprisonment in debtor's jail, destroyed marriages and families and succumbed to suicidal ideation [3, 6]. These accounts are insightful in describing the phenomenology associated with 'compulsive' urges driving an individual motivated by the desire to win to persist despite incurring substantial losses and severe emotional distress. The 'addictiveness' of the behaviour indicated by the presence of tolerance [8] and impaired control and preoccupation comparable to alcohol addiction [9] has been frequently described in the popular literature prior to the twentieth century. Exemplary descriptions of the powerful processes inherent in gambling are contained in Pushkin's *The Queen of Spades* [10], Dostoevsky's *The Gambler* [11], Thackeray's *A Gambler's Death* [12] and Saki's *The Stake* [13], a literature base that depicts the phenomenology of the behaviour in comprehensive detail. However, it was not until von Hattinger's [14] psychodynamic description of gambling was published that scientific consideration was given to the idea of excessive gambling representing a clinical phenomenon reflecting the presence of an underlying psychological disorder.

2.3   Gambling Disorder as a Clinical Phenomenon

Between 1914 and 1957, with continuing pockets of interest, psychodynamic explanations were applied to the aetiology of 'compulsive' gambling. Predominantly based on single case or case series reports, the condition was regarded as the symptomatic expression of an underlying psychoneurosis related to pregenital psychosexual phases and Oedipal conflicts, masturbatory complexes and equivalents or the expression of psychic masochism linked to a tendency for self-punishment resulting from unresolved aggressive feelings [15–17]. Although shaping its intervention, the psychodynamic formulation lacked empirical support, retained untestable hypotheses and failed to explain the transitional shift from recreational to impaired control, a process often taking several years. In addition, the gambling was typically not the primary reason for referral, leaving the causal or interactive relationship between the respective conditions unknown.

Derived from experimental manipulations of behaviour, learning theories gained popularity in the 1960s following the seminal studies of Skinner [18] and Pavlov [19] describing operant and classical conditioning paradigms, respectively. This provided an excellent model explaining how overt gambling behaviours were influenced by contingencies of random ratio-delivered schedules of reinforcement. Anderson and Brown [20] advanced a two-factor theory that incorporated operant and classical conditioning principles with individual differences in autonomic/cortical arousal and sensation-seeking personality traits. This theory was predicated on the assumption that certain individuals had a propensity to respond differently to rewards and punishment, with a proclivity to repetitively seek out risky behaviours to maintain optimal levels of hedonic arousal [21].

Jacobs [22] extended these concepts into his general theory of addictions that contained many of the inherent features of Solomon and Corbitt's [23] opponent process model. Briefly, Jacobs [22] argued that chronically hyper- (anxious) or hypo- (depressed) aroused individuals, in combination with psychological states of low self-esteem and experiences of rejection, placed such individuals at risk for pursuing behaviours that fostered homeostatic levels of arousal. Those hyperaroused, it was suggested, gravitate to low-skills games where their attention is narrowed and focussed, resulting in negative reinforcement, that is, escaping from states of emotional distress [22, 24]. For those hypo-aroused, preferences were directed to higher skill games that engaged their interests resulting in excitement, boosting their affective states.

These early theories highlighted the central role played by biologically determined differences in psychophysiological arousal, the influence of positive and negative reinforcement and personality traits as vulnerability factors leading to a gambling disorder. Cognitive and motivational variables were recognized but did not attract the primary focus of attention at this point. However, cognitive theories gained prominence with the identification of consistent distorted and erroneous beliefs surrounding illusions of control, misunderstanding the mathematics and statistical basis of gambling and concepts of randomness and mutual independence of chance events [25–27]. Chasing losses as a motivation is one of the overarching factors defining a gambling disorder as described by Lesieur [28]. Behavioural and cognitive theories are not mutually exclusive but contain behavioural and motivational components that interact with each other to maintain persistence despite serious deleterious consequences.

Given its repetitive persistent nature, it is unsurprising that analogies between gambling and substance addiction have been promulgated. This perspective was formalised in the DSM-IV [29], where the criteria for what was then termed 'pathological gambling' were revised to explicitly draw attention to the presence of many features commonly found in substance use disorders, including withdrawal symptoms, tolerance and preoccupation/dependence and affective disturbances [30].

Irrespective of the explanatory model applied, phenomenological features of emotional dependence on gambling, impaired control over behaviours, concurrent substance use and affective disturbances and persistence in the face of accumulating stresses and distress characterise gambling disorder as a clinical entity. Typical features include the presence of depression, suicidal ideation, anxiety and emotional distress, marital and familial conflicts, impaired work/study productivity, commission of illegal acts to maintain habitual gambling behaviours and substance use. Cognitive distortions result in individuals overestimating personal skills and probabilities of winning and lead to further attempts to recoup losses through continued gambling.

2.4   Current Diagnostic Criteria for Gambling Disorder

Although recognized as a clinical entity for over 40 years since its inclusion within ICD-9 [31] and DSM-III [32], debate regarding inconsistencies in the terminology used, categorization, and criteria used to diagnose a gambling disorder have been prevalent. In particular, gambling disorders have been variably considered to constitute an impulse control disorder, an addictive behaviour or fall on an obsessive-compulsive spectrum (see [33], for an overview). In the following section, the development of the current diagnostic criteria guided by phenomenological features that consolidate gambling as a clinical disorder will be outlined.

With the release of the DSM-5 [34], the following diagnostic criteria were given for the diagnosis now referred to as 'gambling disorder' (the earlier name of 'pathological gambling' was dropped as the term 'pathological' was considered to be pejorative [35]). In order to receive a diagnosis of a gambling disorder, individuals must meet four of the nine criteria over a 12-month period. Their behaviour must also not be better accounted for by a manic episode.

1. Needing to gamble with increasing amounts of money in order to achieve the desired excitement.
2. Feeling restless or irritable when attempting to cut down or stop gambling.
3. Making repeated unsuccessful attempts to control, cut back or stop gambling.
4. Often experiencing preoccupation with gambling (e.g. having persistent thoughts of reliving past gambling experiences, handicapping or planning the next venture, thinking of ways to get money to gamble).

5. Often gambles when feeling distressed (e.g. helpless, guilty, anxious, depressed).
6. After losing money gambling, often returns another day to get even ('chasing' one's losses).
7. Lies to conceal the extent of involvement with gambling.
8. Jeopardising or losing a significant relationship, job or educational or career opportunity because of gambling.
9. Has relied on others to provide money to relieve desperate financial situations caused by gambling.

As well as the aforementioned name change, these criteria represented several changes from the previous DSM-IV-TR criteria for pathological gambling [36]. Firstly, the diagnosis was moved to the section titled 'Substance Use and Related Disorders', where it is the sole member of a grouping titled 'non-substance-related disorders'. The DSM-5 workgroup on gambling cited research that highlighted clinical, neurological, epidemiological and genetic similarities between gambling and substance use disorders as the key reason for the move, although they noted that there were dissenting voices [37]. The research into the similarities and differences between gambling and substance use disorders will be discussed in detail later in this volume (see Chap. 12).

The second change that was made to the criteria in the DSM-5 was the dropping of the criterion included in past editions 'has committed illegal acts such as forgery, fraud, theft, or embezzlement to finance gambling'. The workgroup reported that this criterion had been removed as only a minority of the treatment population endorsed this criterion, and those who did frequently also reported meeting multiple other criteria, thus diminishing this criterion's usefulness in the diagnosis of gambling disorder [37]. Other writers have disputed this change, noting that illegal acts remain relatively common in treatment samples of gamblers, and the retention of this criterion would draw attention to the relationship between gambling disorder and legal issues [38]. Indeed, regardless of the decision made to exclude this criterion, those working with gamblers should remain aware of the high rates of co-occurrence between gambling disorder and illegal activities. Recent evaluations of the new DSM-5 criteria across various treatment and community samples found that over 40% of those engaged in treatment for gambling-related problems reported engaging in illegal activates [39]. Furthermore, previous work has found that those who have experienced arrests or incarceration as a result of gambling-related crime were more likely to display features suggestive of antisocial personality disorder and substance use disorders [40]. It has also been suggested that gamblers who report illegal activities may also require more intensive treatment than those who do not [41]. Thus, the relationship between gambling and illegality should remain a clinical and research focus despite the illegal acts criterion being removed in the DSM-5.

The final change in the diagnostic criteria for the DSM-5 was the reduction of the number of criteria needs for a diagnosis. In the DSM-IV, meeting five out of the ten listed criteria was necessary in order to obtain a diagnosis of pathological gambling. In the DSM-5, this was reduced to four out of nine criteria. The rationale for this reduction was that it would ensure consistency with previous diagnosis rates following the removal of the illegal acts criterion [35]. Empirical studies since then have shown that this change in the threshold for diagnosis resulted in either no change or in a very slight increase in the numbers of individuals meeting criteria for disordered gambling [39, 42, 43]. However, comparisons with other measures of gambling severity have led to the claim that the reduced threshold leads to more consistent diagnosis relative to the previous criteria [37]. Taken together, these findings suggest that there does appear to be sound empirical support for the changes made to the diagnostic criteria in the DSM-5.

2.5   Diagnosis of Subclinical Gambling

For many clinicians, diagnostic issues are of secondary importance: when an individual presents to a service asking for treatment for their gambling, they will receive it, and whether they meet strict diagnostic criteria is purely of academic interest. However, in some treatment settings, particularly in the United States where insurance companies often dictate that a current diagnosis is necessary for treatment coverage, ensuring that those who seek treatment would also meet some formal diagnosis can make the difference between those who are experiencing gambling-related harm receiving treatment or not. It is in this context that researchers and commentators have often proposed further changes or additions to diagnostic systems used for gambling-related behaviours that attempt to capture those who may not meet DSM-5 criteria for gambling disorder but who may nonetheless be experiencing significant distress or harm as a result of their gambling.

There have been various proposals for how to classify such 'subclinical' gamblers. One proposal has been to model the criteria for the DSM-5 on the classification system used for substance use disorders, where the endorsement of only two symptoms is required for a diagnosis [38]. Under such a system, gamblers would then be further classified into subgroups by the number of criteria met. For example, individuals endorsing two to four symptoms could be classified as having 'disordered gambling, moderate', while those meeting more than four criteria could be classified as having 'disordered gambling, severe' [38]. Another, which was proposed when developing the National Opinion Research Center DSM Screen for Gambling Problems (NODS), a commonly used population-based screening tool for gambling problems, was to classify those who meet one or two of the previous DSM-IV criteria as an 'at-risk' gambler, those who meet three or four classified as a 'problem gambler' and those who meet five or more as a 'pathological gambler' [44]. Other classification schemes refer to 'levels' of gambling, which are based on both gambling severity and willingness to seek treatment, ranging from 'level 0' representing those who have never gambled, up to 'level 4' representing those who both meet diagnostic criteria for a gambling disorder and show willingness to enter treatment [45].

These and similar suggestions of incorporating previously undiagnosed less severe categorisations of gamblers were rejected by the DSM-5 workgroup as it would result in a large increase in the rates at which gambling disorder was diagnosed [37]. However, whatever terms are eventually settled on ([46], documented

14 different classification schemes), it appears clear that there is a large group of individuals who do not meet full diagnostic criteria for gambling disorder, and yet have come to the attention of researchers and clinicians. Work with individuals in this subclinical group has shown that of the current diagnostic criteria, they are more likely to endorse the more 'cognitive'-type symptoms (i.e. lying, gambling to escape problems, preoccupation with gambling) than they are to endorse other symptom clusters (with the exception of the 'chasing losses' criteria, which almost all treatment-seeking gamblers meet [47]).

Despite the decision not to include a subclinical diagnosis in the current edition of the DSM, there is evidence that those who fall into this category may benefit from clinical attention. It has been demonstrated that adults who report symptoms of disordered gambling but do not meet full DSM criteria for gambling disorder (or its previous incarnation, pathological gambling) show increased rates of other Axis I psychiatric disorders [48], higher rates of alcohol and substance use problems [49] and higher rates of suicidal thoughts [50] than the general population. Gambling disorder symptoms are also associated with problem behaviour in adolescents [51]. Furthermore, rather than progressing in a linear fashion as had been previously assumed, longitudinal research has shown that individuals' gambling frequently moves between severity levels [52]. Taken together, these findings should serve as a reminder to anyone working in the gambling field to not narrow their focus solely on those who meet current diagnostic criteria for a gambling disorder.

2.6 A Harm-Based Classification: The Concept of 'Problem Gambling'

Given evidence that there are many individuals experiencing gambling-related harms who do not meet strict criteria for gambling disorder, it is unsurprising that in many places around the world, a different conceptualisation of difficulties related to gambling is used. Rather than focussing on behavioural symptoms, as is done with both gambling disorder and its predecessor pathological gambling, the notion of 'problem gambling' instead focusses on harm in an individual's life as a result of the gambling. The term problem gambling is generally held to refer to any pattern of gambling that is resulting in disruptions to an individual's social, occupational or psychological functioning [46]. While the precise definition of the term problem gambling can differ between jurisdictions, a commonly cited definition for problem gambling is that put forward by Ferris and Wynne [53], which defines it as 'gambling behaviour that creates negative consequences for the gambler, others in his or her social network, or for the community' (p. 58). With such a definition of problem gambling, the aforementioned difficulties with a symptom-based approach often excluding some individuals who are experiencing gambling-related harms are avoided, as the harm itself becomes the hallmark of the problem. Similar definitions have been used in public health contexts in the United Kingdom, Canada and Australia (see [46] for a brief review). An advantage of the problem gambling approach in public health contexts is that it is useful in identifying individuals with lower levels of gambling-related harms and encouraging them to seek treatment before they may meet full diagnosis for a gambling disorder or pathological gambling [54].

However, there are also disadvantages of such an approach as well, given its focus on subjective judgements of 'harm'. Walker [55] gave the example of an individual who has with a spouse with strict religious or moral objections to gambling who buys a weekly lottery ticket. While most people would not consider this a behaviour worthy of clinical attention, it is conceivable that such an individual would be experiencing subjective harm as a result of their gambling, if it resulted in arguments with their spouse. Blaszczynski and Nower [54] further note that defining gambling based solely on subjective measures of harm runs the risk of categorising together those with minor levels of gambling-related harm with those with serious difficulties in controlling and regulating their impulses, potentially resulting in a large, heterogeneous group. To overcome such disadvantages, a compromise definition was put forward by Blaszczynski et al. [56], where problem gambling was defined as 'a chronic failure to resist gambling impulses that result in disruption or damage to several areas of a person's social, vocational, familial or financial functioning'. Such a definition includes both the sense of subjective harm, as well as the notion that the individual has a diminished or impaired ability or willingness to resist their impulses to gamble. However, the most important message of this discussion is that researchers, clinicians and policy-makers working in the area need to be aware of the advantages and disadvantages of whatever approach they take to defining gambling-related difficulties and to select that which best suits their purposes.

2.7   Gambling-Related Harm

The centrality of harm to the concept of problem gambling raises obvious questions: How do we define gambling-related harm? And what harms are commonly observed clinically in gamblers? Langham et al. [57] have recently proposed a conceptual framework to assist in answering both of these questions. Based on both a literature review and focus group research with clinical samples of gamblers, a proposed definition of gambling-related harm was given as 'any initial or exacerbated adverse consequence due to an engagement with gambling that leads to a decrement to the health or wellbeing of an individual, family unit, community or population' [57]. Langham et al. [57] then went on to identify seven domains across which gamblers may experience harm: financial, relational, emotional/psychological, health, cultural, work/study and criminal activity. For each of these domains, there is clear evidence of the potential for gambling to cause harms.

Financial harms are one of the easily identified harms as a result of problem gambling, as they are often directly related to gambling losses. They may also contribute to the harms seen in other domains, as financial losses have the potential to result in marital discord, psychological distress, neglect of healthcare, disruptions at work and criminal activity in an attempt to repay debts. For example, gamblers who have declared bankruptcy were significantly more likely to also be experiencing marital, legal, psychological and work-related disruptions [58]. Financial harms should always be investigated by clinicians working with gamblers, given that they are one of the key motivators for gamblers seeking treatment [59] and are one of the key variables associated with gambling-related suicide [60].

The second identified area of harms caused by gambling identified by Langham et al. [57] were relational harms, which include disruptions in the relationships that gamblers have with their spouse, children or other family members or friends. These harms can be a direct result of the gambler neglecting the relationship due to time spent gambling or due to lack of trust as a result of the gambler lying about their behaviour. Several studies have found that gambling is a potential risk factor for marital discord and divorce [61, 62], domestic violence [63] and child maltreatment [64]. The recognition of such harms has led to the suggestion of providing counselling and treatment directed towards the family members of problem gamblers [65] or for treating problem gambling in the context of family issues [66].

Emotional and psychological distress was the next domain of harm identified by Langham et al. [57]. Emotional distress can result from feelings of hopelessness stemming from poorly controlled behaviour, a lack of security as a result of financial or relational disruptions or shame and stigma associated with gambling. Gambling has been correlated with psychiatric diagnoses generally [48] and with depression and other mood disorders specifically [67, 68]. The existence of stigma and shame around problem gambling should also be noted by clinicians working with problem gamblers, as it may constitute a key barrier to individuals seeking treatment for gambling-related problems [59, 69].

Decrements to health were the fourth domain identified by Langham et al. [57] as an area of potential gambling-related harm. Health problems may result from gamblers neglecting their health due to the time and money they spend gambling, from the stress they experience as a result of their gambling, from living a sedentary lifestyle as a result of time spent gambling or through having no financial resources to engage in more health-positive behaviours. Problem gambling has been associated with poorer physical health and greater numbers of reported physical health problems [70–72]. A large epidemiological survey has specifically found that pathological gambling was specifically associated with higher rates of tachycardia, angina, cirrhosis and other liver diseases, even after controlling for demographic and behavioural risk factors [73]. These findings highlight the toll that gambling may take on physical as well as emotional health.

The fifth domain identified by Langham et al. [57] was cultural harms, which related to the proposal that gambling caused disconnections between gamblers and their cultural beliefs, roles and practices. This process may include distress as a result of going against cultural norms or isolation from a cultural community as a result of gambling. While such harms are more difficult to measure due to their more diffuse conceptualisation, problem gambling has been associated with feelings of loneliness and social isolation [74], and clinicians working with problem gambling should be cognizant of how cultural factors may be impacting on a gambler's psychosocial functioning (for a review on this topic, see [75]).

Reduced performance at work or study was also identified by Langham et al. [57] as an area for potential harm caused by gambling. These harms may result from being distracted at school, university or work as a result of gambling activities, increased absenteeism as a result of not being able to pay for transportation or not being able to pay for work or study tools. Problem gambling has been associated with poorer grades in adolescents [51] and in college students [76]. Problem gambling is also associated with poor work productivity in adults [77], as are financial losses resulting from gambling [78]. The potential for gambling to lead to problems at work should be of particular attention to clinicians working with problem gamblers, due to the importance of problem gamblers needing to maintain regular work in order to address some of their gambling-related debts.

The final domain identified by Langham et al. [57] was criminal acts. As noted in the previous discussion on the changes in the DSM criteria for pathological gambling/gambling disorder, criminal acts are often a sign of more severe gambling pathology, as they represent a desperate attempt to pay back gambling-related losses, with 40% of those engaged in treatment for gambling-related problems reporting engaging in illegal activates [39].

While the above classification of gambling harms has focussed on harms experienced by gamblers and those in close familiar or work relationships with them, Langham et al. [57] identified the potential for more community-wide harms resulting from problem gambling, in forms such as increased levels of debt and bankruptcies, reliance on government support, decreased community-wide economic productivity or increases in crime rates. They also suggested that harms related to gambling have the potential to cross generations, as children and/or grandchildren of problem gamblers may potentially be impacted in lasting ways (e.g. children of problem gamblers experiencing ongoing psychological disturbances as a result of neglect or homelessness that follows from a parent's gambling). These wider harms, while necessarily more difficult to quantify and measure, require further attention from future research.

2.8 Conclusions

Although both gambling and efforts to control it have long histories, it has only been a focus of clinical attention since the twentieth century. At present, there are several competing accounts that have been put forward to explain gambling behaviour. Given that there is no universally accepted theoretical account of gambling, it is unsurprising that there is still considerable debate over the most appropriate way to define excess gambling and its associated symptoms. Both the behavioural symptom-based DSM-5 diagnosis of 'gambling disorder' and the harm-focussed concept of 'problem gambling' have their advantages and disadvantages, and researchers, clinicians and policy-makers working in the field should be aware of these differences when selecting which conceptualisation is most appropriate to use in their work. What does not appear to be in debate is the recognition that a proportion of individuals gamble to excess, exhibit features of impaired control and suffer psychological distress, supporting the notion that gambling to excess in this subpopulation represents a clinical condition.

References

1. Scarne J. Scarne's new complete guide to gambling. London: Constable; 1961.
2. Schwartz D. Roll the bones: the history of gambling. New York: Gotham Books; 2006.
3. Steinmetz A. The gaming table: its votaries and victims in all times and countries, especially in England and France. Publication No. 96, Patterson Smith Reprint Series in Criminology Law Enforcement and Social Problems, vols I and II. NJ: Patterson Smith; 1969 (orig. 1870).
4. Wu A, Lau JT. Gambling in China: socio-historical evolution and current challenges. Addiction. 2015;110:210–6.
5. Blakey R. The development of the law of gambling 1776–1976. Washington: National Institute of Law Enforcement and Criminal Justice; 1977.
6. France CJ. The gambling impulse. Am J Psychol. 1902;13:364–76.
7. Peterson VP. Obstacles to enforcement of gambling laws. Ann Am Acad Pol Soc Sci. 1950;269:9–21.
8. Orford J. Excessive appetites: a psychological view of addictions. New York: Wiley & Sons; 1985.
9. Squires P. Fydor Dostoevsky: a psychopathographical sketch. Psychoanal Rev. 1937;24:365–88.
10. Pushkin AS. Russian short stories (trans. R.S. Townsend). London: Everyman's Library; 1982. p. 1–37.
11. Dostoevsky F. The gambler. (trans J. Coulson). Middlesex: Penguin Books; 1978. p. 17–162.
12. Thackeray WM. A gambler's death. 1840. https://ebooks.adelaide.edu.au/t/thackeray/william_makepeace/paris/contents.html. Retrieved 9 Jan 2016.
13. Saki. The stake. Champaign, IL: Project Gutenberg; 1995.
14. von Hattinger H. Analerotik, Angstlust und Eigensinn. Int Z Psychoanal. 1914;2:244–58.
15. Bergler E. The psychology of gambling. London: International Universities Press; 1957.
16. Harris H. Gambling and addiction in an adolescent male. Psychoanal Q. 1964;34:513–25.
17. Herman RD. Gamblers and gambling. New York: Harper Row; 1976.
18. Skinner BF. Science and human behaviour. New York: Free Press; 1953.
19. Pavlov IP. Lectures on conditioned reflexes (translated by W.H. Gantt). London: Allen and Unwin; 1928.
20. Anderson G, Brown RIF. Real and laboratory gambling: sensation-seeking and arousal. Br J Psychol. 1984;75:401–10.
21. Zuckerman M. Sensation seeking: beyond the optimum level of arousal. NJ: Hillsdale; 1979.
22. Jacobs DF. A general theory of addictions: a new theoretical model. J Gambl Behav. 1986;2:15–31.
23. Solomon RL, Corbit JD. An opponent-process theory of motivation: I. Temporal dynamics of affect. Psychol Rev. 1974;81:119–45.
24. Blaszczynski A, McConaghy. Anxiety and/or depression in the pathogenesis of addictive gambling. Int J Addict. 1989;24:337–50.
25. Ladouceur R, Walker M. A cognitive perspective on gambling. In: Salkovskis PM, editor. Trends in cognitive-behavioural therapies. New York: John Wiley & Sons; 1996. p. 89–120.
26. Toneatto T, Blitz-Miller T, Calderwood K, Dragonetti R, Tsanos A. Cognitive distortions in heavy gambling. J Gambl Stud. 1997;13:253–66.
27. Walker MB. The psychology of gambling. Sydney: Pergamon Press; 1992.
28. Lesieur HR. The chase: career of the compulsive gambler. MA: Schenkman; 1984.
29. American Psychiatric Association. DSM-IV: diagnostic and statistical manual of mental disorders. fourth ed. Washington, DC: American Psychiatric Association; 1994.
30. Reilly C, Smith N. The evolving definition of pathological gambling in the DSM-5. National Center for Responsible Gaming. 2013. p. 1–6.
31. World Health Organisation. ICD-9: international classification of diseases: revisions 9. Geneva, Switzerland: World Health Organisation; 1975.
32. American Psychiatric Association. DSM-III: diagnostic and statistical manual of mental disorders. third ed. Washington, DC: American Psychiatric Association; 1980.

33. Petry N. Pathological gambling: etiology, comorbidity, and treatment. Washington, DC: American Psychiatric Publishing; 2005.
34. American Psychiatric Association. DSM-5: diagnostic and statistical manual of mental disorders. fifth ed. Washington, DC: American Psychiatric Association; 2013.
35. Petry NM. Pathological gambling and the DSM-V. Int Gambl Stud. 2010;10:113–5.
36. American Psychiatric Association. DSM-IV-TR: diagnostic and statistical manual of mental disorders (text revision). fourth ed. Washington, DC: American Psychiatric Association; 2000.
37. Petry NM, Blanco C, Auriacombe M, Borges G, Bucholz K, Crowley TJ, Grant BF, Hasin DS, O'Brien C. An overview of and rationale for changes proposed for pathological gambling in DSM-5. J Gambl Stud. 2014;30:493–502.
38. Mitzner GB, Whelan JP, Meyers AW. Comments from the trenches: proposed changes to the DSM-V classification of pathological gambling. J Gambl Stud. 2011;27:517–21.
39. Petry NM, Blanco C, Stinchfield R, Volberg R. An empirical evaluation of proposed changes for gambling diagnosis in the DSM-5. Addiction. 2013;108:575–81.
40. Potenza MN, Steinberg MA, McLaughlin SD, Rounsaville BJ, O'Malley SS. Illegal behaviors in problem gambling: analysis of data from a gambling helpline. J Am Acad Psychiatry Law Online. 2000;28:389–403.
41. Grant JE, Potenza MN. Commentary: Illegal behavior and pathological gambling. J Am Acad Psychiatry Law Online. 2007;35:302–5.
42. Denis C, Fatséas M, Auriacombe M. Analyses related to the development of DSM-5 criteria for substance use related disorders: 3. An assessment of pathological gambling criteria. Drug Alcohol Depend. 2012;122:22–7.
43. Temcheff CE, Derevensky JL, Paskus TS. Pathological and disordered gambling: a comparison of DSM-IV and DSM-V criteria. Int Gambl Stud. 2011;11:213–20.
44. Hodgins DC. Using the NORC DSM Screen for Gambling Problems as an outcome measure for pathological gambling: psychometric evaluation. Addict Behav. 2004;29:1685–90.
45. Shaffer HJ, Hall MN. Estimating the prevalence of adolescent gambling disorders: a quantitative synthesis and guide toward standard gambling nomenclature. J Gambl Stud. 1996;12:193–214.
46. Abbott M, Volberg R, Bellringer M, Reith G. A review of research on aspects of problem gambling. London: Responsibility in Gambling Trust; 2004.
47. Toce-Gerstein M, Gerstein DR, Volberg RA. A hierarchy of gambling disorders in the community. Addiction. 2003;98:1661–72.
48. Bischof A, Meyer C, Bischof G, Kastirke N, John U, Rumpf HJ. Comorbid axis I-disorders among subjects with pathological, problem, or at-risk gambling recruited from the general population in Germany: results of the PAGE study. Psychiatry Res. 2013;210:1065–70.
49. Blanco C, Hasin DS, Petry N, Stinson FS, Grant BF. Sex differences in subclinical and DSM-IV pathological gambling: results from the National Epidemiologic Survey on Alcohol and Related Conditions. Psychol Med. 2006;36:943–53.
50. Feigelman W, Gorman BS, Lesieur H. Examining the relationship between at-risk gambling and suicidality in a national representative sample of young adults. Suicide Life Threat Behav. 2006;36:396–408.
51. Potenza MN, Wareham JD, Steinberg MA, Rugle L, Cavallo DA, Krishnan-Sarin S, Desai RA. Correlates of at-risk/problem Internet gambling in adolescents. J Am Acad Child Adolesc Psychiatry. 2011;50:150–9.
52. LaPlante DA, Nelson SE, LaBrie RA, Shaffer HJ. Stability and progression of disordered gambling: lessons from longitudinal studies. Can J Psychiatry. 2008;53:52–60.
53. Ferris J, Wynne H, Single E. Measuring problem gambling in Canada. Draft final report for the Inter-Provincial Task Force on Problem Gambling. Canada: Canadian Centre for Substance Abuse; 1998.
54. Blaszczynski A, Nower L. A pathways model of problem and pathological gambling. Addiction. 2002;97:487–99.
55. Walker M. On defining pathological gambling. National Association of Gambling Studies Newsletter. 1998;10:5–6.

56. Blaszczynski AP, Steel ZP, McConaghy N. Impulsivity and pathological gambling. Addiction. 1997;92:75–87.
57. Langham E, Thorne H, Browne M, Donaldson P, Rose J, Rockloff M. Understanding gambling related harm: a proposed definition, conceptual framework, and taxonomy of harms. BMC Public Health. 2016;16:1.
58. Grant JE, Schreiber L, Odlaug BL, Kim SW. Pathological gambling and bankruptcy. Compr Psychiatry. 2010;51:115–20.
59. Evans L, Delfabbro PH. Motivators for change and barriers to help-seeking in Australian problem gamblers. J Gambl Stud. 2005;21:133–55.
60. Blaszczynski A, Farrell E. A case series of 44 completed gambling-related suicides. J Gambl Stud. 1998;14:93–109.
61. Abbott DA, Cramer SL, Sherrets SD. Pathological gambling and the family: practice implications. Fam Soc. 1995;76:213.
62. Wenzel HG, Øren A, Bakken IJ. Gambling problems in the family—a stratified probability sample study of prevalence and reported consequences. BMC Public Health. 2008;8:412.
63. Muelleman RL, DenOtter T, Wadman MC, Tran TP, Anderson J. Problem gambling in the partner of the emergency department patient as a risk factor for intimate partner violence. J Emerg Med. 2002;23:307–12.
64. Afifi TO, Brownridge DA, MacMillan H, Sareen J. The relationship of gambling to intimate partner violence and child maltreatment in a nationally representative sample. J Psychiatr Res. 2010;44:331–7.
65. Lorenz VC, Yaffee RA. Pathological gamblers and their spouses: problems in interaction. J Gambl Behav. 1989;5:113–26.
66. McComb JL, Lee BK, Sprenkle DH. Conceptualizing and treating problem gambling as a family issue. J Marital Fam Ther. 2009;35:415–31.
67. Clarke D. Impulsivity as a mediator in the relationship between depression and problem gambling. Personal Individ Differ. 2006;40:5–15.
68. Kim SW, Grant JE, Eckert ED, Faris PL, Hartman BK. Pathological gambling and mood disorders: clinical associations and treatment implications. J Affect Disord. 2006;92:109–16.
69. Hing N, Holdsworth L, Tiyce M, Breen H. Stigma and problem gambling: current knowledge and future research directions. Int Gambl Stud. 2014;14:64–81.
70. Burge AN, Pietrzak RH, Molina CA, Petry NM. Age of gambling initiation and severity of gambling and health problems among older adult problem gamblers. Psychiatr Serv. 2004;55:1437–9.
71. Desai RA, Desai MM, Potenza MN. Gambling, health and age: data from the National Epidemiologic Survey on Alcohol and Related Conditions. Psychol Addict Behav. 2007;21:431.
72. Erickson L, Molina CA, Ladd GT, Pietrzak RH, Petry NM. Problem and pathological gambling are associated with poorer mental and physical health in older adults. Int J Geriatr Psychiatry. 2005;20:754–9.
73. Morasco BJ, Pietrzak RH, Blanco C, Grant BF, Hasin D, Petry NM. Health problems and medical utilization associated with gambling disorders: results from the National Epidemiologic Survey on Alcohol and Related Conditions. Psychosom Med. 2006;68:976–84.
74. Trevorrow K, Moore S. The association between loneliness, social isolation and women's electronic gaming machine gambling. J Gambl Stud. 1998;14:263–84.
75. Raylu N, Oei TP. Role of culture in gambling and problem gambling. Clin Psychol Rev. 2004;23:1087–114.
76. Winters KC, Bengston P, Door D, Stinchfield R. Prevalence and risk factors of problem gambling among college students. Psychol Addict Behav. 1998;12:127.
77. Collins D, Lapsley H. The social costs and benefits of gambling: an introduction to the economic issues. J Gambl Stud. 2003;19:123–48.
78. Garman ET, Leech IE, Grable JE. The negative impact of employee poor personal financial behaviors on employers. J Financ Couns Plan. 1996;7:157.

The Epidemiology of Gambling Disorder

Donald W. Black and Martha Shaw

This chapter reviews the epidemiology of gambling disorder (GD) including age at onset, prevalence, gender distribution, course and outcome, patterns of comorbidity, and subtypes.

3.1 Prevalence and Gender Distribution

Gambling is a recreational behavior found worldwide and is normative behavior in North American culture. A 1999 survey showed that 86% of the general population reported participating in some form of gambling [1], but other surveys show participation rates exceeding 90%, especially for gambling involving instant lotteries, slot machines, office pools, and card games [2, 3]. While most persons gamble responsibly, a small percentage develop problematic gambling behavior, which includes problem gambling ("at-risk") and its more severe variant, pathological gambling, renamed "gambling disorder" (GD) in the *Diagnostic and Statistical Manual of Mental Disorders, Fifth Edition* (DSM-5 [4]).

3.1.1 Prevalence

Approximately 4–7% of the adult US general population develops problematic gambling behavior [5]. Lifetime prevalence estimates of GD range from 0.42% to 4.0% in the USA [6–8]. Estimates of problem gambling are greater with lifetime prevalence estimates ranging from 3.5% to 5.1% [9]. The wide range in prevalence

D. W. Black (✉) · M. Shaw
Department of Psychiatry, University of Iowa Roy J. and Lucile A. Carver College of Medicine, Iowa City, IA, USA
e-mail: donald-black@uiowa.edu; martha-shaw@uiowa.edu

© Springer Nature Switzerland AG 2019
A. Heinz et al. (eds.), *Gambling Disorder*, https://doi.org/10.1007/978-3-030-03060-5_3

reported in the literature could be due to differences in survey methods, population sampled, or measures used to assess problem gambling and GD.

Two large epidemiologic surveys have been conducted in the USA that report prevalence rates for problem gambling and GD. In a probability subsample of 3435 respondents participating in the National Comorbidity Survey Replication, Kessler et al. [6] reported problem gambling in 2.3% and GD in 0.6%. In the National Epidemiologic Survey on Alcohol and Related Conditions (NESARC), a probability survey involving over 43,000 adult Americans, problem gambling was reported in 0.60% and GD in 0.42% [7, 10].

Problem gambling and GD have been reported wherever gambling is available. For example, a survey in Sweden reported a rate of 3.9% for problem gambling and 0.6% for GD [11]. A Hong Kong survey [12] reported that 4.0% and 1.8% of the respondents could be classified as lifetime problem or pathological gamblers, respectively. Based on results from the National Epidemiologic Survey of Psychiatric Disorders in South Korea, Park et al. [13] reported rates of 3.0% and 0.8%, respectively, for lifetime problem gambling and GD. In New Zealand, rates of lifetime problem and pathological gambling have been reported at 1.9% and 1.0% [14], respectively. In addition to different methods and assessments, these widely varying rates could reflect cultural differences in gambling acceptance and behavior.

The frequency of GD may be even higher among adolescents with a range up to 8% and college students with rates up to 14%. Among persons 18–21 years of age, the prevalence ranges as high as 14.4% [15, 16]. Rates may be lower in those over 60 years [8].

3.1.2   Gender Differences

The prevalence of GD is considerably higher in men than in women. Surveys and clinical data suggest that rates in men are nearly two to three times than for women [3]. For example, in the National Comorbidity Survey Replication, Kessler et al. [6] reported that the odds of GD were significantly higher in men than in women (OR = 4.5). In the NESARC study [17], 72% of people with GD were men and 28% were women. In a sample of psychiatric outpatients reported by Zimmerman et al. [18], 67.5% of persons with GD were men and 33.5% were women. The disorder has a later age at onset in women in whom the disorder progresses more rapidly, as is detailed below. This phenomenon ("telescoping") has been found in women with alcohol use and cannabis use disorders [19].

3.2   Age at Onset

GD has an age at onset ranging from the mid-20s to the late 30s but can occur for the first time even during senescence. In clinical studies, the age at onset range has been relatively narrow. For example, Black et al. [20] reported a mean age of onset of 36.4 years in 31 subjects enrolled in a pilot family study, 38.3 years for 19 persons enrolled in an escitalopram trial [21], and 35.8 years for 39 subjects in a bupropion trial [22]. Grant and Kim [23] reported a mean age at onset among 131 treatment-seeking people with GD of 36.8 years, while Grant et al. [24] found that 207 GD subjects assigned to one of four treatment cells in a medication trial had a mean age at onset ranging from 34.2 years to 36.9 years.

Epidemiological surveys have tended to report an earlier onset. In a general population study in Edmonton, Bland et al. [25] reported a mean age at onset of 25 years for people with "heavy betting." Blanco et al. [17], in reporting data from the NESARC, calculated an earlier mean age at onset for men (29.6 years) than women (34.9 years). Kessler et al. [6] reported data from the National Comorbidity Survey Replication indicating that GD has a bimodal distribution with a peak in the late teens/early 20s with a smaller secondary peak in the late 30s/early 40s. In a study of 287 individuals with GD, Black et al. [26] reported that age at onset ranged from 8 to 87 years with a mean of 34.3 years. Fifty percent of the sample had an onset by age 30, 70% by age 40, and 84% by age 50. Mean age at onset was earlier in men (28.6 years) than women (41.8 years). For women, age at onset was bimodal, with peaks appearing at the 20–24 year age range and the 40–44 year age range. For men, age at onset peaked for the 15–24 year age range and had a smaller spike in the 35–39 year age range. Age at onset is shown in Fig. 3.1.

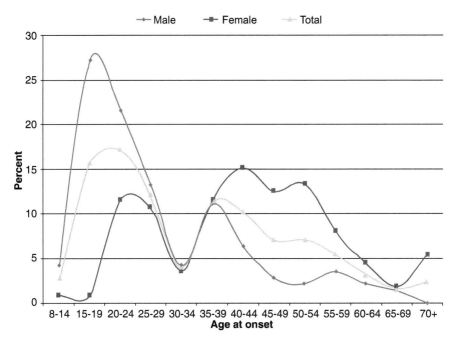

Fig. 3.1 Age at onset in male and female subjects with GD. Source: Black DW, Coryell WH, Crowe RR, et al. (2015) Age at onset of DSM-IV pathological gambling in a nontreatment sample: early- versus later-onset. Compr Psychiatry 60: 40–46

3.3   Course and Outcome

The DSM-5 [4] states that GD is chronic and deteriorating. This view was first articulated by Custer [27], who described GD as a progressive, multistage illness that began with a winning phase, followed by a losing phase, and, finally, a desperation phase. The initial or "winning" phase conferred feelings of status, power, and omnipotence. Fantasies of winning and thoughts of great successes were proposed to be common in this phase. A string of bad luck or an unexpected loss was proposed to then lead to the second or "losing" phase. This phase centers on the behavior known as "chasing," in which the gambler desperately attempts to recover lost money. Wagering is more frequent and often in larger amounts. The uncontrollable spiraling of losing and chasing of losses was proposed to lead the gambler to the third or "desperation" phase. Here, the gambler may engage in illegal activities such as fraud, embezzlement, writing bad checks, or stealing to support his gambling problem. Illegal behaviors are rationalized, often with the intent to pay back what is taken after the "big win" that is thought by the gambler to be in their imminent and eminent future. Fantasies of escape and thoughts of suicide are reported to be common during this phase [28]. Custer's phases of PG gained wide acceptance despite the absence of confirmatory data.

More recent data has challenged the notion of GD as intractable. Instead, GD appears to have a natural ebb and flow with many individuals moving toward reduced gambling involvement or experiencing spontaneous remission. LaPlante et al. [29] showed that most individuals with GD and at-risk gamblers move toward a lower (or less intensive) level of gambling behavior over time, while those who gamble recreationally, or do not gamble, are unlikely to move to more severe level of gambling activity (or to take up gambling). They reviewed five studies [30–34] that met their criteria of reporting longitudinal data pertaining to gambling that did not involve a treatment sample. These studies used various assessment points (between 2 and 4), widely varying populations (US general population, casino employees, college freshmen, adult gamblers, and scratch-card buyers), and used different measures of gambling severity (South Oaks Gambling Screen, Diagnostic Interview Schedule). LaPlante et al. [29] reported that level 3 gamblers (i.e., persons with GD) improved, with most moving toward a lower level. Results were similar for level 2 (i.e., "at-risk") gamblers. Those who were level 0–1 (no gambling and recreational gambling, respectively) at baseline were unlikely to progress to a higher (i.e., more severe) level of gambling behavior.

Other follow-up data are pertinent. Russo et al. [35] reported that 1-year remission rates following a treatment program for veterans were associated with less depression. Taber et al. [36] conducted a 6-month follow-up on 57 of 66 patients (86%) who completed a comprehensive treatment program; 56% reported total abstinence and had improved on measures of alcohol abuse, suicidal behavior, and overall distress. In a cross-sectional study, Westermeyer et al. [37] compared groups of remitted and non-remitted Hispanic and Native Americans with GD and concluded that gamblers with an Axis I disorder were less likely to remit. Goudriaan et al. [38] compared a group of persons with GD who had relapsed and a group that had not and found that those who relapsed performed worse on indicators of disinhibition (stop signal reaction time) and decision-making (card playing task), suggesting that neurocognitive measures may be important tools in predicting progression and relapse.

Hodgins and Peden [39] reinterviewed individuals with "active" GD in Canada after a mean of 40 months. They began with a cohort of 63 subjects; 55 (87%) agreed to an interview, and 40 (63%) were eventually interviewed. Nearly one-third had sought treatment for GD; half had experienced a depressive episode and one-fourth alcohol or drug abuse in the interim. They found that, while most had made an effort to quit or reduce their gambling, over 80% were still gambling problematically, and 34% had a current mood disorder. Hodgins and Peden acknowledged their poor follow-up rate and recommended more frequent contacts to improve participation and minimize "memory problems." Oei and Gordon [40] assessed 75 Australian Gamblers Anonymous (GA) attendees in an attempt to assess psychosocial predictors of abstinence and relapse. They measured social support, gambling cognitions and behavior, religious belief, and involvement in GA. Those achieving abstinence were more involved in GA ("attendance and participation") and reported better social support.

Slutske [41] found that over one-third of persons reporting lifetime GD in the Gambling Impact and Behavior [1] and NESARC studies [7] did not experience gambling-related problems in the past year, and only 7–12% had received treatment or attended Gamblers Anonymous. The absence of past-year symptoms in one-third of the individuals was characterized as "natural recovery," leading her to conclude that GD is not always chronic. Sartor et al. [42] evaluated gambling characteristics retrospectively in 1343 men from the Vietnam Era Twin Registry; 268 developed symptoms suggestive of GD, and 35 met criteria for GD. Those with GD first met criteria at age 21 and first sought treatment at age 29. They experienced five or more gambling "phases" defined as a "consistent pattern of gambling behavior." Seventeen percent of these persons also reported periods of abstinence, and 43% reported five or more symptom-free gambling phases.

Black et al. [43] systematically rated the gambling behaviors of three groups of individuals every 6 months for a mean of 2.6 years: 53 individuals with GD 60 years or older, 72 individuals with GD under 40 years, and 50 controls 60 years or older. Week-by-week gambling activity levels showed a significant downward trend for older and younger individuals with GD. Elder controls had no change in their level of gambling activity.

In summary, data suggest that GD has a natural ebb and flow and tends to improve or, in some cases, remit. The oscillation of gambling behavior in the relative absence of formal treatment suggests that individual and societal factors come into play. The data also suggest that those with comorbid disorders and lack of social support do worse. Gamblers Anonymous attendance may help encourage improvement and maintain gains. The data also suggest that it may be unrealistic to focus treatment efforts on abstinence and that efforts may be more successful if they focus on risk reduction.

3.3.1   Suicidal Ideations and Behaviors

People with GD tend to consider suicide and attempt suicide at rates much higher than in the general population with completed suicide perhaps the most worrisome outcome [44, 45]. Much evidence supporting a link to suicide comes from clinical samples. In a sample of 114 consecutive admissions to a Veterans Administration gambling treatment program, Kausch [46] concluded that nearly 40% of subjects had past suicide attempts, with two-thirds prompted by gambling-related problems. Petry and Kiluk [45] reported that 49% of 342 persons seeking treatment for disordered gambling had lifetime suicidal ideations and 17% reported making a suicide attempt. Those with suicidal ideations or a history of attempts also appeared to have more severe symptoms of GD than those without. Ledgerwood and Petry [47] found that of 125 persons, 48% had a history of gambling-related suicidal ideation, while 12% reported a past gambling-related suicide attempt. In another treatment-seeking sample, Battersby et al. [48] reported even higher rates of suicide ideations and attempts among 43 treatment-seeking people with GD (81% and 30%, respectively).

Data from a recent study show that suicidal ideations and suicide attempts occur at rates substantially greater than among controls [49]. Ninety-five GD subjects, 91 controls, and 1075 relatives were assessed as part of this family study. There were significant differences in the prevalence of lifetime suicidal ideations (27% vs. 9%) and lifetime suicide attempts (36% vs. 4%) between GD subjects and controls. Thirty-five (37%) GD subjects had no history of suicide ideation or attempts, 26 (27%) had a history of only suicide ideations, and 34 (36%) had a history of past suicide attempts. Half of those who attempted suicide made a single attempt, while the other half made more than one attempt. Suicide attempt(s) preceded the onset of GD in 13 subjects (38.2%); in 14 subjects (41.2%), the suicide attempt(s) occurred during the course of GD. In seven subjects (20.6%), the suicide attempts occurred both prior to PG onset and during its course. The study also found that suicide attempts were more frequent among GD offspring compared to control offspring (8.7% versus 0.8%).

3.4   Race and Ethnicity

Rates of disordered gambling may vary among racial and ethnic groups. Studies have found this effect in the USA, Canada, New Zealand, Australia, and Sweden [50]. In the USA, Native Americans, Asians, African-Americans, and Hispanics have shown a greater prevalence of disordered gambling than whites. In the NESARC study [50], prevalence rates of disordered gambling (problem gambling and GD combined) were higher among African-Americans (2.2%) and Native/ Asian Americans (2.3%) than among whites (1.2%). In a 1998 survey, 4.2% of African-Americans were classified as Level 2–3 gamblers, compared with 1.7% of other respondents [1].

3.5 Psychiatric Comorbidity

Psychiatric comorbidity is the rule and not the exception for persons with GD. In community surveys and clinic-based reports, mood/anxiety disorders, substance use disorders (SUDs), attention deficit/hyperactivity disorder (ADHD), impulse control disorders (ICDs), and personality disorders are frequently comorbid with GD [51, 52]. Findings from research studies are reported in Tables 3.1 and 3.2.

3.5.1 Substance Use Disorders

Lifetime alcohol or drug dependence is the best documented group of comorbid disorders in persons with GD. Two large studies have addressed this issue, showing a strong association between GD and substance use disorders. Welte et al. [8] found that 28% of persons with GD had current alcohol dependence compared to a rate of 1% for people without GD. The National Opinion Research Center study [1] found that among persons with GD, the rate of alcohol or drug abuse was nearly seven times higher than that among non-gamblers or recreational gamblers. Other surveys have shown that rates of alcohol abuse and dependence being four or more times higher among persons identified as having a gambling disorder compared to those without GD [25, 58, 72]. In a nationally representative sample, almost three quarters (73.2%) of individuals with GD had an alcohol use disorder [7]. As many as 30–50% of persons with GD seeking treatment have lifetime histories of alcohol or other substance abuse [73]. Rosenthal [74] observed that the use of alcohol or illicit drugs while a person gambles can lead to deterioration in cognitive abilities and judgment which, Rosenthal believes, may cause GD to progress more rapidly. While in some cases GD may predate the onset of substance misuse, psychopathology typically precedes the onset of GD [6].

The National Opinion Research Center study [1] found that 8.1% of persons with GD and 16.8% of persons with problem gambling reported illicit drug use in the past year, compared to 4.2% of recreational gamblers and 2% of non-gamblers. Bland et al. [25] similarly found that the prevalence of illegal drug abuse and dependence for individuals with GD were about four times higher than for people who do not gamble. In the study of Cunningham-Williams et al. [58], 15.5% of individuals with GD evidenced illegal drug use disorders, compared to 7.8% of recreational gamblers and 3.5% of non-gamblers. The lifetime prevalence rate for any drug use disorder in the national survey reported by Petry et al. [7] was 38.1% among GD respondents. Conversely, from 9% to 16% of substance abusers are likely to have GD [73, 75].

The frequency of addictions is also high in treatment-seeking individuals with GD. Zimmerman et al. [18] found that 67.5% of treatment-seeking individuals with GD had a substance use disorder as compared with 40.1% of psychiatric outpatients without GD. Among research subjects, Black et al. [62] reported that 68% of treatment-seeking individuals with GD had a lifetime substance use disorder compared with 27% of controls. A number of differences emerge from looking at treatment-seeking individuals with GD with and without a history of substance misuse.

Table 3.1 Comorbid major psychiatric disorders in persons with gambling disorder

Study	Sample size	Assessment method	Mood disorders	Psychotic disorders	ADHD	OCD	Substance use disorders	Eating disorders	Impulse control disorders	Anxiety disorders	No disorder
McCormick et al. [53]	50	RDC	76%	N/A	N/A	N/A	36%	N/A	N/A	N/A	N/A
Linden et al. [54]	25	SCID	72%	N/A	N/A	20%	48%	N/A	N/A	28%	N/A
Bland et al. [25]	30	DIS	33%	0%	N/A	17%	63%	N/A	N/A	27%	N/A
Specker et al. [55]	40	Operationalized diagnostic interview for ADHD; MIDI	N/A	N/A	20%	N/A	N/A	N/A	35%	N/A	N/A
Specker et al. [56]	40	SCID	78%	3%	N/A	3%	60%	N/A	N/A	38%	8%
Black and Moyer [57]	30	DIS	60%	3%	40%	10%	63%	7%	43%	40%	n/a
Cunningham-Williams et al. [58]	161	DIS	MDD (9%); dysthymia (4%)	4%	N/A	1%	Alcohol (45%); illicit drugs (40%)	N/A	N/A	Panic disorder (23%); GAD (8%); phobias (15%)	N/A
Hollander et al. [59]	10	N/A	30% Bipolar I and II		20%	10%	Current	N/A	N/A	N/A	50%
Hollander et al. [60]	10	N/A	50%	N/A	N/A	10%	10%	N/A	N/A	20%	N/A

Grant and Kim [23]	131	SCID-IV	34%	N/A	N/A	0%	35%	N/A	18%	9%	N/A
Zimmerman et al. [61]	15	SCID-IV; DID; BDI	53% mania		N/A	N/A	Current	N/A	N/A	20%	N/A
Petry et al. [7]	195	AUDADIS-IV	50%	N/A	N/A	N/A	73% alcohol use disorder	N/A	N/A	41%	N/A
Zimmerman et al. [18]	40	SCID-IV	62.5% MDD	5%	5%	10%	67.5%	17.5%	20%	42.5% panic disorder	N/A
Kessler et al. [6]	21	CIDI	56%	N/A	13%	N/A	76%	N/A	42%	60%	N/A
Park et al. [13]	43	DIS	12%	N/A	N/A	N/A	70%	N/A	N/A	14%	N/A
Black et al. [62]	95	SCID-IV	72%	N/A	N/A	13%	68%	14%	N/A	51%	N/A

Note. ADHD attention deficit/hyperactivity disorder, *BDI* Beck Depression Inventory, *DID* Diagnostic Interview for Depression, *DIS* Diagnostic Interview Schedule, Version III, *GAD* generalized anxiety disorder, *MDD* major depressive disorder, *MIDI* Minnesota impulsive disorders interview, *N/A* not available, *OCD* obsessive-compulsive disorder, *RDC* research diagnostic criteria, *SCID* Structured Clinical Interview for DSM-III, *SCID-IV* Structured Clinical Interview for DSM-IV, *CIDI* Composite International Diagnostic Instrument

Table 3.2 Comorbid personality disorders in persons with gambling disorder

Study	Sample size	Assessment method	Any PD	Paranoid	Schizoid	Schizotypal	BPD	Histrionic	Narcissistic	Avoidant	OCPD	ASPD	Dependent	Unspecified
Blaszczynski et al. [63]	109	DSM-III criteria	N/A	N/A	N/A	N/A	14%	N/A	N/A	N/A	N/A	N/A	N/A	14%
Lesieur and Blume [64]	7	N/A	71%	N/A	N/A	28%	N/A	N/A	N/A	N/A	N/A	N/A	N/A	49%
Bellaire and Caspari [65]	51	N/A	N/A	N/A	N/A	N/A	N/A	N/A	N/A	N/A	N/A	15%	N/A	N/A
Bland et al. [25]	30	DIS	N/A	N/A	N/A	N/A	N/A	N/A	N/A	N/A	N/A	40%	N/A	N/A
Specker et al. [56]	40	SCID-P	25%	3%	3%	0%	3%	0%	5%	13%	5%	0%	5%	3%
Black and Moyer [57]	30	PDQ-R	87%	26%	33%	30%	23%	7%	20%	50%	59%	17%	7%	N/A
Blaszczynski and Steel [66]	82	PDQ-R	93%	40%	21%	38%	70%	66%	57%	37%	32%	29%	49%	N/A
Fernandez-Montalvo and Echeburua [67]	50	IPDE	32%	8%	0%	0%	16%	0%	8%	0%	0%	8%	0%	8%
Petry et al. [7]	195	AUDADIS-IV	N/A	24%	15%	N/A	N/A	13%	N/A	14%	28%	23%	3%	N/A
Bagby et al. [68]	61	SCID-II-PQ/ SCID-II	92%/23%	30%/5%	15%/3%	20%/0	62%/10%	26%/0	53%/0	26%/5%	64%/5%	35%/5%	3%/0	N/A
Pelletier et al. [69]	100	SCID-II	64%	18%	4%	3%	10%	1%	15%	10%	16%	29%	3%	27%
Odlaug et al. [70]	77	SCID-II	46%	3%	1%	0%	7%	4%	5%	10%	27%	3%	4%	0%
Black et al. [71]	93	SIDP	41%	7%	1%	1%	19%	2%	6%	6%	10%	15%	6%	N/A

Note. ASPD antisocial personality disorder, *BPD* borderline personality disorder, *DIS* Diagnostic Interview Schedule, Version III, *N/A* not available, *OCPD* obsessive-compulsive personality disorder, *PD* personality disorder, *PDQ-R* Personality Disorders Questionnaire-Revised, *SCID-P* Structured Clinical Interview for DSM-III Personality Disorders, *IPDE* International Personality Disorders Examination

Those with a history of a substance use disorder suffer greater psychiatric distress, experience more frequent gambling, have more years of disordered gambling, and are more likely to receive mental health treatment [76].

Cunningham-Williams et al. [58] reported, based on data from the Epidemiological Catchment Area survey, that problem gambling occurred within 2 years of the onset of alcoholism in 65% of gambling cases. Individuals with GD may use alcohol or other drugs when they stop gambling; similarly, gambling may serve as a substitute for alcohol and other drugs to prolong feelings of exhilaration from gambling or ameliorate the dysphoria that develops during gambling abstinence [64].

3.5.2 Mood Disorders

Multiple general population surveys have investigated the association of psychiatric comorbidities and disordered gambling, including major depression, dysthymia, bipolar disorder, and suicidality. Bland et al. [25] found elevated rates of mood disorders in individuals with GD (33.3%) compared to non-gamblers (14.2%). Rates of major depression were also higher for individuals with gambling problems in the sample reported by Cunningham-Williams et al. [58]. Interestingly, these investigators also found that recreational gamblers appear at greater risk for major depression and dysthymia than those who have never gambled. Neither of these two surveys found a significant association between GD and mania. In the NESARC survey, 49.6% of persons with GD had a mood disorder [7]. Furthermore, these investigators showed that mania was the mood disorder most strongly related to GD with an odds ratio (OR) of 8. Odds ratios for major depression and dysthymia were each 3.3 and for hypomania 1.8.

Clinical studies also show a relationship between mood disorders and GD. In an early study, 76% of an inpatient sample admitted for treatment of GD met criteria for a current major depressive disorder [53]. In a sample of 25 problem gamblers recruited from a Gamblers Anonymous chapter, Linden et al. [54] found that 72% of subjects had experienced at least one episode of major depression. Bipolar disorder has also been reported at high rates in persons with GD. Linden et al. [54] reported a lifetime prevalence of 24% in persons with GD, while McCormick et al. [53] found current hypomania in 38% of an inpatient sample. Mood disorders are also relatively common in the treatment-seeking segment of the GD population. Stinchfield and Winters [77], for example, found that 12% of their 592 GD treatment-seekers also had a current mood disorder. Black et al. [62] systematically assessed GD subjects for a family study and found that 72% had a lifetime history of a mood disorder compared with 30% of controls. The most common mood disorders were major depression (61%) and bipolar disorder (9%).

3.5.3 Anxiety Disorders

Persons with GD also report high rates of lifetime anxiety disorders, such as panic disorder, phobias, obsessive-compulsive disorder, generalized anxiety disorder, and posttraumatic stress disorder. General population surveys show a strong association between GD and anxiety disorders. Kessler et al. [6] found that 60.3% of their sample had any anxiety disorder, with 52.2% having phobias, 21.9% panic disorder, 16.6% generalized anxiety disorder (GAD), and 14.8% posttraumatic stress disorder. Furthermore, these authors found that GD is temporally predicted by panic disorder, GAD, and phobia. Petry et al. [7] reported that panic disorder with and without agoraphobia was most strongly related to GD; the odds of having phobias or GAD were significant but less so. Cunningham-Williams et al. [58] also found the highest percentage of subjects experiencing panic disorder (23.3%), followed by phobias (14.6%), GAD (7.7%), and obsessive-compulsive disorder (OCD, 7.7%). Likewise, Bland et al. [25] found that persons diagnosed with GD had high rates of anxiety disorders. These authors reported lifetime rates of 26.7% for GAD, 17.7% for phobias, 3.3% for panic disorder, and 16.7% for OCD.

Ibanez et al. [78], in their sample of 43 treatment-seeking outpatients, found a lifetime GAD rate of 7.2%, much lower than the 40% reported by Black and Moyer [57] and Specker et al. [56] at 37.5%. Black and Moyer [57] also found rates of panic disorder and OCD at 10% each, while Specker et al. [56] reported 20% and 2.5%, respectively. While samples and rates differ somewhat, there remains little doubt that GD and anxiety disorders share a relationship, although the relationship with OCD seems less clear.

Some investigators believe that GD falls within the obsessive-compulsive spectrum [79, 80]. They point to similarities between GD and OCD, as exemplified by persistent thoughts and urges followed by repetitive behaviors. There are major differences, however, including the fact that OCD is unwanted, yet GD is generally perceived as pleasurable. Comorbidity studies suggest that from 2.5% [56] to 20% [54] of persons with GD also have OCD. In two family studies of OCD that also looked at GD [81, 82], there were few data to support the existence of a relationship between the two disorders.

3.5.4 Attention Deficit/Hyperactivity Disorder

GD has a number of attributes in common with attention deficit/hyperactivity disorder (ADHD), and clinical data suggest substantial syndromal overlap. Goldstein et al. [83] concluded that the electroencephalographic activation patterns to right and left brain tasks seen in eight men with GD resembled those in unmedicated children diagnosed with ADHD. Carlton and Manowitz [84] compared persons with GD to alcoholic persons and reported excessive and comparable levels of ADHD-related behaviors in childhood than control subjects. Rugle and Melamed [85] compared 33 non-substance-abusing persons with GD with 33 nonaddicted controls on nine attention measures and childhood behavior questionnaires. They reported that persons with GD performed significantly worse than controls on higher-order attentional measures and had more childhood behaviors consistent with ADHD. They concluded that attentional deficits and the behavior problems associated with them are long-standing and may be a risk factor for the development of GD.

Specker et al. [55] reported that 8 of 40 (20%) people with GD met criteria for ADHD, and another 7 (17.5%) had symptoms that were considered subthreshold. These authors hypothesized that ADHD may predispose individuals to either substance abuse or GD and that gamblers with attentional deficits might chose gambling activities that do not require sustained attention or concentration. Finally, Kessler et al. [6] found in their general population survey that 13.4% of persons with GD also had ADHD. Black et al. [86] showed that among 54 individuals with GD, ADHD symptoms were significantly more common than in 65 controls. The most pronounced differences observed for individual items from the ADHD Checklist [87] were "Difficulty sustaining attention" and "Blurts out answers." In a series of medication trials, these investigators also showed that ADHD symptoms subside when GD is successfully treated [21, 22].

Impulsivity, an important attribute of ADHD, is also reported to be common among persons with GD. Castellani and Rugle [88] evaluated 843 subjects admitted to an inpatient addictions unit having a primary diagnosis of GD, alcohol dependence, or cocaine abuse. In contrast to individuals with alcoholism and cocaine abuse, those with GD scored significantly higher on measures of impulsivity, such as coming to quick decisions, moving quickly from impulse to action, and lack of future planning. Similar findings have been reported by DeCaria et al. [89], who found higher levels of impulsivity as measured by the Barratt Impulsiveness Scale [90] in persons with GD, compared to individuals with cocaine abuse, alcoholism, polysubstance abuse, and depression. In the study of Black et al. [86], one-third of individuals with GD were highly impulsive (BIS total $\geq$ 72) compared to 8% of controls. The BIS total score among individuals with GD was highly correlated with gambling severity.

3.5.5   Impulse Control Disorders

Lifetime rates of impulse control disorders (ICDs) also appear to be higher in persons with GD than seen in the general population. Investigators have reported rates ranging from 18% to 43% for one or more ICD [23, 55, 57, 91]. Specker et al. [55] examined frequencies of ICDs in a treatment-seeking sample and found increased levels of compulsive shopping and sexual behaviors, intermittent explosive disorder, and kleptomania. Black and Moyer [57] also found high frequencies of compulsive buying (23%), compulsive sexual behavior (17%), and intermittent explosive disorder (13%) in their sample. Grant and Kim [91] reported lower frequencies with a larger sample, with 9% having compulsive sexual behavior, 8% having compulsive shopping, and just 2% reporting intermittent explosive disorder.

Compulsive shopping appears to be the most frequent comorbid ICD in persons with GD [23, 55, 91, 92], perhaps because, as Specker et al. suggest, both compulsive shopping and GD have shared characteristics of focused attention, monetary gratification, and monetary exchange. In their recent family study, Black et al. [92] found that the presence of GD increased the odds of having compulsive shopping nearly 12-fold.

3.6   Personality Disorders

Personality disorders are relatively common in persons with GD (Table 3.2), but prevalence is highly dependent on the study population and assessment used [93]. Studies that use self-report instruments often yield higher rates for personality disorders than studies using structured or semi-structured interviews. For example, the prevalence estimates for personality disorders among people with GD assessed with self-report instruments ranged from 87% to 93% compared with 25% to 61% for those assessed with a structured or semi-structured interview [68].

In a general population survey [7], a robust association was found between GD and all the personality disorders studied; the odds of having any personality disorder if one also has PG were 8.3 times greater than for the general population. The odds ratio of having histrionic personality disorder was 6.9, avoidant personality disorder 6.5, paranoid personality disorder 6.1, antisocial personality disorder 6.0, dependent personality disorder 5.5, schizoid personality disorder 5.0, and obsessive-compulsive personality disorder 4.6.

Antisocial personality disorder (ASPD), characterized by a pervasive pattern of poor social conformity, deceitfulness, and lack of remorse, occurs at relatively high rates among those with GD, perhaps because the two are associated with criminality [94]. In studies using structured assessments, rates of ASPD have ranged from 3% to 40% [25, 57, 63, 66]. In a large community-based study examining this relationship, Slutske et al. [95] reported that 15% of their sample of GDs also had ASPD, compared with 2% of the comparison sample without GD, leading to an odds ratio of 6.4. Pietrzak and Petry [96] compared treatment-seeking individuals with GD with and without ASPD. Those with ASPD had more severe gambling, more medical and drug-related problems, and higher scores on symptom measures of somatization, paranoid ideation, and phobic anxiety. They were also more likely to be younger, male, less educated, divorced, or separated and to have had a history of substance abuse treatment than their non-ASPD counterparts.

In a recent family study of 93 persons with GD [71], personality disorders were found in over 40% of those assessed using a structured instrument. Those with as compared to without a personality disorder had more severe gambling symptoms, earlier age at GD onset, more suicide attempts, more psychiatric comorbidity, and a more robust family history of psychiatric illness. The antisocial, borderline, dependent, and paranoid types were all significantly more frequent in GD subjects than controls, as were all personality disorder clusters. The most frequent personality disorders were the borderline, antisocial, and obsessive-compulsive types. Cluster B disorders had the greatest odds ratio (OR = 17.2).

Bagby et al. [68] used both a self-report and a semi-structured interview in their study of 204 individuals with GD. As expected, personality disorder prevalence estimates with the self-report measure were high (92%); they were lower with the interview tool (23%). These investigators found that only borderline personality disorder had consistently high and significant prevalence rates in their non-treatment-seeking samples across both types of measures. Fernandez-Montalvo and Echeburua [67] also used a structured clinical interview in their study of 50 non-treatment-seeking individuals with GD. These authors reported that borderline personality disorder was the most prevalent personality disorder at 16%, followed by antisocial, paranoid, narcissistic, and non-specified, which were each observed in 8% of cases. Furthermore, they found that the presence of a personality disorder was associated with greater gambling severity and more severe symptoms of anxiety, depression, and alcohol abuse.

3.7   GD Subtypes

There is little disagreement that GD is heterogeneous. Attempts to identify subtypes of GD have generally not been validated by empirical data. Moran [97] identified five subtypes based on work with 50 individuals with GD: (1) subcultural gambling (14%), in which a person gambles to fit in with a group of his peers but later exhibits difficulty controlling gambling; (2) neurotic gambling (34%), in which gambling is motivated in response to a strained situation or an emotional problem, such as marital conflict, and subsides when it is resolved; (3) impulsive gambling (18%), in which gambling is accompanied by poor behavioral control; (4) psychopathic gambling (24%), in which gambling appears as an antisocial behavioral pattern; and (5) symptomatic gambling (10%), in which gambling is associated with some other mental illness, such as depression, and is considered a secondary phenomenon. While Moran's typology is clinically useful, it has not been empirically validated, and the different subtypes are not discrete.

Steel and Blaszczynski [98] used principal component analysis to investigate the factorial structure of PG. The investigators identified four primary factors: psychological distress, sensation-seeking, crime and liveliness, and impulsive-antisocial. The psychological distress factor was associated with female gender, suicidal ideation and behavior, and family psychiatric history, the sensation-seeking factor with a history of alcohol abuse, the crime and liveliness factor with criminal activity, and the impulsive factor (which was described as clinically most useful) with early onset of gambling, poor job history, separation or divorce due to gambling, and highly impulsive gamblingrelated illegal acts. The investigators concluded that gamblers exhibiting features of impulsivity and ASPD are at greatest risk for developing adverse personal and emotional consequences.

A widely discussed distinction is between "escape-seekers" and "sensation-seekers" [99]. The former group tends to include older persons who gamble out of loneliness/boredom, from depression, or to fill time, and who choose passive forms of gambling (e.g., slots). The former group includes persons—often women—who are reported to gamble to relieve feelings of emotional tension, anxiety, or depression. For such people, gambling may act as an analgesic by providing an escape from unpleasant situations. The latter group includes persons who seek stimulation and arousal to alleviate boredom or hyperarousal. For some, gambling provides an intense thrill or feeling of excitement [27].

Blaszczynski and Nower [100] provide a conceptual framework that integrates biological, developmental, cognitive, and other determinants of disordered gambling. They identified three distinct subgroups of individuals with GD: (a) behaviorally conditioned gamblers, (b) emotionally vulnerable gamblers, and (c) antisocial, impulsive gamblers. The behaviorally conditioned gamblers have no specific predisposing psychopathology and develop PG as a result of distorted cognitions and poor judgments regarding gambling. Depression, alcohol abuse, and anxiety may result from gambling, but are not causal. The emotionally vulnerable gamblers suffer premorbid depression or anxiety and have a history of poor coping, frequent life events, and adverse developmental experiences (e.g., childhood abuse or neglect). For these individuals, gambling serves to modulate affective states or meet other psychological needs. Finally, the antisocial, impulsive gambler is highly disturbed with features of ASPD and impulsivity, suggestive of neurological or neurochemical dysfunction. For these persons, gambling begins early in life and escalates rapidly. The subtyping scheme has received some experimental support [101, 102].

References

1. National Opinion Research Center (NORC). Gambling impact and behavior study. Chicago, IL: University of Chicago; 1999.
2. Volberg R. The prevalence and demographics of pathological gamblers – implications for public health. Am J Public Health. 1994;84:237–41.
3. Welte JW, Barnes M, Wieczorek WF, et al. Gambling participation in the US – results from a national survey. J Gambl Stud. 2002;18:313–37.
4. American Psychiatric Association, editor. Diagnostic and statistical manual of mental disorders. 5th ed. Washington, DC: American Psychiatric Association; 2013.
5. Shaffer HJ, Hall MN, Vander Bilt J. Estimating prevalence of disordered gambling behavior in the United States and Canada: a research synthesis. Am J Public Health. 1999;89:1369–76.
6. Kessler RC, Hwang I, LaBrie R, et al. DSM-IV pathological gambling in the National Comorbidity Survey Replication. Psychol Med. 2008;38:1351–60.
7. Petry NM, Stinson FS, Grant BF. Comorbidity of DSM-IV pathological gambling and other psychiatric disorders: results from the National Epidemiologic Survey on alcohol and related conditions. J Clin Psychiatry. 2005;66:564–74.
8. Welte J, Barnes G, Wieczorek W, et al. Alcohol and gambling pathology among U.S. adults: prevalence, demographic patterns and comorbidity. J Stud Alcohol. 2001;62:706–12.
9. Volberg RA. Prevalence studies of problem gambling in the United States. J Gambl Stud. 1996;12:111–28.
10. Chou KL, Afifi TO. Disordered (problem or pathological) gambling and Axis I psychiatric disorders: results from the National Epidemiologic Survey on Alcohol and Related Conditions. Am J Epidemiol. 2011;173:1289–97.
11. Volberg RA, Abbott MW, Ronnberg S, Munck IME. Prevalence and risks of pathological gambling in Sweden. Acta Psychiatr Scand. 2001;104:250–6.
12. Wong ILK, So EMT. Prevalence estimates of problem and pathological gambling in Hong Kong. Am J Psychiatry. 2003;160:1353–4.
13. Park S, Cho MJ, Jeon HJ, et al. Prevalence, clinical correlations, comorbidities, and suicidal tendencies in pathological Korean gamblers: results from the Korean Epidemiologic Catchment Area Study. Soc Psychiatry Psychiatr Epidemiol. 2010;45:621–9.
14. Abbott MW, Volberg RA, Ronnberg S. Comparing the New Zealand and Swedish National Surveys of gambling and problem gambling. J Gambl Stud. 2004;20:237–58.

15. Lesieur HR, Klein R. Pathological gambling among high school students. Addict Behav. 1987;12:129–35.
16. Westphal JR, Rush J. Pathological gambling in Louisiana: an epidemiologic perspective. J La State Med Soc. 1996;148:353–8.
17. Blanco C, Hasin DS, Petry N, Stinson FS, Grant BF. Sex differences in subclinical and DSM-IV pathological gambling: results from the National Epidemiologic Survey on Alcohol and Related Conditions. Psychol Med. 2006;36:943–53.
18. Zimmerman M, Chelminski I, Young D. Prevalence and diagnostic correlates of DSM-IV pathological gambling in psychiatric outpatients. J Gambl Stud. 2006;22:255–62.
19. Tavares H, Zilberman ML, Beites FJ, Gentil V. Gender differences in gambling progression. J Gambl Stud. 2001;17:151–9.
20. Black DW, Monahan P, Temkit M, Shaw M. A family study of pathological gambling. Psychiatry Res. 2006;141:295–303.
21. Black DW, Arndt S, Coryell WH, et al. Bupropion in the treatment of pathological gambling: a randomized, placebo-controlled, flexible-dose study. J Clin Psychopharmacol. 2007;27:143–50.
22. Black DW, Shaw M, Forbush KT, Allen J. An open-label study of escitalopram in the treatment of pathological gambling. Clin Neuropharmacol. 2007;30:206–12.
23. Grant JE, Kim SW. Demographic and clinical features of 131 adult pathological gamblers. J Clin Psychiatry. 2001;62:957–62.
24. Grant JE, Potenza MN, Hollander E, et al. Multi-center investigation of the opioid antagonist nalmefene in the treatment of pathological gambling. Am J Psychiatry. 2006;163:303–12.
25. Bland RC, Newman SC, Orn H, Stebelsky G. Epidemiology of pathological gambling in Edmonton. Can J Psychiatr. 1993;38:108–12.
26. Black DW, Coryell WH, Crowe RR, et al. Age at onset of DSM-IV pathological gambling in a non-treatment sample: early- versus later-onset. Compr Psychiatry. 2015;60:40–6.
27. Custer RL. Profile of the pathological gambler. J Clin Psychiatry. 1984;45:35–8.
28. Lesicur HR, Rosenthal RJ. Pathological gambling: a review of the literature. J Gambl Stud. 1991;7:5–39.
29. LaPlante DA, Nelson SE, LaBrie RA, Shaffer HJ. Stability and progression of disordered gambling: lessons from longitudinal studies. Can J Psychiatry. 2008;53:52–60.
30. Abbott MW, Williams MM, Volberg RA. A prospective study of problem and regular non-problem gamblers living in the community. Subst Use Misuse. 2004;39:855–84.
31. DeFuentes-Merillas L, Koeter MW, Schippers GM, van den Brink W. Temporal stability of pathological scratchcard gambling among adult scratchcard buyers two years later. Addiction. 2004;99:117–27.
32. Shaffer HJ, Hall MN. The natural history of gambling and drinking problems among casino workers. J Soc Psychol. 2002;142:405–24.
33. Slutske W, Jackson KM, Sher KJ. The natural history of problem gambling from age 18 to 29. J Abnorm Psychol. 2003;112:263–74.
34. Winters KC, Stinchfield RD, Botzet A, Anderon N. A prospective study of youth gambling behaviors. Psychol Addict Behav. 2002;16:3–9.
35. Russo AM, Taber JI, McCormick RA, Ramirez LF. An outcome study of an inpatient program for pathological gamblers. Hosp Community Psychiatry. 1984;35:823–7.
36. Taber JI, McCormick RA, Russo AM, et al. Follow-up of pathological gamblers after treatment. Am J Psychiatry. 1987;144:757–61.
37. Westermeyer J, Canive J, Thuras P, et al. Remission from pathological gambling among Hispanics and Native Americans. Community Ment Health J. 2006;42:537–52.
38. Goudriaan AE, Oosterlaan J, de Beurs E, van den Brink W. The role of self-reported impulsivity and reward sensitivity versus neurocognitive measures of disinhibition and decision-making in the prediction of relapse in pathological gamblers. Psychol Med. 2008;38:41–50.
39. Hodgins DC, Peden N. Natural course of gambling disorders: forty month follow-up. J Gambl Iss. 2005;14:1–15.

40. Oei TPS, Gordon LM. Psychosocial factors related to gambling abstinence and relapse in members of Gamblers Anonymous. J Gambl Stud. 2008;24:91–105.
41. Slutske W. Natural recovery and treatment-seeking in pathological gambling: results of two national surveys. Am J Psychiatry. 2006;163:297–302.
42. Sartor CE, Scherrer JF, Shah KR, et al. Course of pathological gambling symptoms and reliability of the Lifetime Gambling History measure. Psychiatry Res. 2007;152:55–61.
43. Black DW, Coryell W, McCormick B, Shaw M, Allen J. A prospective follow-up study of younger and older subjects with pathological gambling. Psychiatry Res. 2017;256:162–8.
44. Blaszczynski A, Farrell E. A case series of 44 completed gambling-related suicides. J Gambl Stud. 1998;14:93–109.
45. Petry NM, Kiluk BD. Suicidal ideation and suicide attempts in treatment-seeking pathological gamblers. J Nerv Ment Dis. 2002;190:462–9.
46. Kausch O. Suicide attempts among veterans seeking treatment for pathological gambling. J Clin Psychiatry. 2003;64:1031–8.
47. Ledgerwood DM, Petry NM. Gambling and suicidality in treatment-seeking pathological gamblers. J Nerv Ment Dis. 2004;192:711–4.
48. Battersby M, Tolchard B, Scurrah M, Thomas L. Suicide ideation and behavior in people with pathological gambling attending a treatment service. Int J Ment Health Addict. 2006;4:233–46.
49. Black DW, Coryell WH, Crowe RR, et al. Suicide ideation, suicide attempts, and completed suicide in persons with DSM-IV pathological gambling and their first-degree relatives. Suicide Life Threat Behav. 2015;45:700–9.
50. Alegria AA, Petry NM, Hasin DS, et al. Disordered gambling among racial and ethnic groups in the US: Results from the National Epidemiologic Survey on Alcohol and Related Conditions. CNS Spectr. 2009;14:132–42.
51. Argo T, Black DW. The characteristics of pathological gambling. In: Grant J, Potenza M, editors. Understanding and treating pathological gambling. Washington, DC: American Psychiatric Publishing Inc.; 2004. p. 39–53.
52. Crockford ND, el-Guebaly N. Psychiatric comorbidity in pathological gambling: a critical review. Am J Psychiatry. 1999;43:43–50.
53. McCormick RA, Russo AM, Ramirez LF, Taber JI. Affective disorders among pathological gamblers seeking treatment. Am J Psychiatry. 1984;141:215–8.
54. Linden RD, Pope HG Jr, Jonas JM. Pathological gambling and major affective disorder: preliminary findings. J Clin Psychiatry. 1986;47:201–3.
55. Specker SM, Carlson GA, Christenson GA, Marcotte M. Impulse control disorders and attention deficit disorder in pathological gamblers. Ann Clin Psychiatry. 1995;7:175–9.
56. Specker SM, Carlson GA, Edmonson KM, et al. Psychopathology in pathological gamblers seeking treatment. J Gambl Stud. 1996;12:67–81.
57. Black DW, Moyer T. Clinical features and psychiatric comorbidity of subjects with pathological gambling behavior. Psychiatr Serv. 1998;49:1434–9.
58. Cunningham-Williams RM, Cottler LB, Compton WM III, Spitznagel EL. Taking chances: problem gamblers and mental health disorders – results from the St. Louis epidemiologic catchment area study. Am J Public Health. 1998;88:1093–6.
59. Hollander E, DeCaria CM, Mari E, et al. Short-term single-blind fluvoxamine treatment of pathological gambling. Am J Psychiatry. 1998;155:1781–3.
60. Hollander E, DeCaria CM, Finkell JN, et al. A randomized double-blind fluvoxamine/placebo crossover trial in pathologic gambling. Biol Psychiatry. 2000;47:813–7.
61. Zimmerman M, Breen RB, Posternak MA. An open-label study of citalopram in the treatment of pathological gambling. J Clin Psychiatry. 2002;63:44–8.
62. Black DW, Coryell WC, Crowe RR, et al. A direct, controlled, blind family study of pathological gambling. J Clin Psychiatry. 2014;75:215–21.
63. Blaszczynski A, Mcconaghy N, Frankova A. Crime, antisocial personality, and pathological gambling. J Gambl Behav. 1989;5:137–52.

64. Lesieur HR, Blume SB. Evaluation of patients treated for pathological gambling in a combined alcohol, substance abuse and pathological gambling treatment unit using addiction severity index. Br J Addict. 1991;86:1017–28.
65. Bellaire W, Caspari D. Diagnosis and therapy of male gamblers in a university psychiatric hospital. J Gambl Stud. 1992;8:143–50.
66. Blaszczynski A, Steel Z. Personality disorders among pathological gamblers. J Gambl Stud. 1998;14:51–70.
67. Fernandez-Montalvo J, Echeburua E. Pathological gambling and personality disorder: an exploratory study with the IPDE. J Pers Disord. 2004;18:500–5.
68. Bagby RM, Vachon DD, Bulmash E, et al. Personality disorders and pathological gambling: a review and re-examination of prevalence rates. J Pers Disord. 2008;22:191–207.
69. Pelletier O, Ladouceur R, Rheaume J: Personality disorders and pathological gambling: comorbidity and treatment dropout predictors. Int Gambl Stud. 2008;8:299–313.
70. Odlaug BL, Schreiber LRN, Grant JE. Personality disorder and dimensions in pathological gambling. J Pers Disord. 2012;26:381–92.
71. Black DW, Coryell WH, Crowe RR, et al. Personality disorders, impulsiveness, and novelty seeking in persons with DSM-IV pathological gambling and their first-degree relatives. J Gambl Stud. 2015;31:1201–14.
72. Smart RG, Ferris J. Alcohol, drugs and gambling in the Ontario adult population. Can J Psychiatry. 1994;41:36–45.
73. Lesieur HR, Blume SB, Zoppa RM. Alcoholism, drug abuse, and gambling. Alcohol Clin Exp Res. 1986;10:33–8.
74. Rosenthal RJ. Pathological gambling. Psychiatric Ann. 1992;22:72–8.
75. Spunt B, Dupont I, Lesieur H, et al. Pathological gambling and substance misuse: a review of the literature. Subst Use Misuse. 1998;33:2535–60.
76. Ladd GT, Petry NM. A comparison of pathological gamblers with and without substance abuse treatment histories. Exp Clin Psychopharmacol. 2003;11:202–9.
77. Stinchfield RD, Winters KC. Outcome of Minnesota's gambling treatment programs. J Gambl Stud. 2001;17:217–45.
78. Ibanez A, de Castro IP, Fernandez-Piqueres J, et al. Pathological gambling and DNA polymorphic markers at MAO-A and MAO-B genes. Mol Psychiatry. 2001;5:105–9.
79. Blaszczynski A. Pathological gambling and obsessive compulsive spectrum disorders. Psychol Rep. 1999;84:107–13.
80. Hollander E, editor. Obsessive-compulsive related disorders. Washington, DC: American Psychiatric Press; 2003.
81. Bienvenu OJ, Samuels JF, Riddle MA, et al. The relationship of obsessive-compulsive disorder to possible spectrum disorders – results from a family study. Biol Psychiatry. 2000;48:387–93.
82. Black DW, Stumpf A, McCormick B, et al. A blind re-analysis of the Iowa family study of obsessive-compulsive disorder. Psychiatry Res. 2013;209:202–6.
83. Goldstein L, Manowitz P, Nora R, et al. Differential EEG activation and pathological gambling. Biol Psychiatry. 1985;20:1232–4.
84. Carlton PL, Manowitz P. Behavioral restraint and symptoms of attention deficit disorder in alcoholics and pathological gamblers. Neuropsychobiology. 1992;25:44–8.
85. Rugle L, Melamed L. Neuropsychological assessment of attention problems in pathological gamblers. J Nerv Ment Dis. 1993;181:107–12.
86. Black DW, Smith M, Forbush K, et al. Neuropsychological performance, impulsivity, symptoms of ADHD, and Cloninger's personality traits, in pathological gambling. Addict Res Ther. 2013;21:216–26.
87. Achenbach TM. The Achenbach behavior checklist. Burlington, VT: University of Vermont; 1991.
88. Castellani B, Rugle L. A comparison of pathological gamblers to alcoholics and cocaine misusers on impulsivity, sensation-seeking, and craving. Int J Addict. 1995;30:275–89.

89. DeCaria C, Hollander E, Grossman R, et al. Diagnosis, neurobiology, and treatment of pathological gambling. J Clin Psychiatry. 1996;57(Suppl 8):80–4.
90. Barratt EE. Anxiety and impulsiveness related to psychomotor efficiency. Percept Mot Skills. 1959;9:191–8.
91. Grant JE, Kim SW. Comorbidity of impulse control disorders in pathological gamblers. Acta Psychiatr Scand. 2003;108:203–7.
92. Black DW, Coryell WH, Crowe RR, et al. The relationship of DSM-IV pathological gambling to compulsive buying and other possible spectrum disorders: results from the Iowa PG family study. Psychiatry Res. 2015;226:273–6.
93. Vaddiparti K, Cottler LB. Personality disorders and pathological gambling. Curr Opin Psychiatry. 2017;30:45–9.
94. Brown RIF. Pathological gambling and associated patterns of crime: a comparison with alcohol and other drug addictions. J Gambl Behav. 1987;3:98–114.
95. Slutske WS, True WR, Goldberg J, et al. A twin study of the association between pathological gambling and antisocial personality disorder. J Abnorm Psychol. 2001;110:297–308.
96. Pietrzak RH, Petry NM. Antisocial personality disorder is associated with increased severity of gambling, medical, drug, and psychiatric problems among treatment-seeking pathological gamblers. Addiction. 2005;100:1183–93.
97. Moran E. Varieties of pathological gambling. Br J Psychiatry. 1970;116:593–7.
98. Steel Z, Blaszczynski A. The factorial structure of pathological gambling. J Gambl Stud. 1996;12:3–20.
99. Blaszczynski A, McConaghy N. Anxiety and/or depression in the pathogenesis of addictive gambling. Int J Addict. 1989;24:337–50.
100. Blaszczynski A, Nower L. Pathways model of problem and pathological gambling. Addiction. 2002;97:487–99.
101. Ledgerwood D, Petry NM. Pathological experience of gambling and subtypes of pathological gamblers. Psychiatry Res. 2006;144:17–27.
102. Nower L, Martins SS, Lin KH, Blanco C. Subtypes of disordered gamblers: results from the National Epidemiologic Survey of Alcohol and Related Conditions. Addiction. 2012;108:789–98.

4

Cognitive Distortions in Disordered Gambling

Adam S. Goodie, Erica E. Fortune, and Jessica J. Shotwell

Cognitive distortions are a central feature in the development and maintenance of gambling disorder (GD), despite the fact that they are not a diagnostic criterion [1–5], including longitudinal demonstration that cognitive distortions predict gambling problems rather than the reverse [6]. In this chapter we review the generally positive literature of clinical interventions targeted at correcting cognitive distortions and then critically review the current state of the literature for measuring cognitive distortions.

A primary inspiration for studying cognitive distortions in GD is the heuristics and biases program of cognitive psychology (e.g., [7, 8]). A vast literature supports the conclusion that the errors discovered in this program are broad-based in the population, including not only problem gamblers but non-problem gamblers and non-gamblers as well. However, the distortions are posited to occur with greater severity or in situations of greater importance among those with GD. Blaszczynski and Nower [9] included cognitive distortions as part of the "learning" pathway to GD, and many studies reveal that irrational cognitions play a central role in the maintenance of disordered gambling [10]. This impact has been shown to be distinct from other disorders, even those that have been identified as markedly similar to GD such as video gaming [11].

A. S. Goodie (✉)
Department of Psychology, University of Georgia, Athens, GA, USA
e-mail: goodie@uga.edu

E. E. Fortune
Department of Psychology, Arcadia University, Glenside, PA, USA
e-mail: fortunee@arcadia.edu

J. J. Shotwell
Department of Health Promotion and Behavior, University of Georgia, Athens, GA, USA
e-mail: j.shotwell@uga.edu

© Springer Nature Switzerland AG 2019
A. Heinz et al. (eds.), *Gambling Disorder*, https://doi.org/10.1007/978-3-030-03060-5_4

There are several existing instruments for measuring gambling-related distortions, but the field lacks consensus on not only which instrument is the best but what the specific purposes of such an instrument should be. For example, there is not a single error or process that defines "cognitive distortions." Rather, the term refers in different contexts to many different errors, including some (mainly the illusion of control and gambler's fallacy) that enjoy widespread acceptance as relevant distortions and a larger number of errors that are targeted in only some of the instruments. Interestingly, whereas gambler's fallacy enjoys a seemingly universal definition, the illusion of control has been the subject of several definitions, often overlapping but seldom accompanied by attempts at full reconciliation (see box below).

The illusion of control is cited regularly as a cognitive distortion among gamblers, but there is widespread inconsistency within the literature on its exact definition. First coined by Ellen J. Langer [12], the illusion of control was defined as an expectancy of personal success that is higher than the actual objective probability of occurrence. Applied to gambling the illusion of control sometimes refers to:

- Beliefs about skills and strategies used to control game outcomes [13, 14].
- A skill orientation toward gambling [15].
- Rituals and behaviors used to increase chances of winning [16].
- A bidimensional construct with distortions related to *primary control* (i.e., strategies aimed at physically changing the environment) and *secondary control* (i.e., attempts to align with higher power [1], which was validated with confirmatory factor analysis).

Given the many different conceptualizations of the illusion of control, it seems likely that it is multidimensional in nature. Further attempts to examine the illusion of control's structure would be advantageous for clarifying what this distortion actually is.

In this chapter, we first review the clinical literature on the success of various means of addressing cognitive distortions as a component of treating GD. We then briefly describe some issues that can limit the utility of measurement instruments and review the current literature on the cognitive distortions themselves, evaluating several instruments that are currently used for their measurement and recommending future steps.

4.1 Addressing Cognitive Distortions in Therapy for Gambling Disorder

Gambling-related cognitive distortions are such an integral feature of GD that their presence, and specifically their change from pre- to posttreatment, has at times been used as an inherent measure of treatment success (e.g., [17, 18]). Likewise, their continued presence has also been posited as being a predictor of treatment failure [19, 20] as well as a predictor of gambling relapse in Gamblers Anonymous members [16, 21]. Further, a naturalistic investigation of the differential characteristics between recovered and non-recovered gamblers' posttreatment provides evidence for three primary factors that separate these two groups: decision-making style, negative affectivity, and cognitive distortions, such that those disordered gamblers who recovered made vast improvements on the Gambler's Beliefs Questionnaire (GBQ [15]), while those who did not recover showed little to no improvement in GBQ [20]. This body of evidence, with seemingly strong ecological validity, naturally draws question to the usefulness of targeting cognitive distortions as a component of the treatment process for disordered gambling. In fact, some reviews of gambling treatment have indicated that correction of cognitive distortions could be a key to therapeutic success [22–24].

Given that some of the most predominate cognitive distortions are rooted in the understanding of statistical concepts—for example, the gambler's fallacy is a failure to recognize the meaning of randomness and the independence of chance events—one might conclude that simply educating gamblers on these statistical concepts would result in less gambling behavior. However, there are two main problems with this conclusion. First, previous findings have shown that gambling severity is not determined or significantly correlated with mathematical ability, nor has it been shown to be specially related to the aforementioned cognitive distortions [25]. Second, even though a math education intervention focused specifically on gambling concepts led to better performance by college students in a testing environment, the actual gambling behavior of the participants (including money spent, frequency, and severity) was no different from the control group after the intervention [26]. Based on this, it appears the targeting of cognitive distortions must go beyond simple education and incorporate some of the more complex components used in various therapies. Cognitive behavioral therapy (CBT) is often viewed as the gold standard in treatment for a wide variety of psychological disorders, including GD. With the predominant goal of CBT being to assist patients in identifying and restructuring maladaptive thought processes in an attempt to modify the associated maladaptive behaviors, the targeting of cognitive distortions in the treatment of GD is indeed inherent to the CBT process. It is with no surprise, then, that CBT is currently considered by many to be the most effective and efficacious therapy for GD [23, 27]. Numerous researchers have explored the effectiveness of CBT in gambling populations, and pooled evidence from these studies support long-term CBT success at follow-up intervals spanning up to 24 months [23]. Of particular interest for our purposes is the question of how CBT might incorporate and directly affect the nature and quantity of cognitive distortions in gamblers.

As one research team well stated, "…if the gambler's erroneous perceptions and understanding of randomness can be corrected, then the motivation to gamble should decrease dramatically" ([28], p. 1116). While CBT inherently focuses on cognitive elements, the vocalization and correction of erroneous thoughts in a therapeutic setting is often achieved through the process of cognitive restructuring (CR), which may also include the thinking-aloud method [29]. Two distortions that have been predominant in research and theorizing about gambling disorder are the illusion of control and the gambler's fallacy, and they have correspondingly been emphasized within CR for gamblers. The goal of the CR process is to help gamblers identify errors in their gambling-related cognitions and understand why they are errors. This process requires therapists to explain and discuss statistical concepts such as randomness and the independence of successive random events, prior to the therapist correcting the previously tape-recorded verbalizations of the gamblers. The thinking-aloud approach encourages patients to recognize erroneous thoughts, as they relate to their gambling behaviors, and in some cases challenges the participants to correct a certain percentage of these thoughts on their own before treatment is terminated. While CR might be administered independently, it might also be used in conjunction with other treatment approaches, including motivational therapy (e.g., [18]), exposure therapy (e.g., [30]), or relapse prevention (e.g., [30]). Therapists might also include problem solving, social skills, or various types of educational components. These practices have resulted in successful outcome measures, such as a reduction in gambling severity and urges, up to 24 months posttreatment [28, 31–33].

In the earliest of these studies, Bujold et al. [31] used a combination of CR, including thinking aloud, response prevention, and problem solving, and while they did not track changes in cognitive distortions, all participants reported better control over urges and less severe gambling behaviors after roughly 20 h of treatment. Sylvain, Ladouceur, and Boisvert [33] used a similar approach, with the same three therapeutic elements plus social skills training for their treatment group ($n = 14$), but they used the more rigorous methods of a randomized controlled trial (RCT), which also included a waitlist control group ($n = 15$). The treatment led to clinically significant change, based upon percentage in change and end state functions. This change was still apparent albeit slightly attenuated at both 6- and 12-month follow-up for the treatment group, whereas only one person in the control group showed clinically significant change. Significant group-level improvement was seen in all five outcome measures (DSM criteria, perception of control, desire to gamble, self-efficacy, and South Oaks Gambling Screen [34] scores) for the treatment group at posttest, but not for the waitlist control.

Similar results were seen when combining CR and response prevention. Individual therapy sessions, lasting an average of 11 h over several weeks, led to a significant decline in the rate of GD, with 14% of treated participants meeting criteria for GD compared to 86% waitlisted controls [35]. The researchers also reported clinically significant change at posttreatment for the majority of their treated participants. The treatment group also reported a significant improvement in perceived control over their gambling urges and reduced gambling frequency and expenditure, which was not observed in the waitlisted group. The response prevention component in this study also incorporated the influence of cognitive distortions by having participants recall events that might lead to relapse and the distortions that might contribute to this. For example, participants were asked to identify how certain erroneous thoughts (e.g., *If I gamble, I will succeed in controlling myself.*) could be the catalyst for gambling relapse. Ladouceur et al. [32] later replicated these findings with a group-administered CR-plus-response prevention approach. Eighty-eight percent of the treatment group no longer met the GD criteria at posttreatment, compared with 20% of the waitlist control group. 6-, 12-, and 24-month follow-ups revealed majorities maintaining their recovery. Similarly, Myrseth, Litlerè, Støylen, and Pallesen [36] found that 86% of their group-administered treatment participants made clinically significant change from pre- to posttreatment, while none of the control group did. This result was achieved with 12 h of treatment (six weekly 2-h sessions), with the third session focusing exclusively on cognitive distortions. Those who received individual therapy exhibited greater success rates than those in group therapy at posttreatment (92% no longer GDs vs. 65%), and this difference was maintained at 6-month follow-up [37].

The inclusion of multiple therapeutic components makes it difficult to assess the specific contribution of CR to therapeutic success. To fill this gap, some studies have used CR in isolation or as a separate treatment condition for comparison purposes. Ladouceur et al. [28] investigated the success of a CR approach that focused on cognitive distortions and corrections, without any additional therapeutic elements. In this comparatively simplistic therapeutic design, lasting no more than 20 h, four of the five participants displayed more control over gambling urges and no longer met DSM criteria for GD at posttreatment or at 6-month follow-up. Another study allows direct comparison among therapeutic strategies, with an RCT including individual exposure therapy and response prevention, group CR, and a combination of these two approaches, in comparison to a waitlisted group [30]. Treatment conditions were completed with six 1-h sessions over a 6-week period, such that the combined group received 12 h of therapy in comparison to the 6 h for the other groups. The three treatment conditions had combined rate of success (defined as gambling no more than twice during 6- and 12-month periods) of 59% at 6 months, compared with 25% for the waitlisted group. The group CR condition had the greatest focus on cognitive distortions, including sessions in which participants discussed gambling-relevant distortions, such as illusion of control and memory bias. The individual and group conditions showed similar success rates at 6 months (75% and 62%, respectively), which was maintained at 12-month follow-up better for the individual condition (69%) than the group conditions (37%). The combined treatment condition had 38% success at both 6- and 12-month follow-up. Based on these results, Echeburúa et al. [30] concluded that "less is more" in the sense that the more complex therapeutic design resulted in less success overall.

4.1.1 Treatment with Measured Change in Cognitive Distortions

Clinical studies that focus on cognitive distortions in their treatment protocol have typically not measured the change in the distortions themselves, alongside measures of therapeutic gain. This is in part due to the fact that much of the development and validation of modern cognition scales occurred after many of the treatment studies were conducted. Fortunately, later studies did include such measures, which allows for a more direct investigation of the influence of therapy on changes in cognitive distortions. One of the first studies to do so used both individual and group CBT with veterans in a 28-day inpatient gambling treatment program and found that the participants had a significant reduction in distortions, during the course of treatment, which resulted in them displaying distortion scores similar to those without GD [17].

Another study directly investigating the changes in cognitive distortions from pre- to posttreatment had four conditions: cognitive therapy, behavioral therapy, motivational therapy, and a minimal intervention, where the cognitive therapy condition was intended to focus primarily on the correction of cognitive distortions [18]. Contrary to predictions, the minimal intervention proved to be the most effective in reducing rates of meeting GD criteria. Crucially for our purposes, this was also the group that showed the greatest reduction in cognitive distortions, as measured by the Gambling Related Cognitions Scale (GRCS [16]). These findings are reminiscent of those by Echeburúa et al. [30], indicating that less is in fact more, but these findings go a step further by directly showing that the simplest intervention not only led to the best therapeutic success but also led to the greatest reduction in relevant cognitive distortions. In a similar study comparing cognitive therapy and exposure therapy, both treatments were also successful [38]. Interestingly, while the cognitive therapy group spent roughly half of their 12 sessions addressing cognitive distortions and erroneous beliefs, the exposure therapy group did not focus on distortions at all yet experienced the same therapeutic success, including relative improvements in the GRCS.

Some theorizing has suggested that if cognitive distortions are a key feature of GD onset or maintenance, the traditional processes of CBT and CR might be enhanced by having gamblers move beyond the simple identification and correction of cognitive distortions. In fact, while gamblers are likely to endorse cognitive distortions, they are less likely to understand how they act as a catalyst for their gambling habits [39]. The process of mindfulness, wherein individuals are asked to be fully aware of their cognitions, but without judgment, can lead to deautomatization [40] of related urges and behaviors, and essentially break the chain of cognitive events (erroneous beliefs → urge to gamble → resulting behavior) that contributes to the maintenance of GD. There is empirical evidence to suggest that the use of mindfulness-based interventions for gamblers might be a fruitful path to explore, including the fact that gamblers tend to demonstrate lower levels of trait mindfulness than others [41, 42]. Two separate case studies showed gamblers who benefited from a mindfulness-based intervention, even after CBT had previously been unsuccessful [43, 44], and one pilot study using mindfulness methods with more than a dozen participants [45] also resulted in promising outcomes. Taking a metacognitive approach to treatment, by spending time focusing on cognitions themselves, might be essential for gamblers trying to correct cognitive distortions.

Toneatto et al. [45] used mindfulness-enhanced cognitive behavioral therapy (M-CBT), in which participants received CBT plus mindfulness instruction and practice for five sessions, along with homework of mindfulness practice. The

M-CBT group reported a reduction in GD symptoms from 6.7 to 3.4, compared with no change for the waitlist control, along with reduced gambling urges at posttreatment. Differential positive outcomes were maintained at 3-month follow-up, at which point 3 of 14 participants met criteria of disordered gambling, compared with 17 of 18 in the control group. Individuals who continued mindfulness practices posttreatment had significantly fewer symptoms and gambling urges.

The available evidence suggests that the targeting of cognitive distortions in therapies for disordered gamblers is often successful, leading to significant reductions in DSM symptoms and other clinically significant outcomes that are maintained throughout substantial follow-up periods. Further, cognitive distortions have been identified as a predictor of gambling relapse among Gamblers Anonymous members [16, 21]. However, the greatest success might be not be achieved when focusing solely on cognitive distortions, but achieved when cognitive distortions are targeted in the broader framework of CBT therapy. Many variations of CBT are shown to be effective for treating GD, despite nuances in practice [23], but this diversity of CBT techniques can be problematic when attempting to identify the specific therapeutic elements that best contribute to patient success. Some evidence suggests that CBT alone leads to similar posttreatment outcomes as CBT in combination with other therapeutic elements, like exposure therapy and response prevention, but also results in better treatment adherence and less attrition [46]. When directly comparing the effects of cognitive therapy versus exposure therapy in an RCT, similar results are found—comparable posttreatment success with less attrition for cognitive therapy—but greater relapse was also noted for the cognitive therapy group [38].

Because the success of a therapeutic intervention might depend on other factors, it is important to consider certain demographic and other influences. The naturalistic study by Rossini-Dib et al. [20] found that age, sex, and ethnicity did not play significant roles in predicting treatment success. Several studies report some degree of therapeutic success regardless of the sex ratio, which include all men (e.g., [31]), all women (e.g., [37]), and combined samples (e.g., [20, 30]). However, there is metaanalytical evidence to suggest that the therapeutic gains may be greater in studies with higher proportions of males [23]. Due to homogeneity of the participants, small sample sizes, and lack of analyzing or reporting, we cannot draw firm conclusions regarding possible moderating effects of age and ethnicity.

Also of methodological importance is the size of the samples and the structure of the therapy provided (e.g., total number and type of conditions, group vs. individual designs, and hours in therapy). The studies included in this review range from case studies that focus on the intensive investigation of only a few participants (e.g., [28, 31]) to samples as large as 99 participants (i.e., [18]), but all of the studies reported varying degrees of success. As far as experimental design is concerned, even the most rigorous methodological approaches—a RCT with a waitlist condition—resulted in therapeutic gains for participants. Some of these treatments focused on individual therapies and others relied on a group-therapy approach or a combination of individual and group therapy. Interestingly, there is no clear conclusion as to which approach might be superior. Therapeutic gains are found when delivering the therapy in a group format (e.g., [32]), but these studies do not always include a comparison to an individual-group format. However, studies making direct comparisons of individual vs. group therapy, or even combined therapies, have found that even though all approaches result in significant improvement from baseline, the therapeutic gains are better maintained when therapy was delivered in an individual format [30, 37]. But in contrast, a metaanalysis of studies using CBT with gamblers found greater statistical support for the long-term benefits of group therapy [23].

The literature on CBT for GD indicates that the duration of therapy does not play a significant role [23]: interventions lasting as little as 90 min [18] led to successful outcomes, while others lasting much longer—around 20 h and spanning several weeks of time—have also led to success (e.g., [28, 31]). Further, intensive inpatient gambling treatment programs lasting an entire month have also demonstrated successful outcomes and significant decreases in cognitive distortions [17].

The literature is thus clear that cognitive distortions play an important role in the development and maintenance of problem gambling, measured by symptoms, gambling frequency, urges, or expenditures. Likewise, addressing distortions plays an important role in the success of treatment. For future clinical research, we believe the literature supports consistent use of pre- and posttreatment assessment of cognitive distortions. Clearly, this step would be enhanced by the availability of psychometrically strong, agreed-upon instruments. We also believe the literature would benefit from improved understanding of the moderating role of comorbid disorders such as substance use and depressive disorders, particularly as many problem gamblers also experience these disorders [47], and as these comorbid disorders have been identified as potential contributors to nonrecovery [20].

4.2   Measuring Cognitive Distortions

Cognitive distortions were first studied using the "think-aloud" method previously discussed for its application to therapy. In a research context [48, 49], speech was coded into two main categories—rational and irrational—and it was discovered that pathological gamblers displayed greater frequencies of cognitive distortions than social or non-gamblers [29]. Rational forms of speech included reference to odds or probabilities that were correct, descriptions of the game, differentiating between reasonable and unreasonable courses of action, and mentioning strategies that were correct in relation to some aspect of the game [10, 48, 50]. Irrational thoughts often included incorrect links between cause and effect, superstitiously based statements, personification of the machine, reference to personal skill or luck as an explanatory or predictive factor, explaining away losses, and trying to influence game outcomes through inappropriate means [4, 10, 48, 50, 51].

The think-aloud method helped shed light on the presence of cognitive distortions in gamblers, revealing higher frequencies and proportions of irrational beliefs among problem gamblers than among other populations [48, 52, 53], and provided a building block from which researchers have continued to study the influence of cognitive distortions on gambling behavior. However, this approach has been criticized for lack of standardization across studies, making it difficult to quantify cognitive distortions among gamblers [13, 54]. Focus has shifted from measuring frequency of cognitive distortions to the development of psychometrically sound instruments that quantify and differentiate between cognitive distortions. Having statistically reliable and valid measures of cognitive distortions enables researchers to identify which cognitive distortions are most pervasive and influential in GD. The field has moved in a salutary direction, as we shall describe, but the current state of the literature points to clear next steps to develop increasingly reliable, valid, and widely used measures. In the following sections, we (a) describe the principal cognitive distortions that have been studied and their theoretical basis, (b) describe the challenges faced by many of the current generation of instruments for measuring cognitive distortions in GD, and (c) describe both the strengths and the principal challenges faced by each of the most widely cited current instruments.

4.2.1 Cognitive Distortions Implicated in GD

Several cognitive distortions have derived from the heuristics and biases program of research [8], in particular biases associated with the availability and representativeness heuristics. According to the availability heuristic, events are judged to be likely if similar events are easy to retrieve from memory. Under the representativeness heuristic, events are judged to be likely to have been drawn from a particular class to the extent they resemble (or are representative of) a typical member of that class. Distortions based on availability include illusory correlations, inherent memory bias, and the availability of others' wins (for a review, see [22]). In a gambling setting, illusory correlations may exist when gamblers believe there is a relationship between events that are in fact unrelated, such as the idea that their personal luck is an influential factor in their gambling outcomes [55]. Times when a superstitious belief or behavior was coincidentally paired winning are more likely to be recalled [56]. Indeed, the winnings of others, such as by hearing the winning sounds of nearby slot machines, can lead gamblers to believe they are more likely to win [48].

Distortions related to the representativeness heuristic include the gambler's fallacy, overconfidence, and trends in number picking. The gambler's fallacy occurs when individuals believe that even short strings of random events must correspond with their perception of what constitutes randomness, leading to beliefs that particular outcomes are "due" [57]. Overconfidence is a tendency to display degrees of confidence that are unwarranted by one's actual ability [58] and correlates positively with GD [10, 59, 60]. Similar patterns of thinking are apparent in number picking such as choosing lottery numbers, where individuals systematically avoid duplicate numbers and prefer number strings that do not contain neighboring digits [61–63].

A strength that is shared by all of the published instruments of which we are aware is reliability, both in terms of Cronbach's alpha and test-retest reliability. This is a vital strength that has sustained the enterprise of instrument development. However, other facets of instrument success have been less consistently tested or tested but not confirmed.

4.2.2   Content Validity of Current Measures

Measuring General Cognitions Related to Gambling. Content validity refers to the extent to which elements of a given measurement scale are relevant and reflective of the construct they seek to measure [64]. Relevance, defined as the appropriateness of included facets for the measurement scales targeted construct [65], is important because we distinguish between specific cognitive distortions, general cognitive processes, and noncognitive process such as emotions. To the extent that it is useful to measure cognitive distortions specifically, it is important to exclude the other categories, or else the content validity of the scale will suffer. Scales have been identified, which are claimed to be measures of cognitive distortions related to pathological gambling, which include items unrelated to cognitive distortions, compromising their content validity [5].

Relevance and content validity decline if a measurement scale includes facets that are outside or unrelated to the construct in question [64]. Applying this to current measures of cognitive distortions reveals many instruments whose scale relevance may be questioned on these grounds, by including general cognitive processes associated with gambling, which do not measure specific cognitive distortions. We will discuss implications that hinge on this distinction. For example, the Gambling Related Cognitions Scale [16] and the Gambling Attitudes and Beliefs Scale [66] include elements reflecting both cognitive distortions (e.g., belief in personal luck, illusion of control) and general cognitive processes (e.g., motivations to gamble, emotions related to gambling). The Gambler's Beliefs Questionnaire [13] includes subscales unrelated to specific cognitive distortions (e.g., memory bias, biased interpretation of evidence), which decreases the scale's level of content validity. This can be an impediment to research attempting to focus specifically on cognitive distortions.

4.2.3   Non-comprehensive Scales

Including relevant facets in a measurement scale not only means excluding irrelevant facets but also including *all* relevant facets. This means the measures of cognitive distortions that measure only a subset of relevant distortions (e.g., Drakes Beliefs about Chance [14]; Information Biases Scale [67]) have diminished content validity. This issue extends further because the field lacks an agreed-upon measurement tool that specifically targets cognitive distortions in GD. This hinders the identification of distortions that is the most impactful in gambling pathology [2]. In order to advance research and treatment programs, researchers need to develop improved measures that include all relevant cognitive distortions and exclude irrelevant general cognitions related to gambling.

4.2.4   Need for Confirmatory Factor Analysis

Confirmatory factor analysis (CFA) is a statistical procedure that tests how well a proposed measurement model fits with a collected sample [68, 69]. Although related to exploratory factor analysis (EFA), CFA goes beyond EFA in that EFA is data-driven, often used for exploratory or descriptive purposes, and does not require substantive theory, whereas CFA requires a strong theoretical foundation to help guide the specified factor model [68, 69]. In measurement construction, EFA is typically used first to identify the number of factors, and then CFA is employed after the underlying factor structure is discovered, and there is a justified theoretical foundation to support the proposed factor-model structure [70]. Scales of measurement that are supported only by EFA are incomplete; CFA should be conducted to see whether or not the proposed measurement model adequately fits the data. It is not enough to establish a measurement scale's factor structure; researchers also need to examine how well their measurement model replicates in actual data. Most of the instruments discussed here lack CFA-based validation of which we are aware, a significant shortcoming in the literature.

4.2.5 Establishing Measurement Invariance

Measurement invariance (sometimes called measurement equivalence) is a relatively recent methodological advance, and so it may be unsurprising that all of the common cognitive distortion measurement scales lack establishment of measurement invariance across levels of gambling severity. Demonstrating measurement invariance means the measured constructs (in this case cognitive distortions) conjure the same conceptual framework across each comparison group [71]. If there is no evidence to suggest measurement invariance across groups, or if measurement invariance assumptions are violated, then inferences drawn from between group comparisons can be made only with reduced confidence [72]. In other words, if the conceptual frame of reference differs between levels of gambling severity, then the ability to make between group comparisons is compromised. Many studies have examined differences in cognitive distortions across disordered, problem, and non-problem gamblers, but without establishing measurement invariance such comparisons are ambiguous. Because all of the instruments reviewed below lack this form of validation, we do not repeat the critique for each one, although we regard it as uniformly relevant for all.

4.2.6 Summary of Measurement Problems

Many measures of cognitive distortions fall short in terms of content validity—including irrelevant items or failing to address the full scope of distortions—and lacking CFA to support the proposed measurement-model structure. All measurement scales lack establishment of measurement invariance across levels of gambling severity, marking the next frontier in understanding how cognitive distortions operate between those with and without gambling disorders. Content validity can be improved by developing a scale that focuses on all cognitive distortions related to gambling and excludes irrelevant facets. CFA can be employed after EFA has identified the measure's factor structure or when there is a sufficient conceptual background. Finally, tests of measurement invariance can easily be conducted within traditional CFA procedures by running simultaneous confirmatory factor analyses in two or more groups [68]. A measurement scale that follows these procedures will not only be the first of its kind but also serve to advance researchers' and clinicians' understanding of the role cognitive distortions play in GD.

4.3   Instruments for Measuring Cognitive Distortions in GD

4.3.1   Gambling Beliefs and Attitudes Survey (GABS)

The GABS [66] was originally developed as a 35-item Likert style questionnaire (*1 = strongly agree, 4 = strongly disagree*) that is not divided into subscales, but rather is intended "to capture a wide range of cognitive biases, irrational beliefs, and positively valued attitudes to gambling" ([66], p. 1102). Several items bear a resemblance to common distortions, such as gambler's fallacy (e.g., *If I have not won any of my bets for a while, I am probably due for a big win*) and the illusion of control (e.g., *No matter what the game is, there are betting strategies that will help you win*). Still, the GABS score is taken holistically to reflect "gambling affinity." The GABS was designed to be administered only to individuals who are familiar with gambling-related concepts and terms. The GABS showed strong internal reliability with both student ($\alpha = 0.93$) and treatment-seeking individuals with GD ($\alpha = 0.90$). GABS scores correlated with SOGS scores among male college students who gambled ($r = 0.38$).

GABS scores are higher among GDs than nonclinical samples ([73, 74], both using SOGS) and correlate with SOGS scores [73, 75]. 10- and 15-item revisions of the GABS correlate with PGSI scores ([76], Studies 1 and 2 [77]), and a 23-item version has been validated and revealed a 5-factor structure [78] relating to strategies, chasing, attitudes, luck, and emotions. Strategies refer to beliefs in illusory gambling strategies supposed to increase one's chances of winning, chasing refers to persistent gambling when losing or winning within a gambling session, attitudes are the conviction in gambling attitudes thought to increase one's chance of winning, luck is the belief in good/bad luck as well as superstition, and emotions refer to the emotional excitement provided by gambling.

The GABS predicts attentional bias in non-problem gamblers [79], and has been successfully translated in Italian [80]. However, it includes cognitions unrelated to cognitive distortions.

4.3.2   Beliefs About Control Scale (BAC)

The BAC [81] is a 19-item Likert-type scale (*1 = strongly disagree, 5 = strongly agree*) that assesses 5 factors: illusion of control, need for money, control over gambling, belief in systems, and cynicism about winning. The illusion of control subscale assesses optimistic views about winning and the belief in luck and other superstitious behaviors. The need for money scale reflects the importance of winning money to help with finances. The control over gambling subscale measures an internal locus of control related to gambling, modulating when it is appropriate to gamble and when it is not. The belief in systems subscale reflects one's belief that strategies and systems can be used to improve gambling outcomes. Finally, the cynicism about winning subscale examines the extent to which a person believes winning is unlikely. The BAC is not a comprehensive measure of cognitive distortions and lacks CFA.

4.3.3 Gambler's Beliefs Questionnaire (GBQ-1)

Two different scales share a single acronym, GBQ, despite having been developed independently and with differing items. We term these "GBQ-1" and "GBQ-2," reflecting the chronological order in which they were published.

The GBQ-1 [15] is a 21-item Likert-type scale (*1 = strongly agree, 7 = strongly disagree*) with two subscales reflecting categories of beliefs: luck/perseverance (13 items) and the illusion of control (8 items). The illusion of control items focus on perceived knowledge and skill related to gambling, and the luck/perseverance items focus on specific beliefs and strategies that might be utilized while gambling. Several of the luck/perseverance items appear to reflect the gambler's fallacy (e.g., *If I continue to gamble, it will eventually pay off and I will make money*). The GBQ-1 shows good test-retest reliability ($r = 0.77$), as well as strong convergent validity with GD measures. Internal reliability indices are strong [82] with $\alpha = 0.93$ for the scale as a whole, 0.89 for illusion of control, and 0.94 for luck/perseverance. GBQ-1 total and subscale scores were significantly higher among DSM-IV-based pathological gamblers (PGs) than among non-pathological gamblers (NPGs), as identified by both the Massachusetts Gambling Screen DMS-IV Questionnaire [83] and the SOGS. However, the GBQ-1 did not differentiate between probable PGs and problem gamblers (those scoring a 3 or 4) on the SOGS. The GBQ-1 was similarly validated in a treatment-seeking sample [84], in which scores improved across treatment, and in a translation into Spanish [85] and in Chinese language with CFA validation [86]. It has also been validated in an English-speaking community with ethnic Chinese culture [87]. GBQ-1 distortions appear to be greater among online than offline poker players [88]. However, these differentiations should be viewed with caution, as measurement invariance has not been established.

Scores on the GBQ-1 decline with improved cognition in VLT players at moderate risk who receive prevention interventions and correlate positively with gambling pathology scores ([82, 89], both using SOGS [90], using CPGI); a control group that did not have improved cognition did not change in GBQ-1 scores [91]. Similarly, reduced distortions are correlated with better recovery from gambling problems [20].

Although the GBQ-1 has been referenced a great deal in the literature, it includes measurement items that are not relevant to specific cognitive distortions (e.g., *My losses aren't as bad if I don't tell my loved ones*).

4.3.4 Perceived Personal Luck Scale (PPLS)

The PPLS [92] consists of ten items from the GBQ-1 [15], with 5-point Likert format (*1 = strongly disagree, 5 = strongly agree*, altered from the 7-point format of the GBQ-1), which represent a "skill orientation toward gambling." The PPLS has strong internal consistency ($\alpha = 0.88$; replicated by [93], $\alpha = 0.90$). Low- and high-risk undergraduate problem gamblers, identified by the Problem Gambling Severity Index (PGSI; a subscale of the CPGI), both had greater perceived personal luck than non-problem gamblers [94]. Furthermore, individuals who preferred games with both skill and chance components, also had greater perceived personal luck than those who preferred chance games [92]. The PPLS arguably lacks content validity because it includes items irrelevant to specific cognitive distortions.

4.3.5 Gambler's Beliefs Questionnaire (GBQ-2)

The GBQ-2 [13] is a 65-item questionnaire designed to measure irrational and distorted cognitions in social and problem gamblers. It is scored on a 5-point Likert scale (*0 = not at all, 4 = very much*) and includes 12 subscales: illusion of control (9 items), erroneous beliefs of winning (4 items), entrapment/gambler's fallacy (12 items), superstition (8 items), impaired control (5 items), near miss (3 items), memory bias (3 items), biased evaluation (equivalent to self-serving bias; 7 items), positive state (3 items), relief (5 items), money equals a solution to problems (4 items), and denial (2 items).

The overall scale shows excellent internal reliability ($\alpha = 0.97$), but subscale reliability indices were not reported. GBQ-2 scores also differ between groups defined by gambling severity. Problem gamblers, defined as a SOGS score of 10 or higher, had significantly higher scores than social gamblers on all subscales except denial. Subsequent studies utilized a 48-item version (i.e., [95]), which lacks published validation, as well as a briefer 24-item version [96]. EFA conducted on the 24-item version revealed 5 factors [96], with 6 items each for coping, personal illusory control, and general illusory control and three items apiece for winning expectancy and rational beliefs. This version correlates significantly with SOGS scores ($r = 0.58$) and has strong internal reliability ($\alpha = 0.89$). However, CFA has not been employed to examine how well the 5-factor structure holds in the data. Both the 65-item [13] and 24-item [96] GBQ-2 scales lack subscales of relevant cognitive distortions and lack CFA validation of the factor structure.

4.3.6 The Information Biases Scale (IBS)

The IBS [67] assesses various distortions rating 25 items on a 7-point Likert scale (*1 = don't agree at all, 7 = strongly agree*). The measure has good internal reliability ($\alpha = 0.92$) and correlates with both the South Oaks Gambling Screen (SOGS [34]; $r = 0.48$) and the National Opinion Research Center DSM-IV Screen for

Gambling Problems ([97]; $r = 0.38$). The SOGS was developed as a research screen and does not reflect a diagnostic symptom count. The DSM-IV screen was symptom-based. The IBS was developed in reference to video lottery terminal (VLT) play, and so it cannot be administered to non-gamblers to compare across groups. The IBS is a single-factor questionnaire, which nevertheless taps into several different distortions, including the illusion of control (e.g., *I would rather use a VLT that I am familiar with than one that I have never used before*), the gambler's fallacy (e.g., *The longer a VLT has gone without paying out a large sum of money, the more likely are the chances that it will pay out in the very near future*), illusory correlations (e.g., *I know some VLT users who are just plain lucky*), and the availability heuristic (e.g., *Hearing about other people winning on VLTs encourages me to keep on playing*). Scores on the IBS decreased among moderate-risk VLT players (using the Canadian Problem Gambling Index; CPGI [98]) with prevention interventions, but not in a control group [91], and mediated a link between low conscientiousness and gambling severity [99]. Scores were lower among non-problem-gambling college students who received educational animation than among those who saw a neutral video [100]. This scale is a non-comprehensive measure of gambling-related cognitive distortions and also lacks CFA to test model-data fit.

4.3.7 The Gambling Related Cognitions Scale (GRCS)

The GRCS [16] is a 23-item questionnaire, assessed on a 7-point Likert scale (*1 = strongly disagree, 7 = strongly agree*), with five subscales defined by a particular cognition: illusion of control (4 items), predictive control (equivalent to gambler's fallacy, 6 items), interpretative bias (4 items), gambling-related expectancies (4 items), and perceived inability to stop gambling (impaired control, 5 items). The illusion of control subscale emphasizes superstitious beliefs (e.g., *I have specific rituals and behaviors that increase my chances of winning*), and the predictive control subscale focuses on probability errors such as the gambler's fallacy (e.g., *Losses while gambling are bound to be followed by a series of wins*). The interpretive bias subscale items appear to strongly represent self-serving bias (e.g., *Relating my losses to bad luck and bad circumstances makes me continue gambling*). Gambling-related expectancies focus on expected benefits from gambling (e.g., *Gambling makes me happier*), and Perceived inability to quit reflects respondents' confidence in their ability to control their gambling (e.g., *I'm not strong to enough to stop gambling*).

The GRCS shows strong internal reliability, with overall scale $\alpha = 0.93$ and sub-scale α values ranging from 0.77 to 0.91. It has demonstrated concurrent validity with measures of depression and anxiety, gambling motivation, and SOGS scores, as well as good discriminant validity. The GRCS total score correlates with SOGS scores ($r = 0.43$), and GRCS subscale scores accounted for 27% of SOGS score variance in a regression analysis. Tests of two discriminant functions, one with the subscales as predictors and one with the total score as a predictor, classified participants into two severity groups: 86% of the time for the first function and 85% of the time for the second function. Individuals with SOGS scores of 4 or greater had significantly higher scores on the GRCS total score and on all of the five subscales than those with SOGS scores of 0.

GRSC scores correlate with measures or gambling severity ([16, 101, 102], all using SOGS), and average scores differ between pathology-defined groups ([103], using PGSI) and by factor analysis [104] and Bayesian structural equation modeling [105]. In cross-cultural comparisons, Chinese and Caucasian participants had similar subscale scores, except for the illusion of control and the perceived inability to stop gambling, in which Chinese participants showed more distortion [106]. The authors suggest that these differences may be an artifact of different cultural norms. The GRSC has also been translated successfully into Turkish [107]. It has been widely utilized in studies of the neural bases of cognitive distortions in GD [108, 109] and has been validated in Italian [110] and Japanese [111] language versions. The GRCS predicts gambling problems, but its factor structure is in question [112]. However, the GRCS addresses cognitions unrelated to specific cognitive distortions, lowering the scale's content validity.

4.3.8 The Drake Beliefs About Chance Inventory (DBC)

The DBC [14] consists of 22 Likert-type items (*1 = strongly disagree, 5 = strongly agree*) and is designed to measure gamblers' erroneous beliefs about games of chance. The scale poses a 2-factor structure of items related to superstition and the illusion of control. Similar to the previous measurement problems, this scale does not include all relevant cognitive distortions associated with GD, and it lacks CFA validation.

4.3.9 Gambling-Related Cognitive Distortion (GRCD)

The GRCD [113] is a 12-item Likert-type questionnaire (*1 = never, 5 = always*) used to examine the relationship between the severity of problem gambling and the severity of cognitive distortions. This scale has questionable content validity because not all relevant cognitive distortions are covered, and the GCI includes items not related to a specific distortion. Furthermore, the authors did not conduct CFA.

4.3.10 Personal Luck Usage Scale (PLUS)

The PLUS [114] is an 8-item unidimensional Likert-type questionnaire (*1 = strongly disagree, 5 = strongly agree*) used to measure gambler's erroneous beliefs that they possess personal luck that can be used to influence outcomes while gambling. The PLUS notably utilized CFA and allows researchers who use it to be more confident in its assessment of personal luck. However, this scale lacks comprehensive content validity by focusing on one specific cognitive distortion.

4.3.11 Gambling Cognitions Inventory (GCI)

The GCI [115] is a 33-item Likert-type scale (*0 = strongly disagree, 3 = strongly agree*) that assesses 2 factors: attitude/skill (e.g., *I am a very skilled gambler*) and luck/chance (e.g., *Repeating certain phrases or thoughts to myself will give me good luck*). This scale notably is supported by CFA-based validation.

4.3.12 Scales Not Developed for Gambling

The following questionnaires were not specifically intended to measure cognitive distortions in gambling but warrant mention because they have subsequently been referenced in relation to gambling pathology [5, 116, 117]. Ferland, Ladouceur, and Vitaro [118] created 16-item Likert scale (*1 = I totally disagree, 4 = I totally agree*) to examine knowledge and misconceptions about gambling. Seven questions assessed misconceptions (e.g., *When I play bingo, I have more chances of winning if I bring my lucky charms with me*) and nine assessed knowledge (e.g., *Lottery is a gambling activity*). This scale was used as a pre-post measure to evaluate any change in item endorsement following treatment. The Belief in Good Luck Scale (BIGL [116]) is a 12-item Likert scale (*1 = strongly agree, 6 = strongly disagree*) designed to measure irrational beliefs about luck. The Beliefs Around Luck Scale (BALS [119]) expanded the BIGL scale such that beliefs about bad luck could be measured. This Likert scale consists of 22 items (*1 = strongly agree, 6 = strongly disagree*) and is composed of four constructs—belief in being unlucky, belief in being lucky, rejection of belief in luck, and a general belief in luck. Thompson and Prendergast [120] created the 12-item Likert-type (*1 = strongly disagree, 5 = strongly agree*) Belief in Luck and Luckiness Scale (BILLS). This bidimensional scale contains six items reflecting a general belief in luck and 6 items reflecting a belief in personal luckiness.

4.4 Conclusion

It is now beyond debate that cognitive distortions play a central role in problem gambling behavior and gambling disorder. Clinical studies in this area have consistently shown beneficial effects of including modules to target cognitive distortions in broader therapies, notably CBT, across genders, races, and types of therapy (especially individual versus group), although important research on moderating effects of these variables remains to be entered in the literature. The trend of clinical researchers using increasingly sophisticated measurement techniques for distortions themselves, as such instruments become available, is unmistakable and understandable, and we anticipate that it will continue.

In the domain of instrument development, we believe that the field stands on the precipice of a third generation of instruments. First were think-aloud protocols [29], which introduced cognitive distortions to the field. Second was a generation of instruments that permitted more systematic exploration of specific cognitive distortions [2, 23]. We believe the field stands ready [5] to move to enhanced instruments that demonstrate better content validity by incorporating all relevant distortions and excluding other factors and are supported by fuller psychometric validation, including internal and test-retest reliability, EFA, and CFA.

References

1. Ejova A, Delfabbro PH, Navarro DJ. Erroneous gambling-related beliefs as illusions of primary and secondary control: a confirmatory factor analysis. J Gambl Stud. 2015;31(1):133–60.
2. Goodie AS, Fortune EE. Measuring cognitive distortions in pathological gambling: review and meta-analyses. Psychol Addict Behav. 2013;27:730–43.
3. Hong X, Shah KR, Phillips SM, Scherrer JF, Volberg R, Eisen SA. Association of cognitive distortions with problem and pathological gambling in adult male twins. Psychiatry Res. 2009;160:300–7.
4. Ladouceur R. Perceptions among pathological and non-pathological gamblers. Addict Behav. 2004;29:555–65.
5. Leonard CA, Williams RJ, Vokey J. Gambling fallacies: what are they and how are they best measured? J Addict Res Ther. 2015;6:256.
6. Yakovenko I, Hodgins DC, el-Guebaly N, Casey DM, Currie SR, Smith GJ, Williams RJ, Schopflocher DP. Cognitive distortions predict future gambling involvement. Int Gambl Stud. 2016;2:175–92.
7. Kahneman D, Tversky A. Subjective probability: a judgment of representativeness. Cogn Psychol. 1972;3:430–54.
8. Kahneman D, Tversky A. Judgment under uncertainty: heuristics and biases. Science. 1974;185:1124–31.
9. Blaszczynski A, Nower L. A pathways model of problem and pathological gambling. Addiction. 2002;97:487–99.
10. Walker MB. Irrational thinking among slot machine players. J Gambl Stud. 1992;8:245–61.
11. Delfabbro P, King D. On finding the C in CBT: the challenges of applying gambling-related cognitive approaches to video-gaming. J Gambl Stud. 2015;31(1):315–29.
12. Langer EJ. The illusion of control. J Pers Soc Psychol. 1975;32:311–28.
13. Joukhador J, MacCallum F, Blaszczynski A. Differences in cognitive distortions between problem and social gamblers. Psychol Rep. 2003;92:1203–14.
14. Wood WS, Clapham MM. Development of the drake beliefs about chance inventory. J Gambl Stud. 2005;21:411–30.
15. Steenbergh TA, Meyers AW, May RK, Whelan JP. Development and validation of the gamblers' beliefs questionnaire. Psychol Addict Behav. 2002;16:143–9.
16. Raylu N, Oei TPS. The Gambling Related Cognitions Scale (GRCS): development, confirmatory factor validation and psychometric properties. Addiction. 2004;99:757–69.
17. Breen RB, Kruedelbach NG, Walker HI. Cognitive changes in pathological gamblers following a 28-day inpatient program. Psychol Addict Behav. 2001;15:246–8.
18. Toneatto T, Gunaratne M. Does the treatment of cognitive distortions improve clinical outcomes for problem gambling? J Contemp Psychother. 2009;39:221–9.
19. Daughters SB, Lejuez CW, Lesieur HR, Strong DR, Zvolensky MJ. Towards a better understanding of gambling treatment failure: implications of translational research. Clin Psychol Rev. 2003;23:573–86.
20. Rossini-Dib D, Fuentes D, Tavares H. A naturalistic study of recovering gamblers: what gets better and when they get better. Psychiatry Res. 2015;227(1):17–26.
21. Oei TP, Gordon LM. Psychological factors related to gambling abstinence and relapse in members of gamblers anonymous. J Gambl Stud. 2008;24:91–105.

22. Fortune EE, Goodie AS. Cognitive distortions as a component and treatment focus of pathological gambling: a review. Psychol Addict Behav. 2012;26:298–310.
23. Gooding P, Tarrier N. A systematic review and meta-analysis of cognitive-behavioural interventions to reduce problem gambling—hedging our bets? Behav Res Ther. 2009;47:592–607.
24. Tavares H, Zilberman ML, el-Guebaly N. Are there specific cognitive and behavioral approaches specific to the treatment of pathological gambling? Can J Psychiatr. 2003;48(1):22–7.
25. Lambos C, Delfabbro P. Numerical reasoning ability and irrational beliefs in problem gambling. Int Gambl Stud. 2007;7:157–71.
26. Williams RJ, Connolly D. Does learning about the mathematics of gambling change gambling behavior? Psychol Addict Behav. 2006;20:62–8.
27. Rizeanu S. The efficacy of cognitive-behavioral intervention in pathological gambling treatment. Procedia Soc Behav Sci. 2014;127:626–30.
28. Ladouceur R, Sylvain C, Letarte H, Giroux I, Jacques C. Cognitive treatment of pathological gamblers. Behav Res Ther. 1998;36:1111–9.
29. Gaboury A, Ladouceur R. Erroneous perceptions and gambling. J Soc Behav Pers. 1989;4:411–20.
30. Echeburúa E, Báez C, Fernández-Montalvo J. Comparative effectiveness of three therapeutic modalities in the psychological treatment of pathological gambling: long-term outcome. Behav Cogn Psychother. 1996;24:51–72.
31. Bujold A, Ladouceur R, Sylvain C, Boisvert J. Treatment of pathological gamblers: an experimental study. J Behav Ther Exp Psychiatry. 1994;25:275–82.
32. Ladouceur R, Sylvain C, Boutin C, Lachance S, Doucet C, Leblond J. Group therapy for pathological gamblers: a cognitive approach. Behav Res Ther. 2003;41:587–96.
33. Sylvain C, Ladouceur R, Boisvert J. Cognitive and behavioral treatment of pathological gambling: a controlled study. J Consult Clin Psychol. 1997;65:727–32.
34. Lesieur HR, Blume SB. The South Oaks Gambling Screen (SOGS): a new instrument for the identification of problem gamblers. Am J Psychiatr. 1987;144:1184–8.
35. Ladouceur R, Sylvain C, Boutin C, Lachance S, Doucet C, Leblond J, Jacques C. Cognitive treatment of pathological gambling. J Nerv Ment Dis. 2001;189:774–80.
36. Myrseth H, Litlerè I, Støylen IJ, Pallesen S. A controlled study of the effect of cognitive-behavioural group therapy for pathological gamblers. Nord J Psychiatry. 2009;63:22–31.
37. Dowling N, Smith D, Thomas T. A comparison of individual and group cognitive-behavioural treatment for female pathological gambling. Behav Res Ther. 2007;45:2192–202.
38. Smith DP, Battersby MW, Harvey PW, Pols RG, Ladouceur R. Cognitive versus exposure therapy for problem gambling: randomised controlled trial. Behav Res Ther. 2015;69:100–10.
39. Morasco BJ, Weinstock J, Ledgerwood DM, Petry NM. Psychological factors that promote and inhibit pathological gambling. Cogn Behav Pract. 2007;14(2):208–17.
40. Kang Y, Gruber J, Gray JR. Mindfulness and de-automatization. Emot Rev. 2013;5:192–201.
41. Lakey CE, Campbell WK, Brown KW, Goodie AS. Dispositional mindfulness as a predictor of the severity of gambling outcomes. Personal Individ Differ. 2007;43:1698–710.
42. Riley B. Experiential avoidance mediates the association between thought suppression and mindfulness with problem gambling. J Gambl Stud. 2014;30:163–71.
43. de Lisle SM, Dowling NA, Sabura Allen J. Mindfulness-based cognitive therapy for problem gambling. Clin Case Stud. 2011;10:210–28.
44. Toneatto T, Nguyen L. Does mindfulness meditation improve anxiety and mood symptoms? A review of the controlled research. Can J Psychiatr. 2007;52:260–6.
45. Toneatto T, Pillai S, Courtice EL. Mindfulness-enhanced cognitive behavioral therapy for problem gambling: a controlled pilot study. Int J Ment Health Addict. 2014;12:197–205.
46. Jimenez-Murcia S, Aymamí N, Gómez-Peña M, Santamaría JJ, Álvarez-Moya E, Fernández-Aranda F, et al. Does exposure and response prevention improve the results of group cognitive-behavioral therapy for male slot machine pathological gamblers? Br J Clin Psychol. 2012;51:54–71.

47. Shaffer HJ, Martin R. Disordered gambling: etiology, trajectory, and clinical considerations. Annu Rev Clin Psychol. 2011;7:483–510.
48. Griffiths MD. The role of cognitive bias and skill in fruit machine gambling. Br J Psychol. 1994;85:351–69.
49. Yurica CL, DiTomasso RA. Cognitive distortions. In: Encyclopedia of cognitive behavior therapy. New York: Springer; 2005. p. 117–22.
50. Toneatto T, Blitz-Miller T, Calderwood K, Dragonetti R, Tsanos A. Cognitive distortions in heavy gambling. J Gambl Stud. 1997;13:253–66.
51. Delfabbro PH, Winefield AH. Predictors of irrational thinking in irregular slot machine gamblers. J Psychol. 2000;134(2):117–28.
52. Baboushkin HR, Hardoon KK, Derevensky JL, Gupta R. Underlying cognitions in gambling behavior among university students. J Appl Soc Psychol. 2001;31:1409–30.
53. Hardoon KK, Baboushkin HR, Derevensky JL, Gupta R. Underlying cognitions in the selection of lottery tickets. J Clin Psychol. 2001;57:749–63.
54. Coventry KR, Norman AC. Arousal, erroneous verbalizations and the illusion of control during a computer-generated gambling task. Br J Psychol. 1998;89:629–45.
55. Petry NP. Pathological gambling: etiology, comorbidity, and treatment. Washington, DC: American Psychological Association; 2004.
56. Wagenaar WA. Paradoxes of gambling behaviour. London: Lawrence Erlbaum Associates; 1988.
57. Tversky A, Kahneman D. Belief in the law of small numbers. Psychol Bull. 1971;76:105–10.
58. Koriat A, Lichtenstein S, Fischhoff B. Reasons for confidence. J Exp Psychol Hum Learn Mem. 1980;6:107–18.
59. Goodie AS. The role of perceived control and overconfidence in pathological gambling. J Gambl Stud. 2005;21:481–502.
60. Lakey CE, Goodie AS, Lance CE, Stinchfield R, Winters KC. Examining DSM-IV criteria in gambling pathology: psychometric properties and evidence from cognitive biases. J Gambl Stud. 2007;23:479–98.
61. Haigh J. The statistics of the national lottery. J R Stat Soc Ser A Stat Soc. 1997;160:187–206.
62. Holtgraves T, Skeel J. Cognitive biases in playing the lottery: estimating the odds and choosing the numbers. J Appl Soc Psychol. 1992;22:934–52.
63. Rogers P, Webley P. "It could be us!": cognitive and social psychological factors in UK national lottery play. Appl Psychol Int Rev. 2001;50:181–99.
64. Haynes SN, Richard D, Kubany ES. Content validity in psychological assessment: a functional approach to concepts and methods. Psychol Assess. 1995;7(3):238–47.
65. Guion RM. Content validity—the source of my discontent. Appl Psychol Methods. 1977;1:1–10.
66. Breen RB, Zuckerman M. 'Chasing' in gambling behavior: personality and cognitive determinants. Personal Individ Differ. 1999;27:1097–111.
67. Jefferson S, Nicki R. A new instrument to measure cognitive distortions in video lottery terminal users: the informational biases scale (IBS). J Gambl Stud. 2003;19:387–403.
68. Brown TA. Introduction to CFA (Ch. 3). In Brown TA, editor. Confirmatory factor analysis for applied research. 2006. Retrieved from http://www.ophi.org.uk/wp-content/uploads/Brown-Ch-3.pdf.
69. Gorsuch RL. Exploratory factor analysis: its role in item analysis. J Pers Assess. 1997;68:532–60.
70. Brown TA. The common factor model and exploratory factor analysis (Ch. 2). In Brown TA, editor. Confirmatory factor analysis for applied research. 2006. Retrieved from http://www.ophi.org.uk/wp-content/uploads/Brown-Ch-2.pdf.
71. Vandenberg RJ, Lance CE. A review and synthesis of the measurement invariance literature: suggestions, practices, and recommendations for organizational research. Organ Res Methods. 2000;3(1):4–70.
72. Horn JL, McArdle JJ. A practical and theoretical guide to measurement invariance in aging research. Exp Aging Res. 1992;18:117–44.

73. Strong DR, Breen RB, Lejuez CW. Using item response theory to examine gambling attitudes and beliefs. Personal Individ Differ. 2004;36:1515–29.
74. Tochkov K. The effects of anticipated regret on risk preferences of social and problem gamblers. Judgm Decis Mak. 2009;4:227–34.
75. Neighbors C, Lostutter TW, Larimer ME, Takuski RY. Measuring gambling outcomes among college students. J Gambl Stud. 2002;18:339–60.
76. Callan MJ, Ellard JH, Shead NW, Hodgins DC. Gambling as a search for justice: examining the role of personal relative deprivation in gambling urges and gambling behavior. Personal Soc Psychol Bull. 2008;34:1514–29.
77. Strong DR, Daughters SB, Lejuez CW, Breen RB. Using the Rasch model to develop a revised gambling attitudes and beliefs scale (GABS) for use with male college student gamblers. Subst Use Misuse. 2004;39:1013–24.
78. Bouju G, Hardouin JB, Boutin C, Gorwood P, Le Bourvellec JD, Feuillet F, Venisse JL, Grall-Bronnec M. A shorter and multidimensional version of the Gambling Attitudes and Beliefs Survey (GABS-23). J Gambl Stud. 2014;30:349–67.
79. Grant LD, Bowling AC. Gambling attitudes and beliefs predict attentional bias in non-problem gamblers. J Gambl Stud. 2015;31(4):1487–503.
80. Marchetti D, Whelan JP, Verrocchio MC, Ginley MK, Fulcheri M, Relyea GE, Meyers AW. Psychometric evaluation of the Italian translation of the Gamblers' Beliefs Questionnaire. Int Gambl Stud. 2016;16(1):17–30.
81. Moore SM, Ohtsuka K. Beliefs about control over gambling among young people, and their relation to problem gambling. Psychol Addict Behav. 1999;13:339–47.
82. Mattson RE, MacKillop J, Castelda BA, Anderson EJ, Donovick PJ. The Factor structure of gambling-related cognitions in an undergraduate university sample. J Psychopathol Behav Assess. 2008;30:229–34.
83. Shaffer HJ, LaBrie R, Scanlan KM, Cummings TN. Pathological gambling among adolescents: Massachusetts Gambling Screen (MAGS). J Gambl Stud. 1994;10:339–62.
84. Winfree WR, Ginley MK, Whelan JP, Meyers AW. Psychometric evaluation of the Gamblers' Beliefs Questionnaire with treatment-seeking disordered gamblers. Addict Behav. 2015;43:97–102.
85. Winfree WR, Meyers AW, Whelan JP. Validation of a Spanish translation of the Gamblers' Beliefs Questionnaire. Psychol Addict Behav. 2013;27(1):274.
86. Wong SS, Tsang SK. Validation of the Chinese version of the gamblers' belief questionnaire (GBQ-C). J Gambl Stud. 2012;28(4):561–72.
87. Tang CSK, Wu AM. Gambling-related cognitive biases and pathological gambling among youths, young adults, and mature adults in Chinese societies. J Gambl Stud. 2012;28(1):139–54.
88. MacKay TL, Bard N, Bowling M, Hodgins DC. Do pokers players know how good they are? Accuracy of poker skill estimation in online and offline players. Comput Hum Behav. 2014;31:419–24.
89. MacKillop J, Anderson EJ, Castelda BA, Mattson RE, Donovick PJ. Convergent validity of measures of cognitive distortions, impulsivity, and time perspective with pathological gambling. Psychol Addict Behav. 2006;20:75–9.
90. Mitrovic DV, Brown J. Poker mania and problem gambling: a study of distorted cognitions, motivation and alexithymia. J Gambl Stud. 2009;25:489–502.
91. Doiron JP, Nicki RM. Prevention of pathological gambling: a randomized controlled trial. Cogn Behav Ther. 2007;36:74–84.
92. Wohl MJA, Young MM, Hart KE. Untreated young gamblers with game-specific problems: self-concept involving luck, gambling ecology and delay in seeking professional treatment. Addict Res Ther. 2005;13:445–59.
93. Wohl MJA, Young MM, Hart KE. Self-perceptions of dispositional luck: relationship to DSM gambling symptoms, subjective enjoyment of gambling and treatment readiness. Subst Use Misuse. 2007;42:43–63.

94. Young MM, Wohl MJA, Matheson K, Baumann S, Anisman H. The desire to gamble: the influence of outcomes on the priming effects of a gambling episode. J Gambl Stud. 2008;24:275–93.

95. Moodie C. An exploratory investigation into the erroneous cognitions of pathological and social fruit machine gamblers. J Gambl Iss. 2007;19:31–50.

96. Moodie C. Student gambling, erroneous cognitions, and awareness of treatment in Scotland. J of Gambl Iss. 2008;21:30–54.

97. Gerstein DR, Volberg RA, Harwood R, Christiansen EM. Gambling impact and behavior study: report to the national gambling impact study commission. Chicago, IL: National Opinion Research Center, University of Chicago; 1999.

98. Ferris J, Wynne H. The Canadian Problem Gambling Index: final report. Ottawa, Ontario, Canada: Canadian Centre on Substance Abuse; 2001.

99. MacLaren V, Ellery M, Knoll T. Personality, gambling motives and cognitive distortions in electronic gambling machine players. Personal Individ Differ. 2015;73:24–8.

100. Wohl MJ, Gainsbury S, Stewart MJ, Sztainert T. Facilitating responsible gambling: the relative effectiveness of education-based animation and monetary limit setting pop-up messages among electronic gaming machine players. J Gambl Stud. 2013;29(4):703–17.

101. Ciccarelli M, Griffiths MD, Nigro G, Cosenza M. Decision-making, cognitive distortions and alcohol use in adolescent problem and non-problem gamblers: an experimental study. J Gambl Stud. 2016;32(4):1203–13.

102. Oei TP, Lin J, Raylu N. Validation of the Chinese version of the Gambling Related Cognitions Scale (GRCS-C). J Gambl Stud. 2007;23:309–22.

103. Edmond MS, Marmurek HHC. Gambling related cognitions mediate the association between thinking style and problem gambling severity. J Gambl Stud. 2010;26:257–67.

104. Taylor RN, Parker JD, Keefer KV, Kloosterman PH, Summerfeldt LJ. Are gambling related cognitions in adolescence multidimensional?: factor structure of the gambling related cognitions scale. J Gambl Stud. 2014;30(2):453–65.

105. Smith D, Woodman R, Drummond A, Battersby M. Exploring the measurement structure of the Gambling Related Cognitions Scale (GRCS) in treatment-seekers: a Bayesian structural equation modelling approach. Psychiatry Res. 2016;237:90–6.

106. Oei TP, Lin J, Raylu N. The relationship between gambling cognitions, psychological states, and gambling: a cross-cultural study of Chinese and Caucasians in Australia. J Cross-Cult Psychol. 2008;39:147–61.

107. Arcan K, Karanci AN. Adaptation study of the Turkish version of the Gambling-Related Cognitions Scale (GRCS-T). J Gambl Stud. 2015;31(1):211–24.

108. Potenza MN. The neural bases of cognitive processes in gambling disorder. Trends Cogn Sci. 2014;18(8):429–38.

109. Worhunsky PD, Malison RT, Rogers RD, Potenza MN. Altered neural correlates of reward and loss processing during simulated slot-machine fMRI in pathological gambling and cocaine dependence. Drug Alcohol Depend. 2014;145:77–86.

110. Iliceto P, Fino E, Cammarota C, Giovani E, Petrucci F, Desimoni M, et al. Factor structure and psychometric properties of the Italian version of the Gambling Related Cognitions Scale (GRCS-I). J Gambl Stud. 2015;31(1):225–42.

111. Yokomitsu K, Takahashi T, Kanazawa J, Sakano Y. Development and validation of the Japanese version of the Gambling Related Cognitions Scale (GRCS-J). Asian J Gambl Issues Public Health. 2015;5(1):1.

112. Kale S, Dubelaar C. Assessment of reliability and validity of the Gambling Related Cognitions Scale (GRCS). Gambl Res. 2013;25(1):25.

113. Xian H, Shah KR, Phillips SM, Scherrer JF, Volberg R, Eisen SA. The association of cognitive distortions with problem and pathological gambling in adult male twins. Psychiatry Res. 2008;160(3):300–7.

114. Wohl MJA, Stewart MJ, Young MM. Personal luck usage scale (PLUS): psychometric validation of a measure of gambling-related belief in luck as a personal possession. Int Gambl Stud. 2011;11(1):7–11.

115. McInnes A, Hodgins DC, Holub A. The gambling cognitions inventory: scale development and psychometric validation with problem and pathological gamblers. Int Gambl Stud. 2014;14(3):410–31.
116. Darke PR, Freedman JL. The belief in good luck scale. J Res Pers. 1997;31:486–511.
117. Wohl MJA, Enzle ME. The deployment of personal luck: sympathetic magic and illusory control in games of pure chance. Personal Soc Psychol Bull. 2002;28:1388–97.
118. Ferland F, Ladouceur R, Vitaro F. Prevention of problem gambling: modifying misconceptions and increasing knowledge. J Gambl Stud. 2002;18:19–29.
119. Maltby J, Day L, Gill P, Colley A, Wood AM. Beliefs around luck: confirming the empirical conceptualization of beliefs around luck and the development of the Darke and Freeman beliefs around luck scale. Personal Individ Differ. 2008;45:655–60.
120. Thompson ER, Prendergast GP. Belief in luck and luckiness: conceptual clarification and new measure validation. Personal Individ Differ. 2013;54:501–6.

Genetic and Environmental Contributions to Risk for Disordered Gambling

5

Wendy S. Slutske

5.1 Introduction

In this chapter, I will review the literature on the behavioral genetics of disordered gambling (DG), including studies that have focused on (1) estimating the aggregate influence of genetic and environmental factors, as well as studies that have focused on (2) identifying the specific genes that account for the aggregate genetic risk. Other topics that will be covered are (3) DG comorbidity, (4) developmentally relevant studies, (5) identifying the specific environments that account for the aggregate environmental risk, and (6) gene-environment interplay. Throughout this chapter, the term "disordered gambling" will refer to not just pathological gambling or gambling disorder as defined by the DSM but also the full spectrum of gambling-related problems including problem gambling. This is consistent with the recent emphasis in psychiatry on the dimensional nature of many disorders [1] and emerging empirical evidence supporting the conceptualization of DG as dimensional [2].

5.2 Disordered Gambling Runs in Families: Setting the Stage

Numerous studies have reported that gambling involvement and problems run in families, but only two studies have obtained direct interviews with family members [3, 4]. In the largest of the studies, 8% of the first-degree relatives of DG-affected probands, compared to 1% of the first-degree relatives of DG-unaffected controls, had a lifetime history of DG [3]. First-degree relatives of the individuals with a diagnosis of DG were over eight times more likely to be affected with DG themselves

W. S. Slutske (✉)
Department of Psychological Sciences, University of Missouri, Columbia, MO, USA
e-mail: slutskew@missouri.edu

© Springer Nature Switzerland AG 2019
A. Heinz et al. (eds.), *Gambling Disorder*, https://doi.org/10.1007/978-3-030-03060-5_5

than the first-degree relatives of the unaffected controls. Although family studies are invaluable, their results are indeterminate with respect to the mechanisms underlying familial transmission. Although these findings are consistent with the social modeling of gambling behaviors of family members, they are just as consistent with an important role for genetic transmission. Genetically informative research designs, such as twin and adoption studies, are required to disentangle the contributions of genetic and environmental factors (such as social modeling) to the risk for DG.

In a twin study, one compares the similarity of monozygotic (MZ) twins, who share 100% of their genetic information, to the similarity of dizygotic (DZ) twins, who share on average 50% of their genetic information (specifically, the genetic information that varies in the population). (Two unrelated humans share about 99.9% of their genetic information; studies of individual differences are concerned with the 0.1% that varies.) When MZ twin pairs are more similar than DZ twin pairs, one can infer that there is a contribution of genetic factors to a trait. This represents the cumulative aggregated influence of all genes that contribute to trait variation. If the DZ twin similarity is greater than half the MZ twin similarity, then one can infer that shared environmental influences contribute to individual differences in a trait. That is, there are factors other than the sharing of genetic information that is contributing to the similarity of twins. A contribution of unique environmental influences is inferred when the MZ twin similarity is less than 1.0 (this also includes measurement error). This is the contribution to individual differences that is not shared by twins and cannot be explained by genes or shared environments.

5.3   Twin Studies of Disordered Gambling: Shared Genes Rather Than Shared Environments

Compared to other psychiatric disorders, there has been much less genetically informative research on DG, with only two major twin studies and no adoption studies conducted to date[1]. The results of twin studies of DG are presented in Table 5.1. The first large twin study was based on a sample of 3359 twin pairs from the Vietnam Era Twin Registry, a national sample of male twin pairs in which both men served in the US military during the Vietnam Era [6]. Despite the large size of the Vietnam Era twin cohort, there were still relatively few men who met the DSM diagnostic criteria for DG when interviewed in 1991–1993. Of 7869 interviewed men, only 112 (1.4%) met the diagnostic criteria for DG.

In the Vietnam Era twin cohort, the lifetime prevalence of DG was significantly elevated among the monozygotic (23%) and dizygotic (10%) cotwins of men with DG compared to the lifetime prevalence of DG (1.4%) in the full sample [24]. When standard twin structural equation models were fit to the data, it was not possible to discern whether this familial similarity for DG was due to genetic or shared family

---

[1] Davis, C.N., Slutske, W.S., Martin, N.G., Agrawal, A., & Lynskey, M.T. (2018). Genetic and environmental influences on gambling disorder liability: A replication and combined analysis of two twin studies. Psychological Medicine, published online first.

Table 5.1 Summary of twin studies of disordered gambling[a]

Phenotype	Setting	Men			Women			Sample size	Authors
		A	C	E	A	C	E		
Lifetime DSM-III-R [5] diagnosis	Telephone interview US Veterans (men)	0.46	0.16	0.38	–	–	–	3359 twin pairs	Eisen et al. [6]
Lifetime 1+ DSM-III-R [5] symptoms	Telephone interview US Veterans (men)	0.48	–	0.52	–	–	–	3359 twin pairs	Eisen et al. [6]
Past-year 1+ DSM-III-R [5] symptoms	Telephone interview US Veterans (men) 10-year follow-up	0.57	–	0.43	–	–	–	1675 twins	Xian et al. [7]
Lifetime 1+ DSM-IV [8] symptoms	Telephone interview Australia general population	0.49	0	0.51	0.52	0	0.48	4764 twins	Slutske et al. [9]
Lifetime 1+ SOGS [10] symptoms	Telephone interview Australia general population	0.62	0	0.38	0.43	0.06	0.50	4764 twins	Slutske et al. [11]
Lifetime Four categories ranging from 0–24 episodes of gambling to 25+ gambling episodes and 2+ DSM-IV [8] symptoms	Volunteer Web-based survey	0.83	0	0.17	0.83	0	0.17	912 twin and sibling pairs	Blanco et al. [12]
Past-year SOGS-RA [13] symptom count	On-site questionnaire Minnesota general population (age 18)	0.05	0.29	0.66	0.37	0.19	0.44	756 twin pairs	King et al. [14]
Past-year SOGS-RA [13] symptom count	On-site questionnaire Minnesota general population (age 25)	0.19	0.09	0.72	0.19	0.17	0.64	756 twin pairs	King et al. [14]

Note: A = proportion of variation due to genetic influences; *C* = proportion of variation due to shared environmental influences; *E* = proportion of variation due to unique environmental influences; DSM-III-R = Diagnostic and Statistical Manual of Mental Disorders, Third Edition, Revised; DSM-IV = Diagnostic and Statistical Manual of Mental Disorders, Fourth Edition; SOGS = South Oaks Gambling Screen; SOGS-RA = South Oaks Gambling Screen Revised for Adolescents. [a]The following study was not included because it was improperly represented as a study of DG and the analyses were flawed: Beaver et al. [15]. The reanalyzed data are listed in Table 5.4 as a study of non-disordered gambling by Slutske et al. [22, 23]

environmental factors, but it was possible to estimate that the total percentage of variation in the risk for DG that was accounted for by all familial factors, both genetic and environmental, was 62%.

A model commonly used in psychiatric genetics for estimating the influence of genetic and environmental factors underlying the risk for categorical disorders, and used in the two twin studies of DG, is the liability threshold model. This model makes the assumption that underlying the categorical diagnosis of DG is a normally distributed latent liability dimension in which being affected with DG corresponds to surpassing a threshold on the continuous latent liability. The liability threshold model assumes that the causes of variation in risk will be the same at any point along the liability distribution and for any threshold imposed [25]. A recent study provided empirical support for the liability threshold model as applied to DG [22]. This suggests that it is likely that the results obtained for a narrower and more stringent DG definition, such as meeting the DSM diagnostic criteria, will be the same as the results obtained for broader definitions of DG, such as experiencing one or more DG symptoms. The benefit of the latter approach is that it yields more cases and has greater statistical power for detecting genetic influences.

In the Vietnam Era twin cohort, firmer evidence for genetic influences on the risk for DG was obtained when a broader phenotype was used. When DG was defined as having one or more DSM symptoms, the heritability was estimated at 48%, with no evidence for a role of shared environmental influences in the familial transmission ([6]; see Table 5.1). The remaining variation in DG risk was due to individual-specific environmental factors that were not shared between twins. A 10-year follow-up was conducted with a selected subsample of 1675 individual twins from the Vietnam Era twin cohort [7]. This longitudinal follow-up allowed for an examination of the stability and change in the genetic and environmental influences to risk for DG from ages 42 to 53 over a time period in which the opportunities to gamble expanded in the United States (1992–2002). The genetic factors that contributed to variation in risk for DG in 1992 completely explained the genetic variation in risk for DG in 2002. On the other hand, most of the individual-specific environmental risk factors for DG in 2002 had not played a role in the risk for DG back in 1992. In other words, the same genes, but largely different environments, contributed to DG risk in 1992 versus 2002 in these middle-aged men.

The other major twin study of DG was based on a sample of 2889 twin pairs (1875 complete and 1014 incomplete pairs) from the national Australian Twin Registry. It differed from the previous US study in several ways: the geographic location, the inclusion of women and opposite-sex twin pairs, the data collection occurring 10+ years later, and the use of multiple measures of DG. Despite these differences, the estimates of genetic and environmental influences contributing to the risk for DSM DG were quite similar in the two studies (see Table 5.1). Perhaps of most interest were the similar estimates of genetic and environmental contributions to DG risk in women and men.

The Australian twin study also incorporated an alternate measure of DG, based on the South Oaks Gambling Screen (SOGS [10]). For many years, this was the most commonly used measure in epidemiologic surveys of DG and is still widely used in treatment settings. There has been a great deal of debate about the relative merits and weaknesses of the two operationalizations of DG. Although many of the SOGS items are not found in the DSM assessment, symptom scores based on the DSM and SOGS are highly correlated with each other. In the Australian twin study, the estimates of genetic and environmental influences in DG risk were similar for the DSM and SOGS (see Table 5.1), and the correlation between the genetic and environmental risk factors for DSM- and SOGS-defined DG was $r_A = 0.86$ and $r_E = 0.54$, respectively [11]. This is important because it suggests that the two measures are largely tapping into the same genetic sources of variation in DG.

A smaller-scale twin study used a novel web-based approach to recruit participants. A website was created that allowed cooperating dyads (including twins) to complete a survey that included an assessment of DG. In addition to monozygotic and dizygotic twin pairs, there were also non-twin sibling, parent-offspring, partner, spouse, and friend pairs included in the sample. All of these dyads were significantly correlated for DG. Of particular interest is that the non-genetically related dyads such as spouses and friends were in many cases as strongly correlated as genetically-related dyads such as dizygotic twin, parent-offspring, and siblings [26]. The similarity of spouse and friendship dyads suggests a role for processes such as social selection or social influence (or both). Formal biometric models were fit to the data from the twin and siblings pairs [12]; the majority of the 609 twin pairs were same-sex female pairs (72%), monozygotic (72%), and White/Caucasian (85%), and most were 18 years of age or older (85% [26]). The results of these model-fitting analyses are also presented in Table 5.1.

The most recent study was based on two waves from the longitudinal Minnesota Twin Family Study. The participants were 756 male and female same-sex twin pairs identified from state of Minnesota records of births occurring from 1978 to 1982. The twins were first assessed at age 11 and were regularly followed up through age 29. The participants completed past-year assessments of gambling problems at ages 18 and 25. The participants reported very few gambling problems at either age—the mean number of problems on a 12-item scale from the South Oaks Gambling Screen Revised for Adolescents [13] was 0.39 at age 18 and 0.36 at age 25. The estimates of the contribution of genetic influences to gambling problems were much lower in this cohort than in the previous studies listed in Table 5.2. This may be due to the youth of the sample but also may be due the narrower past-year assessment of gambling problems and the sparseness of the data. The authors also report the results from analyses of several measures of non-pathological gambling involvement, which is discussed in Sect. 5.6.

Although the studies are few in number, they largely tell the same story: there are significant and substantial genetic and unique environmental influences contributing to DG liability and less evidence for common environmental influences. These findings should come as no surprise, because they are completely consistent with Turkheimer's [34] "Three Laws of Behavior Genetics." Turkheimer's "First Law" of behavior genetics is "all human behavioral traits are heritable."[2]

---

[2]The second law is "the effect of being raised in the same family is smaller than the effect of the genes," and the third law is "a substantial portion of the variation in complex human behavioral traits is not accounted for by the effects of genes or families."

Table 5.2 Summary of twin studies of disordered gambling comorbidity[a]

Phenotype	Setting	Men			Women			Sample size	Authors
		r_A	r_C	r_E	r_A	r_C	r_E		
Alcohol use disorder									
DSM-III-R [5] alcohol dependence	US Vietnam veterans	**0.43**	–	**0.18**	–	–	–	8169 twins	Slutske et al. [24]
DSM-IV [5] alcohol dependence	AU community	**0.46**	–	**0.35**	**0.39**	–	0.25	4764 twins	Slutske et al. [23]
DSM-5 [27] AUD	AU community	**0.30**	–	**0.42**	**0.28**	–	**0.27**	4764 twins	Slutske et al. [23]
DSM-IV [8] AUD symptom count	AU community	**0.41**	–	**0.25**	**0.29**	–	**0.20**	4764 twins	Slutske et al. [23]
Nicotine dependence									
Fagerstrom test for nicotine dependence (FTND) [28]	Web survey	0.29	1.00	0.29	0.29	1.00	0.29	912 twin and sibling pairs	Blanco et al. [12]
DSM-III-R [5] nicotine dependence	US Vietnam veterans	**0.22**	0	**0.24**	–	–	–	7869 twins	Xian et al. [29]
Other substance use disorders									
DSM-III-R [5] cannabis abuse/dependence	US Vietnam veterans	**0.32**	0	**0.36**	–	–	–	7869 twins	Xian et al. [29]
DSM-III-R [5] stimulant abuse/dependence	US Vietnam veterans	**0.58**	0	0	–	–	–	7869 twins	Xian et al. [29]
Antisocial behavior disorders									
DSM-III-R [5] conduct disorder	US Vietnam veterans	**0.47**	–	0.09	–	–	–	7869 twins	Slutske et al. [30]
Adult antisocial behavior	US Vietnam veterans	**0.43**	–	0.29	–	–	–	7869 twins	Slutske et al. [30]
DSM-III-R [5] ASPD	US Vietnam veterans	**0.40**	–	0.30	–	–	–	7869 twins	Slutske et al. [30]
Major depression									
DSM-III-R [5] major depression	US Vietnam veterans	**0.46**	0.05	0.25	–	–	–	7869 twins	Potenza et al. [31]
DSM-III-R [5] major depression	Web survey	0.14	–	0.31	0.14	–	0.31	912 twin and sibling pairs	Blanco et al. [12]
Anxiety disorders									
OCD features	US Vietnam veterans	**0.42**	0	0	–	–	–	1675 twin pairs	Scherrer et al. [32]

Note: Significant parameters are in bold; [a]the following study was not included because there were too few doubly concordant twin pairs to estimate the dizygotic twin correlations: Giddens et al. [33]; r_C = correlation between shared environmental influences; r_A = correlation between genetic influences; r_E = correlation between unique environmental influences; AUD = alcohol use disorder; ASPD = antisocial personality disorder; OCD = obsessive-compulsive disorder

5.4 Twin Studies of Disordered Gambling Comorbidity: Specific and Non-specific Genetic Risks

Individuals with a history of DG are likely to suffer from other psychiatric disorders. Significant associations have been observed between lifetime DG and every other disorder assessed in the largest psychiatric epidemiologic survey conducted to date [35]. The strongest associations were with the substance use and personality disorders, but there were also substantial associations with mood and anxiety disorders.

Multivariate twin modeling has been applied to the question of DG comorbidity. The logic of multivariate twin modeling is similar to that of univariate twin modeling (the analysis of a single trait). With multivariate twin modeling, one is interested in the cross-trait as well as the within-trait similarity. For example, one might examine the within-pair similarity of a diagnosis of DG in one twin with alcohol use disorder in the other twin. If the MZ cross-trait cross-twin similarity is greater than the DZ cross-trait cross-twin similarity, then one infers that genetic factors are contributing to the association between DG and alcohol use disorder. In other words, there is at least one gene that is a risk factor for both DG and alcohol use disorder. If the DZ cross-trait cross-twin similarity is greater than half the MZ cross-trait cross-twin similarity, then one infers that shared environmental factors are contributing to the association between DG and alcohol use disorder. Unique environmental factors are implicated when the MZ cross-trait cross-twin similarity is less than the within-twin correlation between DG and alcohol use disorder.

A series of multivariate twin modeling analyses using data from the Vietnam Era and Australian twin studies have suggested that DG may have common genetic underpinnings with the substance use disorders, including alcohol [22–24], nicotine, cannabis, and stimulant use disorders ([29]; see Table 5.2). Also consistent with the epidemiologic evidence is the substantial genetic overlap between DG and antisocial behavior disorders [30]. Given the substantial comorbidity between substance use and antisocial behavior disorders, these models were elaborated to determine whether the genetic overlap between DG and alcohol use disorders and between DG and the antisocial behavior disorders was being driven by the same or distinct sets of genetic risk factors. When both adult antisocial personality disorder, childhood conduct disorder, and DG were included in the same model, about one-quarter of the genetic variation in the risk for DG was explained by genetic influences on antisocial behavior disorders that were onboard in childhood (via their influence on childhood conduct disorder). These genetic influences in the risk for antisocial behavior disorders also completely explained the genetic association between alcohol dependence and DG [24]. This study suggests that DG, antisocial behavior disorders, and alcohol dependence have common genetic influences that are already manifested in childhood. The most likely explanation for these findings is that there are susceptibility genes that are common to these disorders.

Although DG is often pigeonholed as an externalizing disorder, significant genetic associations between DG and internalizing disorders such as major depression [31] and obsessive-compulsive disorder features [32] have also been reported (see Table 5.2).[3] Factor analyses of diagnostic data from a large representative epi-demiologic survey suggested that DG loaded onto a higher-order "externalizing" factor, along with alcohol dependence, drug dependence, and antisocial personality disorder [36]. However, the factor loading of DG onto this externalizing factor was relatively low, and among women, DG also appeared to load onto the "anxious-misery" factor (a subfactor of a higher-order "internalizing" factor). Clearly, more research is needed to accurately characterize the specific and non-specific risk factors for DG and other addictive and nonaddictive disorders.

Again, the finding of significant genetic correlations between DG and comorbid disorders should come as no surprise. Plomin et al. [37] have commented on the robust finding that correlations between psychological traits, including psychopa-thology, are usually at least partially genetically mediated: "More than 100 twin studies have addressed the key question of comorbidity in psychopathology, and this body of research also consistently shows substantial genetic overlap between common disorders" [37]. Future directions for genetic research on DG comorbidity will be to test more extensive biometric models that consider more than two or three traits at a time (e.g., [38]) and to examine comorbidity at the level of measured genes, rather than at the level of latent aggregated genetic risk estimated in a twin study (e.g., [39]). For example, there is recent molecular genetic evidence from a genome-wide association study (described below) confirming the genetic overlap between DG and alcohol use disorder [40].

5.5   Molecular Genetic Research on Disordered Gambling: Finding the Genetic Risk Factors

The evidence from twin studies (reviewed above) has consistently demonstrated an important aggregate influence of genetic factors in the risk for DG among both men and women. One of the major challenges ahead will be to identify the specific indi-vidual genetic variants that confer this risk. Research into the genetic underpinnings of DG is lagging far behind other mental health disorders.

Candidate genetic association studies. To date, there have been 16 published candidate gene association studies based on nine distinct samples, including a total of 2740 participants and focusing on 43 different candidate genes (selected from the ~20,000 genes found in the human genome). This (albeit limited) research base has not yet led to any consistent, replicated findings (for reviews, see [22, 23, 41, 42]). A summary of the results of candidate gene association studies of DG is presented in Table 5.3. Although there are too few studies to draw any conclusions, the dopa-mine D3 receptor gene is of particular interest because the most recent positive finding in humans was replicated in a rat model [49].

---

[3] Giddens et al. (2011) reported genetic associations of DG with generalized anxiety and panic disorder. However, because there were too few doubly concordant twin pairs to estimate the dizy-gotic twin correlations, the genetic correlations may have been misestimated.

Table 5.3 Summary of genes associated with disordered gambling

System	Genes	No. of studies conducted	No. of studies reporting significant results	Sample size[a] range (n)	Authors
Dopamine	*Systems involved in pleasure and reward*				
	DAT1 (dopamine transporter)	1	1	175	Gray and MacKillop [43]
	DRD1 (dopamine D1 receptor)	4	2	208–287	Comings et al. [44], Lim et al. [45], Lobo et al. [46, 47]
	DRD2 (dopamine D2 receptor)	4	1	208–287	Comings et al. [48], Lim et al. [45], Lobo et al. [46, 47]
	DRD3 (dopamine D3 receptor)	3	1	208–745	Lim et al. [45], Lobo et al. [47, 49]
	DRD4 (dopamine D4 receptor)	4	1	136–280	Gray and MacKillop [43], Perez de Castro et al. [50], Lim et al. [45], Lobo et al. [47]
Other catecholamines					
	COMT (catechol-O-methyltransferase)	3	2[b]	139–260	Gray and MacKillop [43], Grant et al. [51], Guillot et al. [52]
	MAO-A (monoamine oxidase A)	2	1	136	Ibanez et al. [53], Perez de Castro et al. [54]
Serotonin	*Systems involved in mood*				
	5-HT2a (serotonin 2a receptor)	1	1	136	Wilson et al. [55]
	5-HTT (serotonin transporter)	2	1	136–280	Perez de Castro et al. [56], Wilson et al. [55]
Calcium signaling	*Other systems*				
	CAMKD (calcium-/calmodulin-dependent protein kinase II delta)	1	1	745	Lobo et al. [49]

Note: Only genes for which there was at least one significant finding are included in this table. [a]Includes cases and controls, [b]significant findings were in the opposite direction

A unique investigation of a small sample of 139 DG patients and 139 DG-unaffected controls assessed the aggregate effect of 16 (selected from a larger set of 31) candidate genes primarily related to the dopaminergic, serotonergic, and noradrenergic systems [57]. The portion of variation in DG explained by the combined effect of four dopamine genes (*DAT1*, *DRD1*, *DRD2*, *DRD4*), four serotonin genes (*5-HTT*, *5-HT2c*, *TDO2*, *TPH*), and three norepinephrine genes (*DBH*, *ADRAC2*, *COMT*) was 8%, 7%, and 8%, respectively, and the overall portion of variation in DG explained by the full set of 16 genes was 21%.[4] This early study presages more recent efforts that have successfully used the results from large-scale genome-wide association studies to create polygenic risk scores that are significantly associated with important outcomes, such as nicotine dependence [58] in a completely distinct target sample [59].

Genome-wide association studies. Partially in response to the disappointing yield from targeted candidate gene association studies, psychiatric genomics has largely moved on to hypothesis-free approaches that interrogate the entire genome. To date, there have been two published genome-wide association studies (GWAS) of DG [40, 60]. As expected given their small sample sizes, there were no genome-wide significant SNPs (single nucleotide polymorphisms) or genes detected [40, 60]. There were, however, a number of novel "suggestive" associations detected in both samples that invite further investigation.

The first ever genome-wide study of DG was conducted using data from the 1312 participants in the Australian twin study that had provided a DNA sample for genotyping [60]. A quantitative DG phenotype was based on a factor score extracted from an analysis of the ten DSM diagnostic criteria, the 20 SOGS items, and four additional items related to the frequency and diversity of gambling involvement. There were 2,381,914 SNPs available for the analysis, either based on direct genotyping or imputation based on haplotype information.

A standard analysis failed to identify any SNPs that surpassed the stringent threshold for genome-wide significance ($p = 7.2 \times 10^{-8}$) in their association with DG, but there was suggestive evidence ($p = 1 \times 10^{-5}$) for six novel associations: one SNP in or near the metallothionein IX gene (*MT1X*), two SNPs in or near the very low-density lipoprotein receptor gene (*VLDLR*), one SNP in or near the ataxin-1 gene (*ATXN1*), and two SNPs in or near the frizzled-10 (*FZD10*) gene. Another level of analysis grouped SNPs together based on their proximity to known genes; this test also failed to identify any genes that surpassed the threshold of significance with a correction for multiple tests ($p = 2.8 \times 10^{-6}$). None of the 50 genes that were the most strongly associated with DG in the GWAS had been included in previous candidate gene association studies of DG.

The next level of analysis focused on the significance of sets of genes. The set of 16 genes studied by Comings et al. [57], along with eight additional genes implicated in dopamine-agonist-induced DG, were scrutinized (see "Another clue to the genetic basis of gambling disorder"). Again, none of the 24 genes surpassed the

---

[4]These large estimates are interesting but implausible given what we now know based on the results of genome-wide association studies of complex disorders.

threshold of significance with a correction for multiple tests ($p < 0.0021$), but there were two that yielded a p-value <0.05—the alpha-2c adrenergic receptor gene (*ADRAC2*) and the cyclic adenosine monophosphate responsive element-binding protein 1 (*CREB1*). (*ADRAC2* was the gene most strongly associated with DG in the previous study by Comings et al. [57].) Additionally, a follow-up analysis demonstrated that the combined set of 24 genes were significantly associated with DG compared to randomly selected 24 gene sets ($p = 0.017$). This candidate gene set appeared to be enriched with DG susceptibility genes of small effect.

Consistent with the findings from the twin research on DG comorbidity, there were also three known neurobiological pathways (synaptic long-term potentiation, gonadotropin-releasing hormone signaling, and gap junction) that harbored an excess of genes of small effect that were previously implicated in alcohol and substance use disorders [61]. Synaptic long-term potentiation is the experience-dependent strengthening of synaptic transmission that is essential for synaptic plasticity, considered to be important in learning and memory and which underlies neural adaptation to substances of abuse [62]. This mechanism is thought to occur in the mesolimbic dopamine pathway, a putative brain reward circuit that may be a common pathway through which many substances such as alcohol and behaviors such as gambling have their rewarding effects and potential for addiction [63].

A weakness of the previous DG GWAS is that the sample included many individuals with mild gambling problems, which may have hampered efforts to detect significant genetic associations. A more recent GWAS was based on a sample of 445 cases who met the full DSM DG diagnostic criteria, most of whom were receiving treatment for the disorder (including 280 receiving inpatient treatment), and 986 DG-unaffected controls [40]. Because the cases and controls had been genotyped on different platforms, a consensus set of 595,867 SNPs were used in the analyses.

Like the previous GWAS of the quantitative disorder gambling trait, there were no SNPs or genes that achieved genome-wide significance, none of the top hits corresponded to the top hits from the previous GWAS, and there was not a significant association between DG diagnoses and polygenic risk scores empirically derived from the prior GWAS [40]. When the results were compared to published findings of previous candidate gene association studies, none of the previous candidate genes achieved genome-wide significance, although there were SNPs in the *DAT1*, *DRD3*, *5-HT2a*, and *CAMKD* genes that had small p-values. There were three known neurobiological pathways (Huntington's disease, AMPK signaling, and apoptosis) that harbored an excess of genes of small effect, although they differed from the pathways identified in the previous GWAS [60]. The role of these neurobiological processes is still unclear. Lang et al. [40] speculated that the neural circuits that are affected in Huntington's disease are also involved in the predisposition to DG and may include alterations in impulsivity, sensitivity, and delay of gratification [64]. As noted earlier, this study provided molecular genetic evidence confirming the genetic overlap between DG and alcohol use disorder by predicting DG diagnoses from polygenic risk scores empirically derived from a previous GWAS study of alcohol dependence [40].

To put the molecular genetics of DG in perspective, consider the progress in the molecular genetics of schizophrenia. The first significant finding for the *DRD3* candidate gene was published in 1992, followed by 28 replication attempts and a meta-analysis in 1997 [65]. With the exponential increase in the number of informative genetic markers available after the successful completion of the Human Genome Project in 2002, genome-wide rather than candidate gene association investigations became the state-of-the-art approach to gene identification. Since the first GWAS study of schizophrenia was conducted including 27,085 study participants in 2009, the sample sizes have continued to increase to 150,064 participants in 2014 [66]. Note that these sample sizes were only achieved by cross-institutional collaborations. The number of genetic loci has correspondingly increased from 3 to 108; importantly, 77% of the loci detected had not previously been reported, that is, they were not the usual neurobiological suspects [67]. The *DRD3* gene was not implicated in the most recent GWAS of schizophrenia [68].

In addition to uncovering novel genetic risk factors, additional benefits of large-scale genome-wide investigations have been to confirm that complex disorders (such as schizophrenia and DG) are due to the influence of many genes of very small effect [37, 67] and to identify important networks or pathways of genes. The focus on networks of genes acting in concert is more true to life than focusing on individual genes acting in isolation [67]. Although the results of the pathway analyses presented in Lind et al. [60] and Lang et al. [40] may not always easily map onto established DG findings, they should be considered an enigma to potentially be decoded by future investigators.

Another clue to the genetic basis of gambling disorder. Perhaps the strongest clue to unraveling the genetic underpinnings of DG comes from a series of reports on the incidence of DG among individuals with Parkinson's disease (e.g., [69]) and restless legs syndrome (e.g., [70]) who were being treated with a dopamine agonist medication (that typically demonstrate relative selectivity for dopamine D3 receptors) in combination with or without levodopa (an amino acid precursor of dopamine that shows greater selectivity for dopamine D1 and D2 receptors), whose DG usually resolved with the discontinuation of the dopamine agonist therapy [70, 71]. These correlational findings are supported by experimental evidence from studies of rats and humans demonstrating that administration of a dopamine D2/D3 selective receptor agonist [72] or the administration of levodopa in the presence of the 4/7 *DRD4* genotype [73] increases gambling-like behaviors in the laboratory.

Endophenotypes for gambling disorder. Progress in the search for susceptibility genes for DG will involve a better understanding of the genes that are involved in processes that are causally upstream from DG. The identification of potential *endophenotypes* [74], or *intermediate phenotypes* [75], initially comes from a variety of methods but eventually must be validated using evidence from family studies (to establish that it is also present among individuals unaffected but at risk), twin studies (to establish a genetic association with DG), and longitudinal studies (to establish that it is independent of DG status). The literature on DG contains a number of promising potential DG endophenotypes (many covered in this volume), including decision-making [76] and neural systems [77]. None of these have been evaluated as endophenotypes for DG using family, twin, or longitudinal studies.

Research on endophenotypes aligns well with the National Institute of Mental Health Research Domain Criteria (RDoC) initiative [78]. This initiative was meant to encourage research on more fundamental biobehavioral, transdiagnostic dimensions. The transdiagnostic perspective of the RDoC is consistent with the substantial genetic overlap observed between psychiatric disorders (discussed above with respect to DG) and suggests that many of the endophenotypes identified for comorbid disorders will also apply to DG. For example, impulsivity and compulsivity have been proposed as endophenotypes for several disorders [79], and resting EEG and visual P300 event-related potentials have shown promise as endophenotypes for substance use disorders [80]; these might also warrant investigation as endophenotypes for DG.

5.6 Development of DG: The Roots of DG

Like other addictive disorders, DG requires that one passes through a series of stages, including the initiation of participation in gambling activities and the progression to regular involvement, prior to the eventual development of DG symptoms. Thus, genetic susceptibility for DG will also include those genes related to individual differences in these earlier stages. In Table 5.4 is a summary of the twin studies that have focused on these earlier stages of gambling behavior.

The progression through these stages of gambling involvement often mirrors the progression through stages of development of the individual, that is, from adolescence into adulthood. Comparing the results of twin studies conducted among adolescent [14, 17], emerging-adult [14, 18], young-adult [20], and middle-aged-adult [12, 19] samples raises the possibility that there may be differences in the contributions of genetic and family environmental factors to variation in gambling involvement across the life span. In particular, genetic factors appear to play an increasing role at later developmental stages and also at later stages of gambling involvement progression (i.e., from initiation to frequency of use to gambling disorder). This aligns nicely with findings from the substance use literature demonstrating that the contribution of genetic influences increases and the contribution of shared environmental influences decreases with age [81] and stage of involvement [82].

A longitudinal twin study that measured the frequency of gambling, amount spent when gambling, and gambling problems at ages 18 and 25 [14] was able to directly test these ideas about different contributions of genetic and environmental influences at different ages and stages of gambling involvement. When considered individually, there appeared to be a larger contribution of genetic and a smaller contribution of shared environmental influences at age 25 than at age 18 (see Table 5.4 for the maximum spent and gambling frequency results). On the other hand, this pattern did not emerge for the stages of gambling involvement progression, that is, from the frequency of gambling to gambling problems (the gambling problem results are presented in Table 5.1). The contributions of genetic, shared, and unique environmental factors were also estimated for latent gambling factors that were derived from combined analyses of the different indicators of gambling involvement measured at ages 18 and 25 (incorporating measures of both non-problem and problem gambling involvement [14]). The contribution of genetic factors to these latent gambling

Table 5.4 Summary of twin studies of non-disordered gambling involvement[a]

Phenotype	Setting	Age range[b]	Men			Women			Sample size	Authors
			A	C	E	A	C	E		
Age of gambling initiation	AU	32–43[b]	0.36	0	0.64	0.06	0.28	0.66	4532 twins	Richmond-Rakerd et al. [16]
Gambling initiation	US (1962)	17	0.01	0.60	0.39	0.26	0.42	0.42	839 twin pairs	Slutske [17]
Gambling initiation	US	18–26	0	0.45	0.55	0	0.54	0.46	440 twin pairs	Slutske et al. [18]
Gambling initiation[c]	AU	32–43	0.55	0.21	0.24	0.55	0.21	0.24	4764 twins	Slutske et al. [19]
Number of activities ("versatility")[c]	AU	32–43	0.56	0.01	0.43	0.56	0.01	0.43	4764 twins	Slutske et al. [19]
Maximum spent	US (MN)	18	0.24	0.35	0.42	0.19	0.40	0.41	756 twin pairs	King et al. [14]
Maximum spent	US (MN)	25	0.42	0.13	0.45	0.30	0.17	0.53	756 twin pairs	King et al. [14]
Maximum spent[c]	AU	32–43	0.43	0.09	0.47	0.43	0.09	0.47	4764 twins	Slutske et al. [19]
Gambling frequency	US (MN)	18	0.24	0.29	0.48	0.37	0.22	0.41	756 twin pairs	King et al. [14]
Gambling frequency	US (MN)	25	0.40	0.03	0.57	0.30	0.07	0.63	756 twin pairs	King et al. [14]
Gambling frequency[c]	AU	32–43	0.47	0	0.53	0.47	0	0.53	4764 twins	Slutske et al. [19]
Gambling frequency[c]	web survey	??	0.42	0.32	0.25	0.42	0.32	0.25	912 twin and sibling pairs	Blanco et al. [12]

Note: A = proportion of variation due to genetic influences; *C* = proportion of variation due to shared environmental influences; *E* = proportion of variation due to unique environmental influences. [a]The following two studies were not included: Winters and Rich [20] because estimates of genetic and environmental influences were not provided and Vitaro et al. [21] because the frequency of gambling measure was highly skewed and only 20% of the 13-year-old participants had ever gambled. [b]Retrospectively reported age first gambled; [c]sex differences not examined factors was much greater (0.57 versus 0.21), and the contribution of shared environmental factors was much smaller (0.10 versus 0.55) at age 25 than at age 18.

Multivariate twin models have been developed to capture the stage-like nature of the genetic contributions to substance use disorders [83]. For example, Maes et al. [84] fit a three-stage model to tobacco use: from initiation to regular use to nicotine dependence. When examined individually, all three outcomes were substantially heritable. However, a trivariate analysis revealed that most of the genetic influences on regular tobacco use were due to genetic influences on the previous stage (tobacco use initiation). Similarly, most of the genetic influences on nicotine dependence were due to genetic influences on the previous stages (tobacco use initiation and regular use). Similar two-stage modeling has been applied to the progression from the initiation of alcohol use to heavy alcohol use [85], from the initiation of illicit drug use to drug use disorder [86], and from binge eating to bulimia nervosa [87]. Application of such models to the stages of gambling involvement would be informative about the extent to which there are overlapping versus specific genetic and environmental risk factors for gambling initiation, frequency of gambling, and gambling disorder. Based on the previous research on substance use and eating disorders, it is likely that a large portion of the genetic and environmental risk for gambling disorder is shared with the genetic and environmental influences contributing to the initiation and frequency of gambling and that a smaller portion is specific to the risk for DG. Such a result would suggest that the findings from previous twin studies of DG are ambiguous; it is not clear how much of the genetic variation is specific to the progression to DG versus the genetic variation associated with the uptake of and regular involvement in gambling. Disentangling and understanding these different sources of genetic variation will provide a more complete picture of the underpinnings of DG.

Two more points about the results presented in Table 5.4 are worth noting. First, the only gambling behavior in which a sex difference in the contribution of genetic factors has been established is in the age of gambling initiation, wherein genetic factors significantly contributed to variation among men but not among women, and shared environmental factors significantly contributed to variation among women but not among men [16]. This suggests that familial context exerts greater influence over females' than males' decision to initiate gambling. This leads to the second point. Although it's hard to draw conclusions from so few studies, it appears that the estimates of the contribution of genetic factors may be higher in Australia than in the United States. This may be because the main driver of gambling in the United States is differences in availability; when availability is more ubiquitous, such as in Australia, genetic differences will be more likely to be expressed.

5.7 Environment: An Important Piece of the Puzzle

The fact that monozygotic twins are not perfectly correlated for DG[5] is an indication that, in addition to genetic factors, environmental factors are also important in the development of DG. Other evidence comes from cross-national variation in the

---

[5] The monozygotic twin correlations for DG in the Vietnam Era and Australian twin studies ranged from $r = 0.48$ to 0.63 [6, 9, 11].

Table 5.5 Putative environmental risk factors associated with disordered gambling

Environment	Nongenetically informed studies	Genetically informed studies
Non-specific risk factors		
Childhood maltreatment (neglect, abuse)	Afifi et al. [90], Black et al. [91], Hodgins et al. [92], Petry et al. [93]	Scherrer et al. [94]
Stressful life events	Blanco et al. [95]	
Poverty	Welte et al. [96]	
Neighborhood disadvantage	Barnes et al. [97], Martins et al. [98], Pearce et al. [99], Welte et al. [100]	Slutske et al. [101]
Gambling-specific risk factors		
Exposure to parental gambling	Gupta and Derevensky [102], Oei and Raylu [103]	Slutske et al. [104]
Exposure to peer gambling	Fortune et al. [105], Meisel et al. [106]	
Early age of gambling initiation (early exposure)	Lynch et al. [107], Kessler et al. [108]	Slutske et al. [109]
Exposure to gambling advertising	Derevensky et al. [110], Planzer et al. [111]	
Proximity to casino	Gerstein et al. [89], Welte et al. [100]	
Density of gambling outlets	Pearce et al. [99], Storer et al. [112], Slutske et al. [101]	
Number of legal forms of gambling in a region	Planzer et al. [111], Welte et al. [113]	

prevalence of DG [88] and within-national differences across regions within the United States [35, 89]. These cross-national and cross-state differences suggest that the environment plays an important role in the etiology of DG. Table 5.5 includes a list of putative environmental factors that have been studied in relation to DG.

These are considered "putative" environmental factors because the extent to which they are truly environmental has not been empirically established. One can establish that a risk factor is truly environmental by examining whether the relation between a risk factor and DG persists after controlling for genetic factors or by examining whether the risk factor is heritable. In the right column of Table 5.5 are listed four genetically informed studies that have tackled this issue. These four studies are briefly reviewed below.

First, experiencing maltreatment as a child appears to have far-ranging effects in adulthood [114], including suffering from DG [115]. When examined within a genetically informed discordant monozygotic twin design in the Vietnam Era twin study, however, the established relations between DG and having a history of being molested, physically abused, or seriously neglected as a child were nonsignificant [94]. In other words, the twin who had experienced maltreatment was not more likely to later develop DG than the identical cotwin who did not experience maltreatment. This suggests that the association may be due to genetic or environmental differences between families that are related to both exposure to maltreatment and the risk for DG.

Second, it has been suggested that being exposed to parental gambling role models might lead offspring to be more likely to take up the habit [102, 103]. This is a mechanism that has been proposed to explain why DG runs in families. When examined within a genetically informed discordant twin design in the Australian twin study, however, the twin affected with DG was not significantly more likely to have gambled with the parents than was the unaffected cotwin, and the same was true for twins discordant for frequent gambling [104]. This suggests that the familial transmission of DG is probably due to something other than modeling of parental gambling.

Third, beginning to gamble at a young age is commonly cited as an important risk factor for DG (e.g., [116]), and there is some empirical evidence to support this [107, 108]. When examined within a genetically informed discordant twin design in the Australian twin study, however, the twin who had initiated gambling at an earlier age was not more likely to later develop DG than the cotwin who initiated gambling at a later age [109]. Again, this suggests that the association may be due to genetic or environmental differences between families that are related to both early gambling initiation and the risk for DG. Beginning to gamble at a younger age may be a marker of genetic risk for DG, rather than a direct cause of DG.

Fourth, a number of studies have reported an association between living in a disadvantaged neighborhood and suffering from DG [97–100]. It may come as a surprise to some, but living in a disadvantage neighborhood is partially heritable [101, 117, 118]. For example, in the Australian twin study, the level of neighborhood disadvantage where adult twins lived was correlated with the level of neighborhood disadvantage where the cotwin lived: $r = 0.46$ among monozygotic and $r = 0.32$ among dizygotic twin pairs. When standard biometric twin models were fitted to these data, genetic, shared environmental, and unique environmental factors explained 25%, 20%, and 55% of the variation in exposure to neighborhood disadvantage, respectively. Consistent with previous studies, there was a significant association between living in a disadvantaged neighborhood and DG (and the frequency of gambling). These modest associations were mostly explained by genetic factors that were related to exposure to neighborhood disadvantage [101].

These four examples illustrate the danger of making assumptions about measures of the environment, because many of them are partially heritable [37, 119]. It is important to recognize that life is not an experiment in which environments are randomly assigned to people. Rather, our environments (a) arise from genetically influenced choices based on our abilities, interests, talents, and proclivities, (b) are evoked based on reactions of others to our genetically influenced characteristics, and (c) are inherited along with our genes from our parents. Because environmental factors are as important as genetic factors in the etiology of DG, they deserve as much research attention. Unfortunately, establishing that a risk factor is environmental requires more sophisticated research designs (such as natural experiments, treatment studies, and genetically informed designs; see [120]) than have typically been employed in the study of DG.

5.8   Gene-Environment Interplay: Putting the Pieces Together

The examples listed above also illustrate the idea of one form of gene-environment interplay, that is, gene-environment correlation (see Fig. 5.1). Gene-environment correlation is the process by which one's genetic predisposition affects the likelihood of being exposed to environmental risks [121, 122]. One way that this occurs early in life is when we inherit from our birth parents both our genes and our rearing environments. Gene-environment correlation makes the interpretation of associations between parental behavior and offspring outcomes ambiguous because genes and environments are confounded with each other. For example, one can simultaneously inherit from one's parents a genetic predisposition to develop DG along with an environment in which gambling behavior is modeled. One natural experiment in which genes and environments are "un-confounded" is an adoption study in which birth parents provide genes and adoptive parents provide environments. An association between adoptive parent gambling behavior and adoptee gambling would provide strong support for a social modeling interpretation.

In addition to modeling gambling behavior, there is research suggesting that parents with a gambling disorder may be more likely to abuse or neglect their children [115]. Therefore, it is also possible that one can simultaneously inherit from one's parents a genetic predisposition to develop DG along with an environment in which there is abuse or neglect. Gene-environment correlation can also occur later in life through a more active process whereby one seeks out or creates environments based on genetic propensities. This can apply to who we choose as friends, who we marry, the activities that we select (that might expose us to stresses), and where we choose to live.

In addition to genetic and environmental effects being correlated with each other, the effects of genes and environments can also *interact*. Gene-environment interaction is the process by which one's genetic predisposition affects one's sensitivity to environmental risks ([123–125]; see Fig. 5.2). That is, one's genotype may influence the impact of an environmental risk factor. A corollary of this is that the effects of genes might only be revealed in samples that are exposed to the known environmental risks for a particular disorder [126]. For example, the possibility raised earlier that the contribution of genetic factors to gambling frequency may be higher in Australia than in the United States may be due to gene-environment interaction.

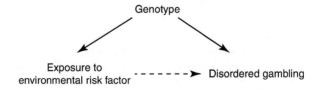

Fig. 5.1 Gene-environment correlation: genes controlling environmental exposure. In the figure, genes impact on disordered gambling indirectly by influencing the probability that an individual becomes exposed to an environmental risk factor

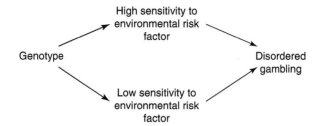

Fig. 5.2 Gene × environment interaction: genes controlling environmental sensitivity. In the figure, genes impact on disordered gambling indirectly by making an individual more sensitive to the DG-ogenic effect of an environmental risk factor

Gene-environment correlation and interaction can be studied at the level of inferred aggregated genetic effects obtained from twin and adoption studies or at the level of measured genes from candidate gene studies or sets of genes obtained from a GWAS. For example, gene-environment interaction in a twin study would be reflected in differences in heritabilities for an outcome observed in different environments (e.g., [127]). Gene-environment interaction in a candidate gene association study would be reflected in different genotype-outcome associations observed in different environments (e.g., [128]). Gene-environment interaction based on GWAS information would be reflected in different associations between polygenic risk scores and an outcome observed in different environments (e.g., [129]). All of the putative non-specific environmental risk factors listed in Table 5.5 have previously been included as environments in a large number of gene-environment interaction studies that have focused on a variety of outcomes such as crime and antisociality, depression, intelligence, and alcohol and substance use. Only one study has focused on gene-environment interaction and DG.

Gene-environment correlation and interaction for gambling frequency and DG were studied at the level of inferred aggregated genetic effects in the Australian twin study [101]. The environment of interest was neighborhood disadvantage, which was based on a census-based composite indicator of disadvantage that was matched to each twin's place of residence. Consistent with previous studies [97–100], the frequency of gambling and the prevalence of DG were higher in more disadvantaged neighborhoods. For example, the prevalence of past-year DG was nearly eight times higher among those living in the highest decile of area disadvantage (3.3%) compared to those living in the lowest decile (0.4%).

After taking into account gene-environment correlation between exposure to neighborhood disadvantage and the gambling outcomes (described in the previous section), differences in the heritability of gambling frequency and DG were examined as a function of the level of disadvantage in the neighborhood where each twin lived. The genetic (and also unique environmental) variation in the frequency of gambling was greater with increasing levels of neighborhood disadvantage, and the same was also found for DG among women. The finding of significant gene-environment correlation and gene-environment interaction suggests that the genetic risk for excessive and disordered gambling makes one more likely to be exposed to settings in which there is greater disadvantage and that the genetic risk for excessive and disordered gambling is more likely to be actualized within settings in which there is greater disadvantage.

Follow-up analyses were conducted to better understand the mechanisms underlying this neighborhood disadvantage effect [101]. Based on previous research (conducted in the United States, Canada, England, New Zealand, and Australia) showing that there is a greater density of gambling outlets in relatively disadvantaged neighborhoods [99, 100, 130–132], the association between neighborhood disadvantage and gambling frequency and DG was examined as a function of the state-level density of local gambling venues in Australia. There are six states and two territories in Australia, and (like the United States) gambling activities and the gambling industry are regulated at the state level. The effects of neighborhood disadvantage and gambling outlet density were "pulled apart" by comparing Western Australia with the remainder of Australia; Western Australia has no local gambling venues, whereas the remainder of Australia has many. There was no association between neighborhood disadvantage and the frequency of electronic machine gambling and DG in Western Australia, but significant associations for the remainder of Australia. At least in Australia, it appears that accessibility to gambling outlets plays a pivotal role in the neighborhood disadvantage effect.

5.9   Summary

Disordered gambling runs in families, and studies of twins suggest that this is due to shared genes rather than shared environments. Genetic factors in aggregate appear to account for about 50% of the risk for developing DG, and unique non-familial environmental factors in aggregate appear to account for the other 50% of the risk. This appears to be the case for both men and women. The specific genes that account for the aggregate genetic risk have not yet been identified; knowledge gained from over a decade of GWAS of psychiatric disorders suggests that there are likely to be many genes of very small effect contributing to the risk for DG. Several promising leads from different sources implicate the dopamine D3 receptor gene as one. The specific environmental factors that account for the aggregate environmental risk have also not yet been identified. There are many candidates, but none have been verified as being truly environmental. Some of the aggregate genetic risk for DG overlaps with the genetic risk for substance use disorders, antisocial behavior disorders, depression, and some anxiety disorders, as do the unique environmental risk factors. Genetic factors appear to be the primary contributor to comorbidity of DG with other mental disorders. In contrast to DG, common familial environmental factors may play a role in earlier stages in the development of DG, such as initiating gambling involvement and the age at which this first occurs. This might differ for men and women. Finally, there is evidence that the genetic risk for DG may put one at risk for being exposed to high-risk environments (such as living in a disadvantaged neighborhood with greater access to gambling outlets) and that the genetic risk for DG is more likely to be expressed in high-risk environments.

5.10   Recommendations for the Way Forward

In addition to drawing out general conclusions about the contributions of genetic and environmental factors to the risk for DG, this review revealed many places where the existing research base is scant or nonexistent.[6] Some of the areas in which there is a need for more research include: longitudinal twin studies, multivariate twin studies focused on identifying endophenotypes, identification of environmental risk factors, and studies of gene-environment interplay.

Longitudinal twin research would be especially informative about possible changes in the genetic underpinnings of DG over the life span and across the different stages of gambling involvement. Multivariate twin research can continue to investigate the causes of comorbidity but could also be extended to include potential behavioral and neurobiological endophenotypes. The identification of potential endophenotypes would be especially valuable in that they might lead to more fruitful targets in the hunt for DG susceptibility genes.

Behavioral genetic research can contribute as much to our understanding of the environmental risk factors as to the genetic risk factors for DG, but there are few putative environmental risk factors that have been through the lens of a genetically informed research design. Another area that has been nearly unexplored is the interplay of genetic and environmental factors. Success here will rest upon identifying both genetic and environmental risk factors. Gene-environment interplay should be examined at the molecular genetic as well as at the aggregate level, but this will require more progress in cataloging genotype-DG associations in GWAS.

I will conclude this chapter with four more sweeping recommendations for the way forward. First, the era of candidate gene association studies for gene identification is over. It will be critical to adopt the more hypothesis-free approach of GWAS in order to think outside the "candidate gene box." Progress in GWAS will require worldwide cooperation and collaboration of many research teams to amass the sample sizes required to detect genes of very small effect [133, 134].

Second, it has been suggested that general population epidemiologic studies of DG "have matured sufficiently for this strategy to be no longer fruitful" (p. 514, [135]). However, there would be substantial value added if such studies were to add biological data collection for genotyping (especially among those exposed to a high-risk environment) and to also include neuroimaging and neurocognitive measures (perhaps in a smaller sub-study). Eventually data from multiple studies that have included genotyping and neuroimaging measures could then be combined (e.g., [136]).

Third, although it may be infeasible for all investigators to redesign their research program to one that is conducted as a twin study, it may not be as difficult to also include same-sex close-in-age siblings (or parents) into laboratory and survey studies of DG. This approach was undertaken in a study of siblings discordant for stimulant dependence in an effort to identify important endophenotypes (e.g., [137]).

---

[6]This may partially be explained by gambling disorder research being a low priority for funding at the US National Institutes of Health. This might change in the future.

Fourth, there are many good reasons to focus on continuous gambling phenotypes, not least of which is increased statistical power [138] and the ability to conduct research on a disorder that is not very common. This returns us to an important issue that was raised at the beginning of this chapter, that is, the dimensional nature of psychiatric disorders, including gambling disorder. Assuming that DG is dimensional at the latent liability [22, 23] and phenotypic [139] levels, studies that identify risk factors for continuous DG symptom counts will further our understanding of the risk factors for gambling disorder because the only differences between the outcomes would be that more or less (but not different) risk factors are involved. In addition, following the lead of previous research on substance use disorders, including dimensional measures of normative gambling involvement such as the frequency or quantity of gambling in studies of DG, one can examine the extent to which the genetic risk for DG is in part explained by genetic influences on earlier stages in the gambling career.

Acknowledgement *Funding*: Preparation of this chapter was funded in part by a Center of Excellence in Gambling Research grant from the National Center for Gaming Research.

References

1. Helzer JE, Kraemer HC, Krueger RF, Wittchen H, Sirovatka PJ, Regier DA. Dimensional approaches in diagnostic classification: refining the research agenda for DSM-V. Arlington, VA: American Psychiatric Association; 2008.
2. Shaffer HJ, Martin R. Disordered gambling: etiology, trajectory, and clinical considerations. Annu Rev Clin Psychol. 2011;7:483–510.
3. Black DW, Coryell WH, Crowe RR, McCormick B, Shaw MC, Allen J. A direct, controlled, blind family study of DSM-IV pathological gambling. J Clin Psychiatry. 2013;75(3):215–21.
4. Black DW, Monahan PO, Temkit MH, Shaw M. A family study of pathological gambling. Psychiatry Res. 2006;141(3):295–303.
5. American Psychiatric Association. Diagnostic and statistical manual of mental disorders: DSM-III-R (rev. ed. 3). Washington, DC: American Psychiatric Association; 1987.
6. Eisen SA, Lin N, Lyons MJ, Scherrer J, Griffith K, True WR, Goldberg J, Tsuang MT. Familial influences on gambling behavior: an analysis of 3,359 twin pairs. Addiction. 1998;93:1375–84.
7. Xian H, Scherrer JF, Slutske WS, Shah KR, Volberg R, Eisen SA. Genetic and environmental contributions to pathological gambling symptoms in a 10-year follow-up. Twin Res Hum Genet. 2007;10:174–9.
8. American Psychiatric Association. Diagnostic and statistical manual of mental disorders: DSM-IV (ed. 4). Washington, DC: American Psychiatric Association; 1994.
9. Slutske WS, Zhu G, Meier MH, Martin NG. Genetic and environmental influences on disordered gambling in men and women. Arch Gen Psychiatry. 2010;67:624–30.
10. Lesieur HR, Blume SB. The South Oaks Gambling Screen (SOGS): a new instrument for the identification of pathological gamblers. Am J Psychiatr. 1987;144:1184–8.
11. Slutske WS, Zhu G, Meier MH, Martin NG. Disordered gambling as defined by the DSM-IV and the South Oaks Gambling Screen: evidence for a common etiologic structure. J Abnorm Psychol. 2011;120:743–51.
12. Blanco C, Myers J, Kendler KS. Gambling, disordered gambling and their association with major depression and substance use: a web-based cohort and twin-sibling study. Psychol Med. 2012;42(03):497–508.

13. Winters KC, Stinchfield RD, Fulkerson J. Toward the development of an adolescent gambling problem severity scale. J Gambl Stud. 1993;9:63–84.
14. King SM, Keyes M, Winters KC, McGue M, Iacono WG. Genetic and environmental origins of gambling behaviors from ages 18 to 25: a longitudinal twin family study. Psychol Addict Behav. 2017;31:367.
15. Beaver KM, Hoffman T, Shields RT, Vaughn MG, DeLisi M, Wright JP. Gender differences in genetic and environmental influences on gambling: results from a sample of twins from the National Longitudinal Study of Adolescent Health. Addiction. 2010;105(3):536–42.
16. Richmond-Rakerd LS, Slutske WS, Heath AC, Martin NG. Genetic and environmental influences on the ages of drinking and gambling initiation: evidence for distinct aetiologies and sex differences. Addiction. 2014;109(2):323–31.
17. Slutske WS. Has the genetic contribution to the propensity to gamble increased? Evidence from national twin studies conducted in 1962 and 2002. Twin Res Hum Genet. 2018;21:119–25.
18. Slutske WS, Richmond-Rakerd LS. A closer look at the evidence for sex differences in the genetic and environmental influences on gambling in the National Longitudinal Study of Adolescent health: from disordered to ordered gambling. Addiction. 2014;109(1):120–7.
19. Slutske WS, Meier MH, Zhu G, Statham DJ, Blaszczynski A, Martin NG. The Australian twin study of gambling (OZ-GAM): rationale, sample description, predictors of participation, and a first look at sources of individual differences in gambling involvement. Twin Res Hum Genet. 2009;12:63–78.
20. Winters KC, Rich T. A twin study of adult gambling behavior. J Gambl Stud. 1998;14(3):213–25.
21. Vitaro F, Hartl AC, Brendgen M, Laursen B, Dionne G, Boivin M. Genetic and environmental influences on gambling and substance use in early adolescence. Behav Genet. 2014;44:347–55.
22. Slutske WS, Cho SB, Piasecki TM, Martin NG. Genetic overlap between personality and risk for disordered gambling: evidence from a national community-based Australian twin study. J Abnorm Psychol. 2013;122:250–5.
23. Slutske WS, Ellingson JM, Richmond-Rakerd LS, Zhu G, Martin NG. Shared genetic vulnerability for disordered gambling and alcohol use disorder in men and women: evidence from a national community-based Australian Twin Study. Twin Res Hum Genet. 2013;16(02):525–34.
24. Slutske WS, Eisen SA, True WR, Lyons MJ, Goldberg J, Tsuang MT. Common genetic vulnerability for pathological gambling and alcohol dependence in men. Arch Gen Psychiatry. 2000;57:666–73.
25. Reich T, Cloninger CR, Guze SB. The multifactorial model of disease transmission: I. Description of the model and its use in psychiatry. Br J Psychiatry. 1975;127:1–10.
26. Kendler KS, Myers J, Potter J, Opalesky J. A web-based study of personality, psychopathology and substance use in twin, other relative and relationship pairs. Twin Res Hum Genet. 2009;12(02):137–41.
27. American Psychiatric Association. Diagnostic and statistical manual of mental disorders: DSM-5. ed 5 ed. Washington, D.C.: American Psychiatric Association; 2013.
28. Heatherton TF, Kozlowski LT, Frecker RC, Fagerström KO. The Fagerström test for nicotine dependence: a revision of the Fagerstrom Tolerance Questionnaire. Br J Addict. 1991;86(9):1119–27.
29. Xian H, Giddens JL, Scherrer JF, Eisen SA, Potenza MN. Environmental factors selectively impact co-occurrence of problem/pathological gambling with specific drug-use disorders in male twins. Addiction. 2014;109(4):635–44.
30. Slutske WS, Eisen SA, Xian H, True WR, Lyons MJ, Goldberg J, Tsuang MT. A twin study of the association between pathological gambling and antisocial personality disorder. J Abnorm Psychol. 2001;110:297–308.
31. Potenza MN, Xian H, Shah K, Scherrer JF, Eisen SA. Shared genetic contributions to pathological gambling and major depression in men. Arch Gen Psychiatry. 2005;62:1015–21.

32. Scherrer JF, Xian H, Slutske WS, Eisen SA, Potenza MN. Associations between obsessive-compulsive classes and pathological gambling in a national cohort of male twins. JAMA Psychiatry. 2015;72(4):342–9.
33. Giddens JL, Xian H, Scherrer JF, Eisen SA, Potenza MN. Shared genetic contributions to anxiety disorders and pathological gambling in a male population. J Affect Disord. 2011;132(3):406–12.
34. Turkheimer E. Three laws of behavior genetics and what they mean. Curr Dir Psychol Sci. 2000;9(5):160–4.
35. Petry NM, Stinson FS, Grant BF. Comorbidity of DSM-IV pathological gambling and other psychiatric disorders: results from the National Epidemiologic Survey on Alcohol and Related Conditions. J Clin Psychiatry. 2005;66:564–74.
36. Oleski J, Cox BJ, Clara I, Hills A. Pathological gambling and the structure of common mental disorders. J Nerv Ment Dis. 2011;199(12):956–60.
37. Plomin R, DeFries JC, Knopik VS, Neiderhiser JM. Top 10 replicated findings from behavioral genetics. Perspect Psychol Sci. 2016;11(1):3–23.
38. Kendler KS, Prescott CA, Myers J, Neale MC. The structure of genetic and environmental risk factors for common psychiatric and substance use disorders in men and women. Arch Gen Psychiatry. 2003;60(9):929–37.
39. Nivard MG, Verweij KJH, Minică CC, Treur JL, Derks EM, Stringer S, et al. Connecting the dots, genome-wide association studies in substance use. Mol Psychiatry. 2016;21:733–5.
40. Lang M, Leménager T, Streit F, Fauth-Bühler M, Frank J, Juraeva D, et al. Genome-wide association study of pathological gambling. Eur Psychiatry. 2016;36:38–46.
41. Gyollai Á, D Griffiths M, Barta C, Vereczkei A, Urbán R, Kun B, et al. The genetics of problem and pathological gambling: a systematic review. Curr Pharm Des. 2014;20(25):3993–9.
42. Lobo DS. Genetic aspects of gambling disorders: recent developments and future directions. Curr Behav Neurosci Rep. 2016;3(1):58–66.
43. Gray JC, MacKillop J. Genetic basis of delay discounting in frequent gamblers: examination of a priori candidates and exploration of a panel of dopamine-related loci. Brain Behav. 2014;4(6):812–21.
44. Comings DE, Gade R, Wu S, Chiu C, Dietz G, Muhleman D, Saucier G, Ferry L, Rosenthal RJ, Lesieur HR, Rugle LJ, MacMurray P. Studies of the potential role of the dopamine D1 receptor gene in addictive behaviors. Mol Psychiatry. 1997;2:44–56.
45. Lim S, Ha J, Choi S, et al. Association study on pathological gambling and polymorphisms of dopamine D1, D2, D3, and D4 receptor genes in a Korean population. J Gambl Stud. 2012;28:481–91.
46. Lobo DSS, Souza RP, Tong RP, et al. Association of functional variants in the dopamine D2-like receptors with risk for gambling behaviour in healthy Caucasian subjects. Biol Psychol. 2010;85:33–7.
47. Lobo DSS, Vallada HP, Knight J, Martins SS, Tavares H, Gentil V, Kennedy JL. Dopamine genes and pathological gambling in discordant sib-pairs. J Gambl Stud. 2007;23:421–33.
48. Comings DE, Rosenthal RJ, Lesieur HR, Rugle LJ, Muhleman D, Chiu C, Dietz G, Gade R. A study of the dopamine D2 receptor gene in pathological gambling. Pharmacogenetics. 1996;6:223–34.
49. Lobo DS, Aleksandrova L, Knight J, Casey DM, El-Guebaly N, Nobrega JN, Kennedy JL. Addiction-related genes in gambling disorders: new insights from parallel human and pre-clinical models. Mol Psychiatry. 2015;20(8):1002–10.
50. Perez de Castro I, Ibanez A, Torres P, Saiz-Ruiz J, Fernandez-Piqueras J. Genetic association study between pathological gambling and a functional DNA polymorphism at the D4 receptor gene. Pharmacogenetics. 1997;7:345–8.
51. Grant JE, Leppink EW, Redden SA, Odlaug BL, Chamberlain SR. COMT genotype, gambling activity, and cognition. J Psychiatr Res. 2015;68:371–6.
52. Guillot CR, Fanning JR, Liang T, Berman ME. COMT associations with disordered gambling and drinking measures. J Gambl Stud. 2015;31(2):513–24.

53. Ibanez A, de Castro IP, Fernandez-Piqueras J, Blanco C, Saiz-Ruiz J. Pathological gambling and DNA polymorphic markers at MAO-A and MAO-B genes. Mol Psychiatry. 2000;5:105–9.
54. Perez de Castro I, Ibanez A, Saiz-Ruiz J, Fernandez-Piqueras J. Concurrent positive association between pathological gambling and functional DNA polymorphisms at the MAO-A and the 5-HT transporter genes. Mol Psychiatry. 2002;7:927–8.
55. Wilson D, da Silva Lobo DS, Tavares H, Gentil V, Vallada H. Family-based association analysis of serotonin genes in pathological gambling disorder: evidence of vulnerability risk in the 5HT-2A receptor gene. J Mol Neurosci. 2013;49(3):550–3.
56. Perez de Castro I, Ibanez A, Saiz-Ruiz J, Fernandez-Piqueras J. Genetic contribution to pathological gambling: possible association between a functional DNA polymorphism at the serotonin transporter gene (5-HTT) and affected men. Pharmacogenetics. 1999;9:397-400.
57. Comings DE, Gade-Andavolu R, Gonzalez N, et al. The additive effect of neurotransmitter genes in pathological gambling. Clin Genet. 2001;60:107–16.
58. Belsky DW, Moffitt TE, Baker TB, Biddle AK, Evans JP, Harrington H, et al. Polygenic risk and the developmental progression to heavy, persistent smoking and nicotine dependence: evidence from a 4-decade longitudinal study. JAMA Psychiat. 2013;70(5):534–42.
59. Wray NR, Lee SH, Mehta D, Vinkhuyzen AA, Dudbridge F, Middeldorp CM. Research review: polygenic methods and their application to psychiatric traits. J Child Psychol Psychiatry. 2014;55(10):1068–87. PMID: 25132410
60. Lind PA, Zhu G, Montgomery GW, Madden PA, Heath AC, Martin NG, Slutske WS. Genome-wide association study of a quantitative disordered gambling trait. Addict Biol. 2013;18(3):511–22.
61. Li CY, Mao X, Wei L. Genes and (common) pathways underlying drug addiction. PLoS Comput Biol. 2008;4:e2.
62. Hyman SE. Addiction: a disease of learning and memory. Am J Psychiatr. 2005;162:1414–22.
63. Nestler EJ. Is there a common molecular pathway for addiction? Nat Neurosci. 2005;8:1445–9.
64. Kalkhoven C, Sennef C, Peeters A, Van Den Bos R. Risk-taking and pathological gambling behavior in Huntington's disease. Front Behav Neurosci. 2014;8:103.
65. Dubertret C, Gorwood P, Ades J, Feingold J, Schwartz JC, Sokoloff P. Meta-analysis of DRD3 gene and schizophrenia: ethnic heterogeneity and significant association in caucasians. Am J Med Genet. 1998;81(4):318–22.
66. Flint J, Munafò M. Schizophrenia: genesis of a complex disease. Nature. 2014;511(7510):412–3.
67. Kendler KS, O'Donovan MC. A breakthrough in schizophrenia genetics. JAMA Psychiat. 2014;71(12):1319–20.
68. Ripke S, Neale BM, Corvin A, Walters JT, Farh KH, Holmans PA, et al. Biological insights from 108 schizophrenia-associated genetic loci. Nature. 2014;511(7510):421.
69. Weintraub D, Koester J, Potenza MN, et al. Impulse control disorders in Parkinson disease: a cross-sectional study of 3090 patients. Arch Neurol. 2010;67:589–95.
70. Tippmann-Peikert M, Park JG, Boeve BF, Shepard JW, Silber MH. Pathologic gambling in patients with restless legs syndrome treated with dopaminergic agonists. Neurology. 2007;68:301–3.
71. Dodd ML, Klos KJ, Bower JH, Geda YE, Josephs KA, Ahlskog JE. Pathological gambling caused by drugs used to treat Parkinson disease. Arch Neurol. 2005;62:1377–81.
72. Johnson PS, Madden GJ, Brewer AT, et al. Effects of acute pramipexole on preference for gambling-like schedules of reinforcement in rats. Psychopharmacology. 2011;213:11–8.
73. Eisenegger C, Knoch D, Ebstein RP, et al. Dopamine receptor D4 polymorphism predicts the effect of L-DOPA on gambling behavior. Biol Psychiatry. 2010;67:702–6.
74. Gottesman II, Gould TD. The endophenotype concept in psychiatry: etymology and strategic intentions. Am J Psychiatr. 2003;160:636–45.
75. MacKillop J, Munafò MR. Genetic influences on addiction: an intermediate phenotype approach. Cambridge, MA: MIT Press; 2013.

76. Clark L. Decision-making during gambling: an integration of cognitive and psychobiological approaches. Philos Trans R Soc B. 2010;365:319–30.
77. Potenza MN. The neurobiology of pathological gambling and drug addiction: an overview and new findings. Philos Trans R Soc B. 2008;363:3181–9.
78. Cuthbert BN, Insel TR. Toward the future of psychiatric diagnosis: the seven pillars of RDoC. BMC Med. 2013;11(1):1.
79. Robbins TW, Gillan CM, Smith DG, de Wit S, Ersche KD. Neurocognitive endophenotypes of impulsivity and compulsivity: towards dimensional psychiatry. Trends Cogn Sci. 2012;16(1):81–91.
80. Hall MH, Smoller JW. A new role for endophenotypes in the GWAS era: functional characterization of risk variants. Harv Rev Psychiatry. 2010;18(1):67–74.
81. Kendler KS, Schmitt E, Aggen SH, Prescott CA. Genetic and environmental influences on alcohol, caffeine, cannabis, and nicotine use from early adolescence to middle adulthood. Arch Gen Psychiatry. 2008;65(6):674–82.
82. Rhee SH, Hewitt JK, Young SE, Corley RP, Crowley TJ, Stallings MC. Genetic and environmental influences on substance initiation, use, and problem use in adolescents. Arch Gen Psychiatry. 2003;60(12):1256–64.
83. Heath AC, Martin NG, Lynskey MT, Todorov AA, Madden PA. Estimating two-stage models for genetic influences on alcohol, tobacco or drug use initiation and dependence vulnerability in twin and family data. Twin Res. 2002;5(02):113–24.
84. Maes HH, Sullivan PF, Bulik CM, Neale MC, Prescott CA, Eaves LJ, Kendler KS. A twin study of genetic and environmental influences on tobacco initiation, regular tobacco use and nicotine dependence. Psychol Med. 2004;34(07):1251–61.
85. Fowler T, Lifford K, Shelton K, Rice F, Thapar A, Neale MC, et al. Exploring the relationship between genetic and environmental influences on initiation and progression of substance use. Addiction. 2007;102(3):413–22.
86. Agrawal A, Neale MC, Jacobson KC, Prescott CA, Kendler KS. Illicit drug use and abuse/dependence: modeling of two-stage variables using the CCC approach. Addict Behav. 2005;30(5):1043–8.
87. Wade TD, Bulik CM, Sullivan PF, Neale MC, Kendler KS. The relation between risk factors for binge eating and bulimia nervosa: a population-based female twin study. Health Psychol. 2000;19(2):115.
88. Williams RJ, Volberg RA Stevens RMG. The population prevalence of problem gambling: methodological influences, standardized rates, jurisdictional differences, and worldwide trends. Report prepared for the Ontario Problem Gambling Research Centre and the Ontario Ministry of Health and Long Term Care. 8 May 2012. http://hdl.handle.net/10133/3068.
89. Gerstein D, Murphy S, Toce M, Hoffmann J, Palmer A, Johnson R, et al. Gambling impact and behavior study: report to the National Gambling Impact Study Commission. Chicago: National Opinion Research Center; 1999.
90. Afifi TO, Brownridge DA, MacMillan H, Sareen J. The relationship of gambling to intimate partner violence and child maltreatment in a nationally representative sample. J Psychiatr Res. 2010;44(5):331–7.
91. Black DW, Shaw MC, McCormick BA, Allen J. Marital status, childhood maltreatment, and family dysfunction: a controlled study of pathological gambling. J Clin Psychiatry. 2012;73(10):1293–7.
92. Hodgins DC, Schopflocher DP, el-Guebaly N, Casey DM, Smith GJ, Williams RJ, Wood RT. The association between childhood maltreatment and gambling problems in a community sample of adult men and women. Psychol Addict Behav. 2010;24(3):548.
93. Petry NM, Steinberg KL. Childhood maltreatment in male and female treatment-seeking pathological gamblers. Psychol Addict Behav. 2005;19(2):226.
94. Scherrer JF, Xian H, Kapp JMK, Waterman B, Shah KR, Volberg R, Eisen SA. Association between exposure to childhood and lifetime traumatic events and lifetime pathological gambling in a twin cohort. J Nerv Ment Dis. 2007;195:72–8.

95. Blanco C, Hanania J, Petry NM, Wall MM, Wang S, Jin CJ, Kendler KS. Towards a comprehensive developmental model of pathological gambling. Addiction. 2015;110(8):1340–51.
96. Welte JW, Wieczorek WF, Barnes GM, Tidwell MCO. Multiple risk factors for frequent and problem gambling: individual, social, and ecological. J Appl Soc Psychol. 2006;36(6):1548–68.
97. Barnes GM, Welte JW, Tidwell MO, Hoffman JH. Effects of neighborhood disadvantage on problem gambling and alcohol abuse. J Behav Addict. 2013;2:82–9.
98. Martins SS, Storr CL, Lee GP, Ialongo NS. Environmental influences associated with gambling in young adulthood. J Urban Health. 2013;90:130–40.
99. Pearce J, Mason K, Hiscock R, Day P. A national study of neighborhood access to gambling opportunities and individual gambling behavior. J Epidemiol Community Health. 2008;62:862–8.
100. Welte JW, Wieczorek WF, Barnes GM, Tidwell MC, Hoffman JH. The relationship of ecological and geographic factors to gambling behavior and pathology. J Gambl Stud. 2004;20(4):405–23.
101. Slutske WS, Deutsch AR, Statham DJ, Martin NG. Local area disadvantage and gambling involvement and disorder: evidence for gene-environment correlation and interaction. J Abnorm Psychol. 2015;124:606–22.
102. Gupta R, Derevensky J. Familial and social influences on juvenile gambling behavior. J Gambl Stud. 1997;13(3):179–92.
103. Oei TP, Raylu N. Familial influence on offspring gambling: a cognitive mechanism for transmission of gambling behavior in families. Psychol Med. 2004;34(07):1279–88.
104. Slutske WS, Piasecki TM, Ellingson JM, Martin NG. The family history method in disordered gambling research: a comparison of reports from discordant twin pairs. Twin Res Hum Genet. 2010;13:340–6.
105. Fortune EE, MacKillop J, Miller JD, Campbell WK, Clifton AD, Goodie AS. Social density of gambling and its association with gambling problems: an initial investigation. J Gambl Stud. 2013;29(2):329–42.
106. Meisel MK, Clifton AD, MacKillop J, Miller JD, Campbell WK, Goodie AS. Egocentric social network analysis of pathological gambling. Addiction. 2013;108(3):584–91.
107. Lynch WJ, Maciejewski PK, Potenza MN. Psychiatric correlates of gambling in adolescents and young adults grouped by age at gambling onset. Arch Gen Psychiatry. 2004;61(11):1116–22.
108. Kessler RC, Hwang I, LaBrie R, Petukhova M, Sampson NA, Winters KC, et al. DSM-IV pathological gambling in the National Comorbidity Survey Replication. Psychol Med. 2008;38:1351–60.
109. Slutske WS, Deutsch AR, Richmond-Rakerd LS, Chernyavskiy P, Statham DJ, Martin NG. Test of a potential causal influence of earlier age of gambling initiation on gambling involvement and disorder: a multilevel discordant twin design. Psychol Addict Behav. 2014;28(4):1177.
110. Derevensky J, Sklar A, Gupta R, Messerlian C. An empirical study examining the impact of gambling advertisements on adolescent gambling attitudes and behaviors. Int J Ment Heal Addict. 2010;8(1):21–34.
111. Planzer S, Gray HM, Shaffer HJ. Associations between national gambling policies and disordered gambling prevalence rates within Europe. Int J Law Psychiatry. 2014;37(2):217–29.
112. Storer J, Abbott M, Stubbs J. Access or adaptation? A meta-analysis of surveys of problem gambling prevalence in Australia and New Zealand with respect to concentration of electronic gaming machines. Int Gambl Stud. 2009;9(3):225–44.
113. Welte JW, Tidwell MCO, Barnes GM, Hoffman JH, Wieczorek WF. The relationship between the number of types of legal gambling and the rates of gambling behaviors and problems across US states. J Gambl Stud. 2016;32(2):379–90.
114. Teicher MH, Samson JA. Childhood maltreatment and psychopathology: a case for ecophenotypic variants as clinically and neurobiologically distinct subtypes. Am J Psychiatr. 2013;170(10):1114–33.

115. Lane W, Sacco P, Downton K, Ludeman E, Levy L, Tracy JK. Child maltreatment and problem gambling: a systematic review. Child Abuse Negl. 2016;58:24–38.
116. Wilber MK, Potenza MN. Adolescent gambling: research and clinical implications. Psychiatry. 2006;3(10):40.
117. Marioni RE, Davies G, Hayward C, Liewald D, Kerr SM, Campbell A, et al. Molecular genetic contributions to socioeconomic status and intelligence. Intelligence. 2014;44:26–32.
118. Sariaslan A, Fazel S, D'onofrio BM, Långström N, Larsson H, Bergen SE, et al. Schizophrenia and subsequent neighborhood deprivation: revisiting the social drift hypothesis using population, twin and molecular genetic data. Transl Psychiatry. 2016;6:e796.
119. Kendler KS, Baker JH. Genetic influences on measures of the environment: a systematic review. Psychol Med. 2007;37:615–26.
120. Moffitt TE. Genetic and environmental influences on antisocial behaviors: evidence from behavioral–genetic research. Adv Genet. 2005;55:41–104.
121. Rutter M. Genes and behavior: nature-nurture interplay explained. Malden, MA: Blackwell Publishing; 2006.
122. Scarr S, McCartney K. How people make their own Environments: a theory of genotype → environment effects. Child Dev. 1983;54:424–35.
123. Dick DM. Gene-environment interactions in psychological traits and disorders. Annu Rev Clin Psychol. 2011;7:383–409.
124. Manuck SB, McCaffery JM. Gene-environment interaction. Annu Rev Psychol. 2014;65:41–70.
125. Shanahan MJ, Hofer SM. Social context in gene-environment interactions: retrospect and prospect. J Gerontol B Psychol Sci Soc Sci. 2005;60B:65–76.
126. Moffitt TE, Caspi A, Rutter M. Strategy for investigating interactions between measured genes and measured environments. Arch Gen Psychiatry. 2005;62(5):473–81.
127. Dick DM, Rose RJ, Viken RJ, Kaprio J, Koskenvuo M. Exploring gene-environment interactions: socioregional moderation of alcohol use. J Abnorm Psychol. 2001;110:625–32.
128. Caspi A, McClay J, Moffitt TE, Mill J, Martin J, Craig IW, et al. Role of genotype in the cycle of violence in maltreated children. Science. 2002;297(5582):851–4.
129. Meyers J, Cerdá M, Galea S, Keyes K, Aiello AE, Uddin M, Wildman D, Koenen K. Interaction between polygenic risk for cigarette use and environmental exposures in the Detroit neighborhood health study. Transl Psychiatry. 2013;3(8):e290.
130. Marshall DC, Baker RGV. The evolving market structures of gambling: case studies modelling the socioeconomic assignment of gaming machines in Melbourne and Sydney. Aust J Gambl Stud. 2002;18:273–91.
131. Wardle H, Keily R, Astbury G, Reith G. 'Risky places?': mapping gambling machine density and socio-economic deprivation. J Gambl Stud. 2014;30:201–12.
132. Wilson DH, Derevensky J, Gilliland J, Gupta R, Ross NA. Video lottery terminal access and gambling among high school students in Montreal. Can J Public Health. 2006;97:202–6.
133. Psychiatric GWAS Consortium Steering Committee. Mol Psychiatry. 2009;14:10–7.
134. Sullivan PF. The psychiatric GWAS consortium: big science comes to psychiatry. Neuron. 2010;68(2):182–6.
135. Shaffer HJ, LaBrie RA, LaPlante DA, Nelson SE, Stanton MV. The road less travelled: moving from distribution to determinants in the study of gambling epidemiology. Can J Psychiatry. 2004;49(8):504–16.
136. Thompson PM, Stein JL, Medland SE, Hibar DP, Vasquez AA, Renteria ME, et al. The ENIGMA Consortium: large-scale collaborative analyses of neuroimaging and genetic data. Brain Imaging Behav. 2014;8(2):153–82.
137. Ersche KD, Jones PS, Williams GB, Turton AJ, Robbins TW, Bullmore ET. Abnormal brain structure implicated in stimulant drug addiction. Science. 2012;335(6068):601–4.
138. Kraemer HC, Noda A, O'Hara R. Categorical versus dimensional approaches to diagnosis: methodological challenges. J Psychiatr Res. 2004;38(1):17–25.
139. Strong DR, Kahler CW. Evaluation of the continuum of gambling problems using the DSM-IV. Addiction. 2007;102(5):713–21.

Animal Models of Gambling-Related Behaviour

6

Paul J. Cocker and Catharine A. Winstanley

6.1   Introduction

Gambling or wagering on uncertain outcomes is a widespread and pervasive part of society, as estimates suggest that the vast majority of individuals engage in some form of gambling at least once a year [1, 2]. For most, gambling is a relatively harmless pastime, but for some individuals it can become a maladaptive compulsion akin to drug or alcohol addiction resulting in severe impairments in social and occupational functioning and a significantly elevated risk of suicide [3–5].

The recent reclassification of gambling disorder (GD) as an addictive disorder in the DSM-V reflects a growing recognition that the phenomenology underlying both behavioural and substance addictions may best be considered as equivalent (see [6, 7] for review). However, GD could arguably be conceptualised as a 'pure' addiction, in that the behavioural perturbations observed within GD are not accompanied by ingestion of a psychoactive substance. Consequently, a more complete understanding of GD could offer insight into the motivation underlying the commencement of substance addiction, particularly as precipitating vulnerabilities may be obfuscated in drug addicts following the ingestion of psychoactive substances. Problem gambling may therefore offer an ideal platform from which to make inferences about the development of the cycle of addiction, both cognitively and neurobiologically, independent of any changes induced by the pharmacological actions of drugs themselves [8]. However, problematic engagement with gambling in humans is often co-morbid with affective and substance use disorders, making it difficult to

P. J. Cocker (✉)
Department of Psychology, University of British Columbia, Vancouver, Canada

Department of Psychology, University of Cambridge, Cambridge, UK
e-mail: pcocker@psych.ubc.ca, pc579@cam.ac.uk

C. A. Winstanley (✉)
Department of Psychology, University of British Columbia, Vancouver, Canada
e-mail: cwinstanley@psych.ubc.ca

© Springer Nature Switzerland AG 2019
A. Heinz et al. (eds.), *Gambling Disorder*, https://doi.org/10.1007/978-3-030-03060-5_6

truly remove confounds relating to drug use and other psychiatric issues when examining behaviour [9]. In this regard animal models may offer a solution, in that they offer an invaluable opportunity to elucidate the underlying neurobiological underpinnings of GD without the issues of causality that are endemic to human research. Animal models with sufficient face, construct and predictive validity may not only aid in a better understanding of GD but also facilitate the development of more efficacious treatment options.

However, whether an animal model can completely encapsulate disease states where the aetiology is likely complex and multifactorial, such as addictive disorders, is unclear. Such a consideration is especially pertinent in the case of GD, given that there are a wide range of gambling games that appeal to demonstrably differing demographics [10]. Consequently, the motivation and the associated neurobiological sequelae promoting the formation and persistence of gambling engagement are likely to be diverse. As such, considering different gambling games as potentially subject to independent expression and regulation, rather than assuming a universal pro-gambling phenotype, may be a more efficacious starting point for exploring risk factors for the development of GD. Moreover, such an approach is in line with emerging diagnostic frameworks [11, 12]. To that end animal models that capture different facets of dysfunction commonly observed in GD may be useful in delineating a conceptual framework of precipitating vulnerabilities towards differing forms of gambling.

A number of factors may contribute to the formation and maintenance of problem gambling in human populations, such as the increased presence of cognitive biases or distorted beliefs regarding the outcome of uncertain events [13, 14], increased levels of impulsivity [15–20], perturbations in cost-benefit decision-making [21–23] and augmented cue reactivity [24–27]. Importantly, all of these processes can be modelled in animals. Therefore, this chapter will initially discuss findings indicating that rats, like humans, are susceptible to cognitive biases that may facilitate continued gambling engagement. Subsequently we will briefly discuss multiple paradigms that can be used to measure impulsivity and touch upon a potential role for increased compulsivity in the development of GD. Relatedly, we will also examine several rodent models of decision-making, wherein perturbations in cost-benefit judgements cannot be attributed to a rise in impulsivity—indicating that these two constructs may represent differing vulnerabilities towards the development of GD. Lastly, we will examine increased cue reactivity and how that might contribute towards problem gambling.

For the sake of brevity, we will restrict this discussion to the use of tasks that utilise rodents, as rodent models have been more widely used for both neural and pharmacological characterisation studies. Moreover, all of the tasks discussed herein utilise computer-controlled operant chambers, as the use of such apparatus minimises inter-experimenter variation and allows for multiple behavioural measurements as well as rigid parameter control through greater automation. All the tasks discussed here can be run in standard five-hole operant chambers. These chambers contain an array of five response apertures on one wall, each fitted with an infrared beam capable of detecting nose-poke entries. Along the opposite wall, two retractable levers or other manipulanda can be installed, typically positioned on either side of a food tray into which sugar pellets are delivered via an external dispenser. The paradigms discussed herein are not intended as an exhaustive list, but simply highlight a number of tools that may be beneficial in providing a quantitative measure of several facets of gambling-related behaviour.

6.2   The Rodent Slot Machine Task

There are numerous forms of cognitive biases or distortions within gambling; indeed these perturbations are not only used to probe the severity of problem gambling, but their continued presence following treatment can reliably predict relapse [28–31]. Broadly it appears that rats, like humans, are susceptible to similar biases and distortions (see [32] for a more complete discussion of these biases). Here we intend to focus on one particular distortion that is modelled using the rodent slot machine task (rSMT). Behaviour on the rSMT has consistently demonstrated that the presence of multiple reward-related stimuli presented within a compound stimulus array generates the expectation of future reward [33]. Put more simply, rats like humans appear susceptible to the near-miss effect. Near-misses are unsuccessful outcomes that are visually proximal to a win, such as matching two out of three items on a slot machine payline. Subjectively near-misses are experienced as aversive [34], but these sorts of trials reliably promote continued game play, fostering beliefs of mastery and that winning outcomes are imminent [35–37]. Near-misses have garnered considerable attention as a cognitive distortion in human gamblers and have been suggested to make a key contribution to the particularly virulent form of gambling often associated with slot machines and other electronic gaming machines (EGMs) (see [38] for discussion). EGMs such as slot machines are often reported as the primary game of choice by patients presenting for treatment for GD, and these individuals also show the shortest latency between the onset of recreational play and the development of problematic engagement [39–41].

Imaging studies have demonstrated that near-misses operate in a qualitatively similar way to winning outcomes and enhance activity within frontostriatal circuitry and midbrain reward-related areas [34, 42, 43]. Such data intimate that near-misses promote a positive reward signal encoded by dopaminergic circuits. Dopamine neurons in the midbrain will fire in response to a primary appetitive stimulus, but if this stimulus is preceded with a cue that predicts its appearance, then these neurons will instead respond to this conditioned stimulus (see [44] for discussion). Aberrant dopaminergic signaling is a key component of drug addiction and has been suggested to drive the maladaptive attributions of salience to drug-paired cues that facilitate addiction [45]. Near-misses may be such an associative stimulus due to their structural proximity to a win; thus these sorts of trials may be able to evoke the representation of a win even in the absence of any reward. Although a definitive role for dopamine is currently unclear, there is general evidence that dopamine dysfunction may contribute towards problem gambling [46]. For instance, administration of the psychostimulant amphetamine, which potentiates the actions of dopamine, has been shown to increase motivation to gamble in problem gamblers [47]. Also, polymorphisms of both the dopamine D_2 and D_4 receptors have been associated with increased prevalence of GD [48–52]. Lastly, a key role for dopamine in the pathology of behavioural addictions has been demonstrated by the iatrogenic GD that occurs in a small but significant subset of patients with Parkinson's disease (PD) [53] which arises *de novo* typically following adjunctive therapy with D_2-like agonists and generally abates following the cessation of these treatments [54].

The rSMT was designed specifically to function as an analogue of a simple slot machine. During the rSMT animals respond to a series of three flashing aperture lights, similar to the three wheels of a slot machine, and nose-poke responses in each hole cause the light to set to on or off. A win is signaled by all three lights setting to on, whereas any other light pattern indicates a loss. At the end of a trial, the animal chooses between the 'collect' lever, which delivers ten sugar pellets on winning trials, but a 10-s time-out penalty on losing trials, and the 'roll' lever which allows the animal to begin a new trial immediately. Similar to human gamblers, rats appear to exhibit a near-miss-like effect, responding on the collect lever significantly more when two out of three lights are illuminated. These sorts of trials therefore seem able to generate the expectation of reward, even after extensive training.

Reward expectancy on the rSMT is critically modulated by the dopamine D_2-like receptor family. Systemic administration of the D_2-like agonist quinpirole augments animals' expectations of reward, producing a robust increase in erroneous attempts to collect reward on nonwinning trials [33]. The D_2-like family contains D_2, D_3 and D_4 receptors, and of these the D_4 receptor appears to play the most crucial role in mediating performance on the rSMT. Systemic administration of a highly selective D_4 receptor agonist impairs performance in a similar manner to quinpirole, whereas a D_4 receptor antagonist decreased erroneous collect responses [55]. Thus, a D_4 agonist impairs, whereas an antagonist improves, animals' ability to differentiate winning from nonwinning outcomes on a simple slot machine, ostensibly through modulating animals' responsivity to reward-salient information. Unlike other members of the D_2-like family, D_4 receptors are located predominantly in prefrontal cortical areas engaged with higher-order cognitive processes and as such represent an intriguing target for modulating gambling-related behaviour [56]. Such a supposition has been bolstered by recent findings demonstrating that targeting prefrontal regions relatively rich in D_4 receptors such as the anterior cingulate cortex (ACC) and insular cortex also alters performance on the rSMT [57, 58].

The rSMT has highlighted a potential role for D_4 receptors in controlling salience attribution to reward-related stimuli and indicates that D_4 receptor antagonists might be useful pharmacotherapies for GD. However, such studies were conducted in healthy animals and do not address whether the rSMT can be used to model problematic engagement with gambling. One issue in developing an animal model of GD is that, like other addictive disorders, it is broadly idiopathic. However, iatrogenic gambling has been predominantly described in human patients following dopamine replacement therapy [53]. This particularly compulsive form of GD, along with other impulse control disorders (ICDs), is most often observed in patients with Parkinson's disease (PD), but has also been reported in patients with restless leg syndrome, fibromyalgia and prolactinoma following therapeutic administration of D_2-like agonists [59–61]. Thus these ICDs appear to arise directly as a result of the dopaminergic drugs themselves, as opposed to a consequence of the neurobiological sequelae associated with PD. Therefore, recent investigations have attempted to model this particularly compulsive form of gambling using subcutaneously implanted mini-pumps to chronically deliver the $D_{2/3}$ agonist ropinirole to animals trained on the rSMT.

Chronic administration of ropinirole produced a robust increase in the number of trials animals completed and a reduction in the degree to which reward-related stimuli altered animals' ongoing behaviour [62, 63]. On their face, these behavioural changes resemble the increased desire to gamble observed in iatrogenic GD. These behavioural effects were also concomitant with a dramatic and prolonged increase in the inactive (phosphorylated) form of GSK3β in the dorsal striatum and an increase in the active (phosphorylated) form of CREB in the nucleus accumbens (NAc) [62]. CREB and GSK3β have been implicated in a broad range of functions including modulating learning and memory [64–66]. Both are activated by dopamine and contribute to subjective responsivity to drugs of abuse such as cocaine [65, 67–70]. However, any role for either protein in controlling gambling-related decision-making has, to our knowledge, not been investigated. Targeting one or both of these proteins could represent a novel treatment target for iatrogenic GD. Interestingly, preliminary data suggests that administering the β-adrenoreceptor blocker propranolol, which inhibits the phosphorylation of CREB in the NAC [71], ameliorates the compulsive-like task engagement observed following ropinirole, whereas dietary administration of lithium chloride, a potent GSK3β inhibitor [72], had no effect on task performance [63]. Thus, there is preliminary evidence that propranolol may be an effective therapeutic for iatrogenic gambling, putatively as a result of attenuating pCREB in the NAc.

In addition to the pharmacological data highlighting a role for dopamine in controlling slot machine engagement, recent data has suggested that animals that display increased 'optimism', in that they appear to interpret an ambiguous tone as more closely resembling a positive one, display impaired performance on the rSMT [73]. Such data may indicate that increased endorsement of other gambling-related cognitive biases may also confer susceptibility to increased reward expectancy and hint at a potential role for animal models in investigating the relationship between differing cognitive biases that may operate synergistically to confer vulnerability towards GD.

In summary, the rSMT is a reasonable facsimile of a simple slot machine. The task has repeatedly demonstrated that animals, like humans, are susceptible to win-related stimuli presented within a compound array, the so-called near-miss effect. Moreover, data from the rSMT suggests that D_4 receptors may be critically involved in mediating these attributions of salience to reward-related stimuli [55, 57, 58] and that augmented reward expectancy in response to near-miss-like trials may be indicative of other putatively pro-addictive constructs, such as optimism [73]. Additionally, chronic administration of D_2-like agonists appears to promote a compulsive-like endophenotype on the rSMT, indicating this task may provide a model for investigating problematic engagement with gambling, and inhibition of pCREB within the NAC may be an efficacious starting point for treatments targeting iatrogenic gambling [62, 63].

6.3   Impulsivity

Impulsivity, loosely defined as acting or making decisions without appropriate fore-thought, can in some cases be an adaptive trait. However, in excess, impulsivity inevitably results in deleterious consequences and is associated with a wide range of neuropsychiatric disorders, including the manifestation of both substance and behavioural addictions [74–77]. Impulsivity is a non-unitary construct that one recent model has proposed constitutes a two-factor process: an inhibitory process and an approach impulse process [78]. The inhibitory process, or response impulsivity, tends to be measured by motor disinhibition or impulsive action [79]. The approach process includes increased reward sensitivity and is typically parametrised as impulsive choice. Increases in both processes may confer vulnerability towards GD [79]. Operant behavioural tasks measuring impulsivity have tended to be classified into two similar areas: those that measure motor impulsivity and impulsive decision-making. The five-choice serial-reaction time task (5CSRTT) is perhaps the most widely used paradigm that contains a measure of impulsive action, or motor disinhibition, whereas delay discounting tasks have principally been used to measure impulsive decision-making (see [80] for discussion).

The 5CSRTT was designed as an analogue of the continuous performance time task (CPT), commonly used in human subjects, and the 5CSRTT has even been back-translated in human subjects, further confirming its validity [81, 82]. The CPT requires participants to scan a five-digit sequence and respond to a target sequence. Impulsive responses occur when a participant responds prematurely to a sequence that appears similar to the target. Similarly, the 5CSRTT requires animals to scan a five-hole array in order to accurately detect a brief light presentation (typically 0.5 s) in one of the apertures. The animal must make a 'nose-poke' response in the hole that was illuminated in order to gain food reward, thereby providing a measure of animals' visuospatial attention. Responses made prematurely, before the stimulus light is illuminated, generate an index of motor impulsivity [83]. The 5CSRTT has been widely adopted, and a significant body of work exists delineating pharmacological and neurobiological regulation of the task (see [83] for review). Amphetamine has reliably been shown to increase premature responding, an effect which appears principally mediated by dopamine [84]. However, amphetamine also affects other monoamines such as serotonin (5-HT) and noradrenaline [85], neurotransmitters that also modulate impulsive responding on the 5CSRTT (see [86] for review). Corticostriatal circuits appear to mediate these prepotent motor responses, as lesions to the infralimbic (IL) region of the mPFC, ACC or OFC increase premature responding [87, 88]. Similarly, lesions of the NAc also increase premature responding, but only on trials immediately following an incorrect response [89].

Although the 5CSRTT is arguably the most widely adopted task that includes a metric of impulsive responding, two other tasks that measure distinct aspects of impulsive responding are worth briefly mentioning, namely, the go-no-go and stop-signal tasks. The go-no-go assay measures action restraint, whereas the stop-signal task requires animals to stop a response that has already been initiated, or action cancellation. Both go-no-go and stop-signal tasks generally require animals to perform a specific action, e.g. lever press in response to a 'go' cue, but inhibit this action in response to a no-go, or stop cue. During go-no-go paradigms, the go and no-go cues are never presented within the same trial, whereas in the stop-signal task, the stop signal is presented after some delay following the go signal. Thus, go-no-go requires animals to inhibit a prepotent response—in a similar manner to the 5CSRTT—whereas stop-signal task requires animals to withhold from making a response that has already been initiated. Although all of these tasks measure action restraint and appear superficially similar, there are key differences in both the pharmacological and anatomical underpinnings of these tasks. Broadly, neither task appears to be critically mediated by dopaminergic function [90]. Serotonin depletion impairs action restraint [91], whereas noradrenaline appears to be more involved in action cancellation [92]. However, both action restraint and action cancellation appear to be subserved by the OFC as well as striatal regions ([93, 94], but see [95]). A full discussion of these differences is beyond the scope of this chapter (see [86] for discussion, [96]). Rather, both tasks are mentioned here to highlight that there is considerable heterogeneity in the neurobiology underpinning a construct such as impulsivity, even within subdomains, and that differing neurotransmitter systems are recruited dependent on when the action inhibition signal is presented. Consequently, clarity regarding the cognitive process being tested must be considered when discussing findings from any behavioural test pertaining to measuring multifaceted constructs such as impulsivity.

Delay discounting is arguably the most widely used measure used to assess non-planning or impulsive decision-making. Impulsive choice on such tasks is measured by preference for smaller, immediately available rewards over larger delayed ones. The size of the reward and/or the length of the delays can be varied in order to generate a hyperbolic discounting curve. Steeper discounting curves, i.e. increased preference for smaller-sooner rewards, have been repeatedly shown in subjects with GD [18, 20, 97]. Animal models of delay discounting, like their human counterparts, require subjects to choose between either a small reward delivered immediately or a larger reward delivered after some delay [98]. Although multiple iterations of delay discounting paradigms have been developed for use in laboratory animals, perhaps the most widely used methodology is that based on Evenden and Ryan's original model [99]. In this task, animals choose between a small reward (typically one sugar pellet) delivered immediately and a large reward (typically four pellets) that is delivered after a delay. The delay increases in a stepwise fashion across blocks of trials, for instance, from 0, 10, 20 and 40–60 s. All trials are of an equivalent length, such that selection of the larger reward always results in more reward throughout a session. In a similar manner to premature responses on the 5CSRTT, delay discounting tasks are sensitive to pharmacological agents that potentiate the actions of dopamine. However, in contrast to the pro-impulsive effects on the 5CSRTT, administration of amphetamine, cocaine or a dopamine reuptake inhibitor increases choice of the large delayed reward, i.e. decrease impulsive choice [100–102]. However, it should be noted that amphetamine has also been reported to increase choice of the smaller immediate reward during delay discounting (see [80, 103] for discussion of methodological issues that may explain these seemingly incongruous results). There are also some differences in regard to the neural loci that mediate impulsive choice and impulsive action. In contrast to impulsive responding on the 5CSRTT, ACC lesions do not increase impulsive decision-making during delay discounting [104]. However, the OFC does appear integral to optimal decision-making, in that excitotoxic lesions and inactivations have been shown to both increase and decrease choice of the large reward [105], dependent on task demands and baseline behaviour (see [106, 107] for discussion). Consistent with reports on the 5CSRTT, lesions to the NAc and ventral hippocampus both increase impulsive responding [89, 104, 108, 109].

Impulsivity is broadly considered to enhance vulnerability towards the development of both substance and behavioural addictions [75, 76]. A potentially related construct that has received relatively little attention, at least in regard to its potential role in GD, is compulsivity. The relationship between impulsivity and compulsivity is complex. Traditionally, these multifaceted constructs have been viewed as diametrically opposed, with individuals exhibiting a preponderance of one at the expense of the other, yet more contemporary theories now suggest that the relationship between the two is dynamic and can shift over time (see [110] for discussion). Whether compulsivity definitively constitutes a vulnerability towards GD is unclear. Certainly, the archetypal pathology of aberrant compulsivity, obsessive-compulsive disorder (OCD), is rarely co-morbid with GD, which would argue against such a conclusion [111]. However, gamblers do score higher on self-report measures of compulsivity [112], and the presence of OCD-like symptoms is well correlated with gambling severity [113]. Moreover, many of the cognitive distortions such as an adherence to 'lucky' rituals, which have been suggested as central to the development of GD [13, 14], could be considered compulsive in nature.

Selective serotonin reuptake inhibitors (SSRIs) are the primary pharmacological treatment for OCD and have reliably been shown to be effective at alleviating compulsive behaviours (see [114] for review). Consequently, animal work investigating compulsive-like behaviours has focused on the serotonergic system. The signal attenuation model consists of four stages: firstly, a compound stimulus is established as signal of food delivery, secondly, rats trained to lever press for food that is delivered concomitant with the compound stimulus, thirdly, signal attenuation, during which the ability of the cue to predict reward is attenuated by extinguishing the contingency between the two and, lastly, the test phase, during which rats lever press for the presentation of the stimulus alone [115]. An increase in responding on the lever during this test phase is hypothesised to reflect a failure in response feedback analogous to the inability of patients to cease responding once an action has been successfully completed [116]. Systemic administration of selective serotonin reuptake inhibitors or D_1 receptor antagonists alleviates compulsive-like responding on the lever [116, 117].

Further evidence of a potential role for dopamine in mediating compulsive-like behavioural responding comes from a relatively recent study using the operant observing response task. This paradigm presents animals with two levers, one an active lever that delivers food reward and the other inactive. There is also a third lever that, when pressed, signals which of the other two levers is active by illuminating the light above the active lever [118]. In contrast to the signal attenuation model which intimated that D_1, but not D_2 receptors, may underlie compulsive behaviours, in the operant observing response task, chronic administration of the D_2-like agonist quinpirole significantly increased the number of responses on the 'observing' lever both in order to obtain the cue and also when the cue was already illuminated, potentially indicative of compulsive-like checking [118]. Interestingly, this increase in compulsive-like behaviour following chronic treatment with quinpirole may be related to the invigorated task performance on the rSMT following chronic ropinirole we reported in Sect. 6.2, in that the latter appears to reflect increased task 'focus'; animals on the rSMT were not quicker to make any particular response; therefore the increase in trials completed must have resulted from a decrease in other non-task-related activities, such as grooming or exploration. Furthermore, such an increase in task engagement superficially resembles the attentional narrowing observed in human gamblers, which is thought to reflect a compulsive style of play [119, 120].

In sum, impulsivity is a multifaceted construct that is influenced by multiple neurotransmitter systems. Broadly, dopamine, NE and 5-HT appear to be involved to some degree in action inhibition and impulsive choice, and such duplicity of neurotransmitter involvement may indicate some mechanistic redundancy in the control of these forms of impulsivity, whilst there may be a slightly more selective role for 5-HT and NE in action restraint and action cancellation, respectively. Interestingly, although all forms of impulsivity are sensitive to amphetamine, the direction of these effects varies depending on the form of impulsivity and the task demands, again further highlighting the complex nature of the construct and its measurement. Recent work has highlighted an important role for dopamine in mediating compulsivity, although the recruitment of receptor subtype appears to vary dependent on task parameters, and consequently, much remains to be done with regard to investigating the neurochemical basis of compulsive behaviours in animals. Moreover, chronic administration of dopaminergic agonists may be an effective way of modelling compulsive-like gambling engagement, and consequently these models may represent a potential method for screening novel pharmacotherapies for iatrogenic gambling.

6.4 Deficits in Decision-Making

Gambling broadly involves participants placing themselves at a probabilistic disadvantage for a potential windfall. In this regard, gambling could be considered irrational, insofar as people are generally aware that the odds of winning are stacked against them [121]. Thus the cognitive dysfunction exhibited by problem gamblers does not appear to be related to an inability to perceive or calculate the odds. Consequently, increased risky or dysfunctional decision-making could be considered as a hallmark for problem gambling. Although numerous other personality constructs such as those discussed in this chapter might contribute to the onset of problem (subclinical) gambling and GD, perturbations in cost-benefit decision-making are something of a prerequisite. Gamblers' real-world decision-making deficits extend to the laboratory, with both recreational and pathological gamblers exhibiting deficits in comparison to healthy controls on tasks such as the Cambridge Gambling Task [17], Game of Dice Task [23] and the Iowa Gambling Task (IGT) [122]. These deficits are manifested when subjects are making decisions under both risk—choices between outcomes with explicit probabilities—and ambiguity, choices between outcomes with unknown probabilities, and cannot exclusively be accounted for by increased impulsivity or deficits in cognitive ability [122]. Consequently, decision-making deficits are, to a certain extent, dissociable from other behavioural facets of GD. Amongst these laboratory tasks, the IGT has been the most widely characterised, and consequently several rodent analogues have been developed (see [123] for discussion); in the interest of brevity, we will limit our discussion to the most widely adopted of these, the rodent gambling task (rGT) [124].

The IGT is generally considered as a test of 'real-world' decision-making and requires participants to select from four decks of cards, with the goal of accumulating points [125]. Two of the four decks are advantageous, in that they offer smaller immediate gains, but smaller penalties. In comparison the other two decks offer comparatively larger gains but also larger losses. The optimal strategy is to avoid the superficially alluring but ultimately disadvantageous decks and instead choose from the low-risk, low-reward decks. This strategy along with the relative contingencies for the decks is never made explicitly available to the participant, but healthy subjects learn the optimal strategy over time. Persistent choice of the disadvantageous decks has been linked to frontal lobe dysfunction and has been observed in both GD and drug addiction [22, 122, 125–128]. The rGT, consistent with the IGT, requires animals to choose between four options with established contingencies. Again, two options are disadvantageous, associated with larger gains (food reward) but more frequent and larger punishments (time-out periods), whereas the other two options are advantageous—associated with smaller gains but smaller and less frequent punishments. Animals have 30 min to maximise their 'earnings'; therefore these time-out periods reduce the opportunity to earn reward and were designed to approximate loss. Animals on the rGT show a similar behavioural profile to humans on the IGT, in that selection of the tempting high-risk, high-reward option declines as experience with the contingencies progresses and animals instead develop a clear preference for the smaller but safer rewards. The construct validity of the rGT has been tested by examining whether the neural loci underpinning task performance are comparable across species. Performance on the human IGT has consistently been shown to be critically dependent on brain regions that also putatively play a key role in the formation and maintenance of addictive disorders, namely, the prefrontal cortex and amygdala [125, 129–131]. Likewise, performance of the rGT is mediated by these same regions, lesions of the PFC and agranular insula impair choice behaviour, whilst inactivations of the orbitofrontal cortex and BLA or disconnection of these two areas severely retards learning of the optimal task strategy [132–135].

In contrast to other animal models of cost-benefit decision-making, dopamine does not appear to play a particularly prominent role; rather performance on the rGT is modulated by multiple pharmacological systems. Administration of selective DA reuptake inhibitors, or D_1 or D_2-like agonists, does not alter choice behaviour [124, 136]. In contrast, administration of amphetamine and the 5-HT$_{1A}$ receptor agonist 8-OH-DPAT both impair performance on the rGT [124]. Interestingly, the effect of amphetamine appears to arise as a result of additive effects on multiple monoamine neurotransmitter systems, as selective reuptake inhibitors for 5-HT, dopamine or norepinephrine produce only mild effects when administered in isolation, but any combination of two of the reuptake inhibitors impairs behaviour, potentially indicative of a redundancy in the neurochemical regulation of choice [137]. Furthermore, the effects of amphetamine on choice, unlike on motor impulsivity, cannot be blocked by either a D_1 or a D_2 receptor antagonist [138]. The finding that dopamine does not appear to play a particularly prominent role in the rGT is interesting given the relatively ubiquitous role ascribed for mesolimbic dopamine in cost-benefit decision-making. Much of this work has focused on animals' willingness to exert physical effort in order to obtain a larger reward—such as scaling a barrier or lever pressing. Broadly, blockade of dopamine receptors decreases animals' willingness to work for reward, whereas drugs that potentiate the actions of dopamine, such as amphetamine, increase the choice of the more effortful yet more lucrative option [139–142]. These data suggest that alterations in task demands may differentially recruit dopaminergic systems. Indeed, in contrast to the pronounced role dopamine plays in physical effort, it appears to play only a minor role if the effort required is cognitive [143]. Thus, the relative contributions of neurotransmitters, such as dopamine, to the choice process are critically dependent on task demands.

Probability discounting tasks (PDTs), in a similar manner to delay discounting paradigms, present animals with two levers, one of which delivers a small reward (e.g. one sugar pellet) with 100% likelihood, whilst the other lever yields a larger reward (e.g. four sugar pellets). In contrast to delay discounting, this reward is not devalued by a delay, but rather the likelihood of it being delivered is probabilistic and varies in a stepwise manner across the session. In the original iteration, the likelihood of the larger reward progressed downwards from 100%, 50%, 25% and 12.5–6.25%, although the probabilities can also be presented in ascending order [144]. There are some notable differences between delay and probability discounting, despite some similarities in the task structure. In delay discounting, both the large and small reward are always available, but the valence of the large reward is diminished by accompanying delay; thus the task measures the impulsive choice of immediate gratification over long-term benefits. In contrast, during probability discounting the large reward is not always delivered; thus the animal must decide whether to take the small safe reward or 'play the odds' and risk not receiving anything. During delay discounting, the larger delayed reward is always (at least objectively, if not subjectively) optimal, whereas the best strategy on probability discounting changes throughout the session, requiring animals to respond to shifting contingencies. Thus, preference for the uncertain outcome may not always be maladaptive, and the degree to which this maps on to the construct of impulsive decision-making is open to debate.

Unlike the anti-impulsivity effects amphetamine has on delay discounting, systemic administration of the psychostimulant increases choice of the larger probabilistic reward [142], an effect contingent on amphetamine's ability to potentiate dopamine as indicated by its blockade by prior administration of either a D_1-like or a D_2-like antagonist. Similarly, administration of both D_1-like and D_2-like agonists increased choice of the uncertain option [145]. Similar to data from the delay discounting and 5CSRTT tasks, lesions to the NAc core increase maladaptive behaviour, as exemplified by increased choice of the smaller-certain option [144].

A risk discounting task (RDT) has also been developed that utilised electric shocks as punishments, i.e. the probability of reward was kept the same throughout the blocks, but the chances of a larger reward being accompanied by a footshock increased throughout the blocks (25%, 50%, 75–100%). There is a modest correlation between probability and risk discounting, suggesting some of the same cognitive processes may be implicated in both tasks [146]. In contrast to its effects on the PDT, amphetamine decreases choice of the larger, but potentially punishing option on the RDT, an effect blocked by a D_2-like antagonist. Likewise, a D_2-like agonist decreases risky choice, whereas drugs targeting D_1-like receptors have no effect [147]. Comparing the neurochemical regulation of choice behaviour across the rGT, PDT and RDT suggest that the neurobiology underlying risk-based decision-making may vary contingent on the presence or absence of explicit penalties, as well as the nature of those penalties, further complicating delineating a singular aetiology for human gambling.

One potentially interesting, and relatively underexplored avenue, is what governs decision-making in the absence of optimal choice. In the majority of operant paradigms, the probabilities are such that there is almost always an optimal strategy. Arguably a better measure of biased decision-making would be to examine choice behaviour when options are ultimately equivalent. In the rodent betting task (rBT), the 'bet size' in play is indicated by the illumination of one, two or three response apertures at the start of each trial [148]. The bet size varies between blocks of trials on a pseudorandom schedule. Once the animals have nose-poked at each illuminated aperture, two levers are extended into the chamber. These levers are permanently designated as either the 'safe' or 'uncertain' lever. Responses on the safe lever lead to guaranteed delivery of the bet size at stake (i.e. one, two or three sugar pellets), whereas the uncertain lever leads to either double the safe bet size or no reward with equal probability. Thus, exclusive choice of either option would lead to equivalent reward in the long term. Initial investigations with this task revealed that animals could broadly be split into two sub-groups—one that remained indifferent to the size of the wager (insensitive) or those that began to select the safe lever more as the bet size increased (sensitive).

In contrast to the rGT, choice behaviour on the rBT is acutely sensitive to manipulations of OFC, as inactivations of this region, but not the mPFC increased risky choice in wager-sensitive rats [149]. However, lesions to the basolateral amygdala did not affect performance, regardless of baseline choice patterns [150]. As such, simple preference for uncertain outcomes, as measured by an unbiased paradigm, can be dissociated from the adoption of an optimal choice strategy in which the risks of winning and losing must be integrated.

Systemic administration of amphetamine increased choice of the uncertain lever, but only in wager-sensitive animals, whereas the D_2-like antagonist eticlopride decreased choice of the uncertain lever, but only in wager-insensitive rats. Thus animals' baseline choice behaviour critically mediated the response to dopaminergic ligands. Using micro-PET and autoradiography, a strong relationship was confirmed between increased wager sensitivity and lower levels of $D_{2/3}$ receptors in the striatum [148]. A decreased density of striatal dopamine receptors has been proposed as a canonical biomarker for drug addiction. These results may therefore suggest that mathematically nonnormative decision-making under uncertainty, which is associated with elevated risk for GD, may arise through similar neurobiology as traits which confer vulnerability to drug addiction [151, 152]. Moreover, these results highlight the potential value in exploring individual differences in animal models of decision-making, as differences in subjective choice at baseline can shape later response to pharmacological challenges. Further studies utilising this task have shown that chronic administration of ropinirole increases choice of the uncertain lever and such results not only highlight the critical role played by dopaminergic activity in mediating risk-based decision-making but arguably provide further evidence that chronic $D_{2/3}$ agonism may represent a putative model of problem gambling [153].

Ultimately, perturbations in cost-benefit decision-making are varied, and task demands such as response requirements, the valence/volatility of the outcome and consequences of loss/failure to win can all affect how animals engage with the task. Although broadly the majority of these tasks remain sensitive to dopaminergic and/or serotonergic manipulations, alterations in task design and individual differences can have profound effects on the neurobiology recruited.

6.5   Cue Reactivity

The ability of cues to facilitate ongoing addictive behaviours is a cornerstone of contemporary theories of addiction [45, 154–156]. However, the relevance of cues to GD is less clear. Certainly exposure to gambling-related cues can promote craving in gamblers [24, 25], and removing sound cues reduced both the enjoyment derived from and the desire to continue playing slot machines in problem gamblers [157]. Additionally, problem gamblers have been reported to display attentional bias towards gambling-related stimuli in comparison to controls (see [158] for review), and an increased attentional bias towards salient cues has been suggested to contribute to the transition from recreational to problematic gambling [26]. These data ultimately suggest that cues are an integral part of the gambling milieu, yet the exact role cues play in the formation or maintenance of GD and the contextual specificity of gambling cues remain to be determined (see [159] for discussion).

Relatively few animal tasks have specifically addressed the role of cues on gambling-related decision-making, with the notable exception of a modified version of the rGT, wherein reward delivery resulting from choice of the larger, but riskier, options is associated with more salient and complex audiovisual cues [160]. Interestingly, the presence of cues promotes a more disadvantageous choice profile, with more rats exhibiting a risk-preferring profile at baseline, providing the first evidence in non-human animals that reward-paired audiovisual cues can promote risky decision-making [160]. Moreover, the presence of cues on this modified rGT recruited the dopaminergic system to a greater degree than the uncued version. As mentioned in Sect. 6.4, the rGT does not appear to be greatly influenced by dopaminergic agents, yet choice on the cued rGT appears uniquely sensitive to the administration of compounds specific for the D_3 receptor; a highly selective D_3 agonist increased, whereas a selective antagonist decreased risky choice. These findings are in direct contrast to the lack of effects D_3 ligands produce on the 'standard' rGT [161] and provide novel evidence that D_3 receptors may play a role in controlling responsivity to gambling-related cues. In support of such a supposition, D_3 receptors have previously been demonstrated to mediate cue-induced seeking of addictive drugs and consequently have been suggested to represent a potential pharmacological target for the treatment of drug addiction [162–165]. Given the theory that the phenomenological processes underlying both behavioural and substance addictions may be similar, D_3 receptors may represent something of a common target for controlling certain aspects of behavioural dysfunction.

It is worth noting that in the cued rGT, the cues are concurrent with reward—and absent following a loss. In contrast, cues during the rSMT signal the current status of the apertures and function as predictors of reward (reward-predictive), as opposed to being delivered subsequent to the trial outcome (reward-concurrent). Thus, whilst both tasks contain overt cues, the cues signal very different information and may therefore impact cognition via distinct mechanisms. Certainly, these different cue-mediated behavioural effects appear pharmacologically distinct, as selective D_4, but not D_3, ligands alter performance on the rSMT [55], whereas targeting D_3, but not D_4, receptors modulates behaviour on the cued rGT [160].

In contrast to the relative dearth of empirical investigations examining the role of cues on cost-benefit decision-making, a comparatively larger body of evidence exists using simple behavioural tasks that have been used to delineate the neurobiological underpinnings of cue-guided responding. Similar to both the cued rGT and the rSMT, the role of dopamine in controlling cue reactivity has been the predominant focus of these investigations. Dopaminergic signaling particularly through the D_2-like class of receptors has been generally associated with attributing salience to reward associated stimuli [166]. Indeed, this process plays an important role in some theories of addiction (see [45] for discussion). Relatively simple behavioural paradigms such as autoshaping, as well as a Pavlovian-to-instrumental transfer (PIT) and conditioned reinforcement (CRf), have been used most commonly. Ostensibly all these paradigms measure how reward-paired cues can influence action, but differ slightly in regard to brain areas and neurochemical regulation. These tasks could be considered hierarchical in that the property of the cues increases in behavioural significance, from attracting attention (autoshaping), to influencing ongoing behaviour (PIT) and finally to becoming the goal itself (CRf).

During autoshaping, a classically conditioned stimulus (CS) reliably predicts delivery of an unconditioned stimulus (US), for instance, presentation of a lever and accompanying light (CS+) for 5 s before a food pellet (US) is delivered. Over repeated CS-US pairings, some animals begin to approach and interact with the CS, even though the US is not contingent on any such response. Typically animals vary in the extent to which they respond to the CS and can be separated into those who approach the CS, i.e. 'sign trackers' (ST), and those who orient towards the delivery location of the US, i.e. 'goal trackers' (GT) [167]. The incentive salience assigned to the CS by sign trackers has been linked with increased dopamine release within the NAc [168], and both acquisition and expression of sign tracking can be disrupted by administration of non-selective dopamine antagonists [169]. Whilst sign tracking could be taken as evidence that reward-paired cues are salient and attractive, it does not necessarily imply that they can influence goal-directed action.

PIT measures the degree to which a CS that has previously been classically conditioned with reward can invigorate instrumental responding that has, in separate training sessions, also resulted in reward. PIT begins in a similar manner to autoshaping, in that a CS, e.g. a tone, predicts delivery of a US (food). Subsequently animals are shaped to make an operant response for reward such as lever press. Lastly, during a test session, usually done during extinction (i.e. reward is not delivered), the CS is presented with the supposition that the presentation of the CS will augment animals' operant responding on the lever. The CS is presented intermittently and non-contingently; thus the animals' actions do not affect the presentation of the CS, yet the CS can bias the animal towards actions previously associated with reward delivery. PIT is sensitive to modulation of dopaminergic circuits (see [170] for discussion) and can be disrupted by systemic administration of non-selective dopamine antagonists [171].

In a somewhat similar manner to PIT, CRf begins with classically conditioning a CS to delivery of a US. Yet in contrast to PIT, the subsequent test session determines the degree to which an animal is prepared to perform a novel response, such as lever pressing, that is reinforced solely by the CS. Thus, in contrast to PIT, the presentation of a CS during CRf is entirely contingent on the animals' behaviour. CRf appears to be primarily influenced by dopaminergic activity within the NAc, as infusion of amphetamine into this area potentiates animals' responding for the CS, an effect that is remediated by prior blockade of D_1 or D_2 receptors [172]. Similarly, infusion of non-selective D_1-like or D_2-like agonists into the NAc potentiated responding for the CS, an effect that was mimicked by a systemically administered D_2-like agonist, but not a D_1 receptor agonist [172, 173].

In broad terms, therefore, performance on all three of these tasks has been shown to be sensitive to ligands with selectivity at D_2-like receptors [174–176] and more specifically manipulations of dopaminergic activity within the NAc [177–179]. The NAc receives extensive inputs from cortical and limbic regions and has been suggested to be critically involved in response selection, yet the upstream inputs that might be important for driving behaviour during the performance (rather than the acquisition) of tasks such as autoshaping or CRf remain elusive [180]. Interestingly, recent work from our group showed that a highly selective D_4 agonist had no effect on either CRf or autoshaping [181]. Additionally, mixed results have been observed with partially selective D_3 agonists, and more selective D_3 antagonists are without effect on simple behavioural tasks [176, 182], intimating that D_3 receptors cannot exclusively account for responsivity to CS+. Interestingly, increased cue-driven behaviour on CRf and autoshaping, a putative biomarker for addiction vulnerability, is associated with lower levels of impulsivity [183]. Additionally, we have preliminary evidence that suggests animals' instrumental motivation for cues on a CRf paradigm does not correlate with performance on either the regular or cued version of the rGT (Tremblay, Ferland, Hounjet and Winstanley unpublished observations). Thus, increased cue reactivity, at least as assessed by CRf and autoshaping, is not associated with increases in either impulsivity or perturbations in cost-benefit decision-making, canonical measures of dysfunction in addictive disorders. Clearly, in this regard we are comparing between relatively simple behavioural tasks and much more complex ones. Decision-making on more intricate tasks likely promotes a higher cognitive load; consequently, behaviour is unlikely to be exclusively influenced by stimulus-response relationships. In contrast tasks such as autoshaping, PIT and CRf, although useful insofar as they have reliably intimated that the D_2-like receptor is critically involved in mediating approach behaviour, may be somewhat limited in regard to exploring more complex disorders such as addiction, where the cognitive processes involved are likely complex and multifactorial. The likelihood of approach, or motivation to obtain a CS+, may therefore be a weak facsimile of the more complex role cues play in behavioural or substance addictions.

In sum, unlike the other sections of this chapter that have generally highlighted a complex interaction of the monoamine neurotransmitters in controlling behaviour, cue reactivity appears to be principally mediated by dopamine. This is not all together surprising given the canonical role ascribed [44] to dopamine in signaling the appetitive value of environmental stimuli. However, the role for dopamine in mediating animals' responsivity to cues is nuanced and dependent upon the complexity of the task and the contextual quality of the cues.

6.6 Conclusions

We have argued here that excessive cognitive distortions, impulsivity, compulsivity cue reactivity and impaired cost-benefit decision-making may confer vulnerability towards GD. The criteria discussed here may offer an opportunity to 'deconstruct' some facets of behavioural dysfunction observed in problem gambling. Indeed, it is unlikely, given the heterogeneity of gambling that any human gambler would exhibit perturbations in all of these symptom domains. Thus, a more comprehensive understanding of subtypes within gamblers may be useful in delineating a conceptual framework to explore the underlying neurobiology using animal models and consequently treatment development. However, animal models may also be useful for exploring the relationship between these constructs, given recent data indicating that increased impulsivity is associated with a greater endorsement of gambling-related cognitions [184].

These putative risk factors appear to have overlapping but discrete neurobiological underpinnings. Broadly speaking, a common role can be attributed to the monoamine transmitters dopamine, 5-HT and noradrenaline as well as frontostriatal brain regions. A role for both 5-HT and dopamine in mediating aspects of impulsivity and impaired cost-benefit decision-making is relatively well established. Importantly, the data here offer at least two relatively novel potential lines of enquiry. First, the potential role for D_3 and D_4 receptors in mediating differing behavioural responses to reward associated stimuli has yet to be fully explored. Data from the rSMT indicate that D_4 receptors might control attributions of salience to reward-predictive stimuli, whereas D_3 receptors appear to mediate risky choice in response to reward-concurrent cues. The majority of studies that target D_2-like receptors often attribute their findings to the D_2 receptor itself, potentially due to its relative abundance within the D_2 family [185] and its localisation within reward-related neural structures such as the dorsal striatum and NAc [186]. However, the results highlighted here may be indicative of an increased role for D_3 and D_4 in the more complex cognitions associated with GD.

A common theme throughout this chapter has been that tasks pertaining to measure the same construct can recruit differing neurobiological systems. This variability is by no means a weakness of animal models. In fact, both the inter- and intra-task variability may be invaluable at gaining a more comprehensive understanding of the aetiology underlying behavioural disorders. Moreover, the individual differences within animals could also be extremely beneficial in identifying what forms of interventions may best be used to combat differing behavioural perturbations. These differences, however, do signify considerable variability within constructs such as impulsivity, such that care should be taken not to extrapolate too widely from one paradigm to another. The variability both within and between some of these tasks does lead to questions about reliability. As there is no currently approved pharmacological treatment available for GD, pharmacological isomorphism is not a good measure of assessing these tasks' validity. However, one of the cornerstones of a valid operant measure is reliability. As all of these tasks have been used repeatedly, in most cases by different researchers, the retest reliability of the core behavioural observations discussed herein appears high. However, there are intractable issues with animal models that potentially limit their efficacy, mainly in regard to how both rewards and losses are represented (see [32] for full discussion of these potential limitations).

Ultimately, despite limitations, animal models with high translational validity allow a degree of control and breadth of manipulations that allow inferences about the causality of clinical disorders. This control and range may be invaluable in elucidating a more comprehensive understanding of diseases such as GD where the aetiology is complex and multifactorial.

Acknowledgements This work was supported by operating grants awarded to C.A.W. from the Canadian Institutes of Health Research (CIHR; MOP-89700), Ontario Problem Gambling Research Council, Parkinson Society Canada and the Natural Sciences and Engineering Council of Canada. P.J.C. was funded through a graduate student award from Parkinson Society Canada (PSC). C.A.W. received salary support through the Michael Smith Foundation for Health Research and the Canadian Institutes for Health Research (CIHR) New Investigator Program.

Conflict of interest C.A.W. has previously consulted for Shire on an unrelated matter. Neither P.J.C. nor C.A.W. has any other conflicts of interest or financial disclosures to make.

References

1. Wardle H, Moody A, Spence S, Orford J, Volberg R, Jotangia D, Griffths M, Hussey D, Dobbie F. British Gambling Prevalence Survey 2010. The Gambling Commission. 2010.
2. Gerstein D, Hoffman J, Larison C, Engelam L, Murphy S, Palmer A, Chuchro L, Toce M, Johnson R, Buie T, Hill MA. Gambling Impact and Behavior study. Report to the National Gambling Impact Study Commission. 1999.
3. Black DW, et al. Suicide ideations, suicide attempts, and completed suicide in persons with pathological gambling and their first-degree relatives. Suicide Life Threat Behav. 2015;45(6):700–9.
4. Petry NM, Kiluk BD. Suicidal ideation and suicide attempts in treatment-seeking pathological gamblers. J Nerv Ment Dis. 2002;190(7):462–9.
5. Hollander E, Buchalter AJ, DeCaria CM. Pathological gambling. Psychiatr Clin North Am. 2000;23(3):629–42.
6. Potenza MN. Review. The neurobiology of pathological gambling and drug addiction: an overview and new findings. Philos Trans R Soc Lond Ser B Biol Sci. 2008;363(1507):3181–9.
7. Potenza MN. Should addictive disorders include non-substance-related conditions? Addiction. 2006;101(Suppl 1):142–51.
8. Bechara A. Risky business: emotion, decision-making, and addiction. J Gambl Stud. 2003;19(1):23–51.
9. Martin RJ, et al. Disordered gambling and co-morbidity of psychiatric disorders among college students: an examination of problem drinking, anxiety and depression. J Gambl Stud. 2014;30(2):321–33.
10. Petry NM. A comparison of treatment-seeking pathological gamblers based on preferred gambling activity. Addiction. 2003;98(5):645–55.
11. Kirmayer LJ, Crafa D. What kind of science for psychiatry? Front Hum Neurosci. 2014;8:435.
12. Morris SE, Cuthbert BN. Research Domain Criteria: cognitive systems, neural circuits, and dimensions of behavior. Dialogues Clin Neurosci. 2012;14(1):29–37.
13. Toneatto T, et al. Cognitive distortions in heavy gambling. J Gambl Stud. 1997;13(3):253–66.
14. Ladouceur R, et al. Gambling – relationship between the frequency of wins and irrational thinking. J Psychol. 1988;122(4):409–14.
15. Potenza MN. Impulsivity and compulsivity in pathological gambling and obsessive-compulsive disorder. Rev Bras Psiquiatr. 2007;29(2):105–6.
16. Rodriguez-Jimenez R, et al. Impulsivity and sustained attention in pathological gamblers: influence of childhood ADHD history. J Gambl Stud. 2006;22(4):451–61.
17. Lawrence AJ, et al. Problem gamblers share deficits in impulsive decision-making with alcohol-dependent individuals. Addiction. 2009;104(6):1006–15.
18. Dixon MR, Marley J, Jacobs EA. Delay discounting by pathological gamblers. J Appl Behav Anal. 2003;36(4):449–58.
19. Petry NM. Pathological gamblers, with and without substance use disorders, discount delayed rewards at high rates. J Abnorm Psychol. 2001;110(3):482–7.
20. Michalczuk R, et al. Impulsivity and cognitive distortions in pathological gamblers attending the UK National Problem Gambling Clinic: a preliminary report. Psychol Med. 2011;41(12):2625–35.
21. Linnet J, et al. Dopamine release in ventral striatum during Iowa Gambling Task performance is associated with increased excitement levels in pathological gambling. Addiction. 2011;106(2):383–90.
22. Goudriaan AE, et al. Decision making in pathological gambling: a comparison between pathological gamblers, alcohol dependents, persons with Tourette syndrome, and normal controls. Brain Res Cogn Brain Res. 2005;23(1):137–51.
23. Brand M, et al. Decision-making impairments in patients with pathological gambling. Psychiatry Res. 2005;133(1):91–9.

24. Kushner M, et al. Urge to gamble in a simulated gambling environment. J Gambl Stud. 2008;24(2):219–27.
25. Kushner MG, et al. Urge to gamble in problem gamblers exposed to a casino environment. J Gambl Stud. 2007;23(2):121–32.
26. Grant LD, Bowling AC. Gambling attitudes and beliefs predict attentional bias in non-problem gamblers. J Gambl Stud. 2015;31(4):1487–503.
27. Ciccarelli M, et al. Attentional biases in problem and non-problem gamblers. J Affect Disord. 2016;198:135–41.
28. Lesieur HR, Blume SB. The South Oaks Gambling Screen (SOGS): a new instrument for the identification of pathological gamblers. Am J Psychiatry. 1987;144(9):1184–8.
29. Raylu N, Oei TP. The Gambling Related Cognitions Scale (GRCS): development, confirmatory factor validation and psychometric properties. Addiction. 2004;99(6):757–69.
30. Steenbergh TA, et al. Development and validation of the Gamblers' Beliefs Questionnaire. Psychol Addict Behav. 2002;16(2):143–9.
31. Oei TPS, Gordon LM. Psychosocial factors related to gambling abstinence and relapse in members of gamblers anonymous. J Gambl Stud. 2008;24(1):91–105.
32. Cocker PJ, Winstanley CA. Irrational beliefs, biases and gambling: exploring the role of animal models in elucidating vulnerabilities for the development of pathological gambling. Behav Brain Res. 2015;279:259–73.
33. Winstanley CA, Cocker PJ, Rogers RD. Dopamine modulates reward expectancy during performance of a slot machine task in rats: evidence for a 'near-miss' effect. Neuropsychopharmacology. 2011;36(5):913–25.
34. Clark L, et al. Gambling near-misses enhance motivation to gamble and recruit win-related brain circuitry. Neuron. 2009;61(3):481–90.
35. Walker MB. Irrational thinking among slot machine players. J Gambl Stud. 1992;8(3):245–61.
36. Cote D, et al. Near wins prolong gambling on a video lottery terminal. J Gambl Stud. 2003;19(4):433–8.
37. Clark L, et al. Physiological responses to near-miss outcomes and personal control during simulated gambling. J Gambl Stud. 2012;28(1):123–37.
38. Murch WS, Clark L. Games in the brain: neural substrates of gambling addiction. Neuroscientist. 2016;22(5):534–45.
39. Breen RB, Zimmerman M. Rapid onset of pathological gambling in machine gamblers. J Gambl Stud. 2002;18(1):31–43.
40. Choliz M. Experimental analysis of the game in pathological gamblers: effect of the immediacy of the reward in slot machines. J Gambl Stud. 2010;26(2):249–56.
41. Dowling N, Smith D, Thomas T. Electronic gaming machines: are they the 'crack-cocaine' of gambling? Addiction. 2005;100(1):33–45.
42. Chase HW, Clark L. Gambling severity predicts midbrain response to near-miss outcomes. J Neurosci. 2010;30(18):6180–7.
43. Habib R, Dixon MR. Neurobehavioral evidence for the 'near-miss' effect in pathological gamblers. J Exp Anal Behav. 2010;93:313–28.
44. Schultz W. Predictive reward signal of dopamine neurons. J Neurophysiol. 1998;80(1):1–27.
45. Robinson TE, Berridge KC. The neural basis of drug craving: an incentive-sensitization theory of addiction. Brain Res Brain Res Rev. 1993;18(3):247–91.
46. Potenza MN. How central is dopamine to pathological gambling or gambling disorder? Front Behav Neurosci. 2013;7:206.
47. Zack M, Poulos CX. Amphetamine primes motivation to gamble and gambling-related semantic networks in problem gamblers. Neuropsychopharmacology. 2004;29(1):195–207.
48. Noble EP. Addiction and its reward process through polymorphisms of the D-2 dopamine receptor gene: a review. Eur Psychiatry. 2000;15(2):79–89.
49. Comings DE, et al. A study of the dopamine D2 receptor gene in pathological gambling. Pharmacogenetics. 1996;6(3):223–34.

50. Blum K, et al. The D₂ dopamine receptor gene as a determinant of reward deficiency syndrome. J R Soc Med. 1996;89:396–400.
51. Comings DE, et al. The additive effect of neurotransmitter genes in pathological gambling. Clin Genet. 2001;60(2):107–16.
52. Comings DE, et al. Studies of the 48 bp repeat polymorphism of the DRD4 gene in impulsive, compulsive, addictive behaviors: Tourette syndrome, ADHD, pathological gambling, and substance abuse. Am J Med Genet. 1999;88(4):358–68.
53. Dodd ML, et al. Pathological gambling caused by drugs used to treat Parkinson disease. Arch Neurol. 2005;62(9):1377–81.
54. Kimber TE, Thompson PD, Kiley MA. Resolution of dopamine dysregulation syndrome following cessation of dopamine agonist therapy in Parkinson's disease. J Clin Neurosci. 2008;15(2):205–8.
55. Cocker PJ, et al. A selective role for dopamine D(4) receptors in modulating reward expectancy in a rodent slot machine task. Biol Psychiatry. 2014;75(10):817–24.
56. Van Craenenbroeck K, Rondou P, Haegeman G. The dopamine D4 receptor: biochemical and signalling properties. Cell Mol Life Sci. 2010;67(12):1971–86.
57. Cocker PJ, et al. Activation of dopamine D4 receptors within the anterior cingulate cortex enhances the erroneous expectation of reward on a rat slot machine task. Neuropharmacology. 2016;105:186–95.
58. Cocker PJ, et al. The agranular and granular insula differentially contribute to gambling-like behavior on a rat slot machine task: effects of inactivation and local infusion of a dopamine D4 agonist on reward expectancy. Psychopharmacology (Berl). 2016;233(17):3135–47.
59. Weintraub D, Potenza MN. Impulse control disorders in Parkinson's disease. Curr Neurol Neurosci Rep. 2006;6(4):302–6.
60. Voon V, Potenza MN, Thomsen T. Medication-related impulse control and repetitive behaviors in Parkinson's disease. Curr Opin Neurol. 2007;20(4):484–92.
61. Clark CA, Dagher A. The role of dopamine in risk taking: a specific look at Parkinson's disease and gambling. Front Behav Neurosci. 2014;8:196.
62. Cocker PJ, Tremblay M, Kaur S, Winstanley CA. Chronic administration of the dopamine D2/3 agonist ropinirole invigorates performance of a rodent slot machine task, potentially indicative of a less distractable or compulsive-like gambling behaviour. Psychopharmacology. 2017;234:137–53.
63. Cocker PJ, Lin MY, Tremblay M, Kaur S, Winstanley CA. The ß-adrenoceptor blocker propranolol ameliorates compulsive-like gambling behaviour in a rodent slot machine task: implications for iatrogenic gambling disorder. Eur J Neurosci. 2018.
64. Carlezon WA Jr, Duman RS, Nestler EJ. The many faces of CREB. Trends Neurosci. 2005;28(8):436–45.
65. Beaulieu JM, Gainetdinov RR, Caron MG. The Akt-GSK-3 signaling cascade in the actions of doparnine. Trends Pharmacol Sci. 2007;28(4):166–72.
66. Li YC, Gao WJ. GSK-3 beta activity and hyperdopamine-dependent behaviors. Neurosci Biobehav Rev. 2011;35(3):645–54.
67. Self DW, et al. Involvement of cAMP-dependent protein kinase in the nucleus accumbens in cocaine self-administration and relapse of cocaine-seeking behavior. J Neurosci. 1998;18(5):1848–59.
68. Nestler EJ, Carlezon WA Jr. The mesolimbic dopamine reward circuit in depression. Biol Psychiatry. 2006;59(12):1151–9.
69. Miller JS, Tallarida RJ, Unterwald EM. Cocaine-induced hyperactivity and sensitization are dependent on GSK3. Neuropharmacology. 2009;56(8):1116–23.
70. Enman NM, Unterwald EM. Inhibition of GSK3 attenuates amphetamine-induced hyperactivity and sensitization in the mouse. Behav Brain Res. 2012;231(1):217–25.
71. Kabitzke PA, Silva L, Wiedenmayer C. Norepinephrine mediates contextual fear learning and hippocampal pCREB in juvenile rats exposed to predator odor. Neurobiol Learn Mem. 2011;96(2):166–72.

72. Beaulieu JM, et al. An Akt/beta-arrestin 2/PP2A signaling complex mediates dopaminergic neurotransmission and behavior. Cell. 2005;122(2):261–73.
73. Rafa D, et al. Effects of optimism on gambling in the rat slot machine task. Behav Brain Res. 2016;300:97–105.
74. Winstanley CA, Eagle DM, Robbins TW. Behavioral models of impulsivity in relation to ADHD: translation between clinical and preclinical studies. Clin Psychol Rev. 2006;26(4):379–95.
75. Verdejo-Garcia A, Lawrence AJ, Clark L. Impulsivity as a vulnerability marker for substance-use disorders: review of findings from high-risk research, problem gamblers and genetic association studies. Neurosci Biobehav Rev. 2008;32(4):777–810.
76. Chamberlain SR, Sahakian BJ. The neuropsychiatry of impulsivity. Curr Opin Psychiatry. 2007;20(3):255–61.
77. Moeller FG, et al. Psychiatric aspects of impulsivity. Am J Psychiatry. 2001;158(11):1783–93.
78. Gullo MJ, Loxton NJ, Dawe S. Impulsivity: four ways five factors are not basic to addiction. Addict Behav. 2014;39(11):1547–56.
79. Hodgins DC, Holub A. Components of impulsivity in gambling disorder. Int J Ment Health Addict. 2015;13(6):699–711.
80. Winstanley CA, et al. Insight into the relationship between impulsivity and substance abuse from studies using animal models. Alcohol Clin Exp Res. 2010;34(8):1306–18.
81. Young JW, et al. Reverse translation of the rodent 5C-CPT reveals that the impaired attention of people with schizophrenia is similar to scopolamine-induced deficits in mice. Transl Psychiatry. 2013;3:e324.
82. Voon V, et al. Measuring "waiting" impulsivity in substance addictions and binge eating disorder in a novel analogue of rodent serial reaction time task. Biol Psychiatry. 2014;75(2):148–55.
83. Robbins TW. The 5-choice serial reaction time task: behavioural pharmacology and functional neurochemistry. Psychopharmacology. 2002;163(3–4):362–80.
84. Cole BJ, Robbins TW. Amphetamine impairs the discriminative performance of rats with dorsal noradrenergic bundle lesions on a 5-choice serial reaction time task: new evidence for central dopaminergic-noradrenergic interactions. Psychopharmacology. 1987;91(4):458–66.
85. Sulzer D, et al. Mechanisms of neurotransmitter release by amphetamines: a review. Prog Neurobiol. 2005;75(6):406–33.
86. Winstanley CA. The utility of rat models of impulsivity in developing pharmacotherapies for impulse control disorders. Br J Pharmacol. 2011;164(4):1301–21.
87. Muir JL, Everitt BJ, Robbins TW. The cerebral cortex of the rat and visual attentional function: dissociable effects of mediofrontal, cingulate, anterior dorsolateral, and parietal cortex lesions on a five-choice serial reaction time task. Cereb Cortex. 1996;6(3):470–81.
88. Chudasama Y, Robbins TW. Dissociable contributions of the orbitofrontal and infralimbic cortex to pavlovian autoshaping and discrimination reversal learning: further evidence for the functional heterogeneity of the rodent frontal cortex. J Neurosci. 2003;23(25):8771–80.
89. Christakou A, Robbins TW, Everitt BJ. Prefrontal cortical-ventral striatal interactions involved in affective modulation of attentional performance: implications for corticostriatal circuit function. J Neurosci. 2004;24(4):773–80.
90. Eagle DM, et al. Differential effects of modafinil and methylphenidate on stop-signal reaction time task performance in the rat, and interactions with the dopamine receptor antagonist cis-flupenthixol. Psychopharmacology. 2007;192(2):193–206.
91. Harrison AA, Everitt BJ, Robbins TW. Central serotonin depletion impairs both the acquisition and performance of a symmetrically reinforced go/no-go conditional visual discrimination. Behav Brain Res. 1999;100(1–2):99–112.
92. Chamberlain SR, et al. Neurochemical modulation of response inhibition and probabilistic learning in humans. Science. 2006;311(5762):861–3.
93. Eagle DM, et al. Stop-signal reaction-time task performance: role of prefrontal cortex and subthalamic nucleus. Cereb Cortex. 2008;18(1):178–88.

94. Eichenbaum H, Shedlack KJ, Eckmann KW. Thalamocortical mechanisms in odor-guided behavior. I. Effects of lesions of the mediodorsal thalamic nucleus and frontal cortex on olfactory discrimination in the rat. Brain Behav Evol. 1980;17(4):255–75.
95. Schoenbaum G, et al. Orbitofrontal lesions in rats impair reversal but not acquisition of go, no-go odor discriminations. Neuroreport. 2002;13(6):885–90.
96. Eagle DM, Bari A, Robbins TW. The neuropsychopharmacology of action inhibition: cross-species translation of the stop-signal and go/no-go tasks. Psychopharmacology. 2008;199(3):439–56.
97. Alessi SM, Petry NM. Pathological gambling severity is associated with impulsivity in a delay discounting procedure. Behav Process. 2003;64(3):345–54.
98. Ainslie G. Specious reward: a behavioral theory of impulsiveness and impulse control. Psychol Bull. 1975;82(4):463–96.
99. Evenden JL, Ryan CN. The pharmacology of impulsive behaviour in rats: the effects of drugs on response choice with varying delays of reinforcement. Psychopharmacology. 1996;128(2):161–70.
100. van Gaalen MM, et al. Critical involvement of dopaminergic neurotransmission in impulsive decision making. Biol Psychiatry. 2006;60(1):66–73.
101. Winstanley CA, et al. Interactions between serotonin and dopamine in the control of impulsive choice in rats: therapeutic implications for impulse control disorders. Neuropsychopharmacology. 2005;30(4):669–82.
102. Winstanley CA, et al. DeltaFosB induction in orbitofrontal cortex mediates tolerance to cocaine-induced cognitive dysfunction. J Neurosci. 2007;27(39):10497–507.
103. Winstanley CA, et al. Global 5-HT depletion attenuates the ability of amphetamine to decrease impulsive choice on a delay-discounting task in rats. Psychopharmacology. 2003;170(3):320–31.
104. Cardinal RN, et al. Impulsive choice induced in rats by lesions of the nucleus accumbens core. Science. 2001;292(5526):2499–501.
105. Winstanley CA, et al. Contrasting roles of basolateral amygdala and orbitofrontal cortex in impulsive choice. J Neurosci. 2004;24(20):4718–22.
106. Zeeb FD, Floresco SB, Winstanley CA. Contributions of the orbitofrontal cortex to impulsive choice: interactions with basal levels of impulsivity, dopamine signalling, and reward-related cues. Psychopharmacology. 2010;211(1):87–98.
107. Floresco SB, et al. Cortico-limbic-striatal circuits subserving different forms of cost-benefit decision making. Cogn Affect Behav Neurosci. 2008;8(4):375–89.
108. Abela AR, et al. Inhibitory control deficits in rats with ventral hippocampal lesions. Cereb Cortex. 2013;23(6):1396–409.
109. Abela AR, Chudasama Y. Dissociable contributions of the ventral hippocampus and orbitofrontal cortex to decision-making with a delayed or uncertain outcome. Eur J Neurosci. 2013;37(4):640–7.
110. Fineberg NA, et al. Probing compulsive and impulsive behaviors, from animal models to endophenotypes: a narrative review. Neuropsychopharmacology. 2010;35(3):591–604.
111. Fontenelle LF, Mendlowicz MV, Versiani M. Impulse control disorders in patients with obsessive-compulsive disorder. Psychiatry Clin Neurosci. 2005;59(1):30–7.
112. Blaszczynski A. Pathological gambling and obsessive-compulsive spectrum disorders. Psychol Rep. 1999;84(1):107–13.
113. Scherrer JF, et al. Associations between obsessive-compulsive classes and pathological gambling in a national cohort of male twins. JAMA Psychiatry. 2015;72(4):342–9.
114. Zohar J, Insel TR. Obsessive-compulsive disorder: psychobiological approaches to diagnosis, treatment, and pathophysiology. Biol Psychiatry. 1987;22(6):667–87.
115. Joel D. Current animal models of obsessive compulsive disorder: a critical review. Prog Neuropsychopharmacol Biol Psychiatry. 2006;30(3):374–88.
116. Joel D, Doljansky J. Selective alleviation of compulsive lever-pressing in rats by D1, but not D2, blockade: possible implications for the involvement of D1 receptors in obsessive-compulsive disorder. Neuropsychopharmacology. 2003;28(1):77–85.

117. Joel D, et al. Role of the orbital cortex and of the serotonergic system in a rat model of obsessive compulsive disorder. Neuroscience. 2005;130(1):25–36.
118. Eagle DM, et al. The dopamine D2/D3 receptor agonist quinpirole increases checking-like behaviour in an operant observing response task with uncertain reinforcement: a novel possible model of OCD. Behav Brain Res. 2014;264:207–29.
119. Diskin KM, Hodgins DC. Narrowing of attention and dissociation in pathological video lottery gamblers. J Gambl Stud. 1999;15(1):17–28.
120. Schüll ND. Addiction by design : machine gambling in Las Vegas. Princeton, NJ: Princeton University Press; 2012. xi, 442p
121. Rachlin H. Why do people gamble and keep gambling despite heavy losses. Psychol Sci. 1990;1(5):294–7.
122. Cavedini P, et al. Frontal lobe dysfunction in pathological gambling patients. Biol Psychiatry. 2002;51(4):334–41.
123. de Visser L, et al. Rodent versions of the iowa gambling task: opportunities and challenges for the understanding of decision-making. Front Neurosci. 2011;5:109.
124. Zeeb FD, Robbins TW, Winstanley CA. Serotonergic and dopaminergic modulation of gambling behavior as assessed using a novel rat gambling task. Neuropsychopharmacology. 2009;34(10):2329–43.
125. Bechara A, et al. Insensitivity to future consequences following damage to human prefrontal cortex. Cognition. 1994;50(1–3):7–15.
126. Bechara A, Tranel D, Damasio H. Characterization of the decision-making deficit of patients with ventromedial prefrontal cortex lesions. Brain. 2000;123(Pt 11):2189–202.
127. Petry NM. Substance abuse, pathological gambling, and impulsiveness. Drug Alcohol Depend. 2001;63(1):29–38.
128. Grant S, Contoreggi C, London ED. Drug abusers show impaired performance in a laboratory test of decision making. Neuropsychologia. 2000;38(8):1180–7.
129. Bechara A, et al. Different contributions of the human amygdala and ventromedial prefrontal cortex to decision-making. J Neurosci. 1999;19(13):5473–81.
130. Jentsch JD, Taylor JR. Impulsivity resulting from frontostriatal dysfunction in drug abuse: implications for the control of behavior by reward-related stimuli. Psychopharmacology. 1999;146(4):373–90.
131. Bechara A. Decision making, impulse control and loss of willpower to resist drugs: a neuro-cognitive perspective. Nat Neurosci. 2005;8(11):1458–63.
132. Paine TA, et al. Medial prefrontal cortex lesions impair decision-making on a rodent gambling task: reversal by D1 receptor antagonist administration. Behav Brain Res. 2013;243:247–54.
133. Zeeb FD, Winstanley CA. Lesions of the basolateral amygdala and orbitofrontal cortex differentially affect acquisition and performance of a rodent gambling task. J Neurosci. 2011;31(6):2197–204.
134. Zeeb FD, Winstanley CA. Functional disconnection of the orbitofrontal cortex and basolateral amygdala impairs acquisition of a rat gambling task and disrupts animals' ability to alter decision-making behavior after reinforcer devaluation. J Neurosci. 2013;33(15):6434–43.
135. Pushparaj A, et al. Differential involvement of the agranular vs granular insular cortex in the acquisition and performance of choice behavior in a rodent gambling task. Neuropsychopharmacology. 2015;40(12):2832–42.
136. Baarendse PJ, Vanderschuren LJ. Dissociable effects of monoamine reuptake inhibitors on distinct forms of impulsive behavior in rats. Psychopharmacology. 2012;219(2):313–26.
137. Baarendse PJ, Winstanley CA, Vanderschuren LJ. Simultaneous blockade of dopamine and noradrenaline reuptake promotes disadvantageous decision making in a rat gambling task. Psychopharmacology. 2013;225(3):719–31.
138. Zeeb FD, Wong AC, Winstanley CA. Differential effects of environmental enrichment, social-housing, and isolation-rearing on a rat gambling task: dissociations between impulsive action and risky decision-making. Psychopharmacology. 2013;225(2):381–95.
139. Denk F, et al. Differential involvement of serotonin and dopamine systems in cost-benefit decisions about delay or effort. Psychopharmacology. 2005;179(3):587–96.

140. Salamone JD, et al. Nucleus accumbens dopamine depletions make animals highly sensitive to high fixed ratio requirements but do not impair primary food reinforcement. Neuroscience. 2001;105(4):863–70.
141. Nowend KL, et al. D1 or D2 antagonism in nucleus accumbens core or dorsomedial shell suppresses lever pressing for food but leads to compensatory increases in chow consumption. Pharmacol Biochem Behav. 2001;69(3–4):373–82.
142. Floresco SB, Tse MT, Ghods-Sharifi S. Dopaminergic and glutamatergic regulation of effort- and delay-based decision making. Neuropsychopharmacology. 2008;33(8):1966–79.
143. Hosking JG, Floresco SB, Winstanley CA. Dopamine antagonism decreases willingness to expend physical, but not cognitive, effort: a comparison of two rodent cost/benefit decision-making tasks. Neuropsychopharmacology. 2015;40(4):1005–15.
144. Cardinal RN, Howes NJ. Effects of lesions of the nucleus accumbens core on choice between small certain rewards and large uncertain rewards in rats. BMC Neurosci. 2005;6:37.
145. St Onge JR, Floresco SB. Dopaminergic modulation of risk-based decision making. Neuropsychopharmacology. 2009;34(3):681–97.
146. Simon NW, et al. Balancing risk and reward: a rat model of risky decision making. Neuropsychopharmacology. 2009;34(10):2208–17.
147. Simon NW, et al. Dopaminergic modulation of risky decision-making. J Neurosci. 2011;31(48):17460–70.
148. Cocker PJ, et al. Irrational choice under uncertainty correlates with lower striatal D(2/3) receptor binding in rats. J Neurosci. 2012;32(44):15450–7.
149. Barrus MM, et al. Inactivation of the orbitofrontal cortex reduces irrational choice on a rodent Betting Task. Neuroscience. 2017;345:38–48.
150. Tremblay M, et al. Dissociable effects of basolateral amygdala lesions on decision making biases in rats when loss or gain is emphasized. Cogn Affect Behav Neurosci. 2014;14(4):1184–95.
151. Volkow ND, et al. Imaging dopamine's role in drug abuse and addiction. Neuropharmacology. 2009;56(Suppl 1):3–8.
152. Dalley JW, et al. Nucleus Accumbens D2/3 receptors predict trait impulsivity and cocaine reinforcement. Science. 2007;315(5816):1267–70.
153. Tremblay M, et al. Chronic D2/3 agonist ropinirole treatment increases preference for uncertainty in rats regardless of baseline choice patterns. Eur J Neurosci. 2017;45(1):159–66.
154. Robinson TE, Berridge KC. Addiction. Annu Rev Psychol. 2003;54:25–53.
155. Robinson TE, Berridge KC. Incentive-sensitization and addiction. Addiction. 2001;96(1):103–14.
156. Field M, Cox WM. Attentional bias in addictive behaviors: a review of its development, causes, and consequences. Drug Alcohol Depend. 2008;97(1–2):1–20.
157. Loba P, et al. Manipulations of the features of standard video lottery terminal (VLT) games: effects in pathological and non-pathological gamblers. J Gambl Stud. 2001;17(4):297–320.
158. Honsi A, et al. Attentional bias in problem gambling: a systematic review. J Gambl Stud. 2013;29(3):359–75.
159. Barrus MM, Cherkasova M, Winstanley CA. Skewed by cues? The motivational role of audiovisual stimuli in modelling substance use and gambling disorders. Curr Top Behav Neurosci. 2016;27:507–29.
160. Barrus MM, Winstanley CA. Dopamine D3 receptors modulate the ability of win-paired cues to increase risky choice in a rat gambling task. J Neurosci. 2016;36(3):785–94.
161. Di Ciano P, et al. The impact of selective dopamine D2, D3 and D4 ligands on the rat gambling task. PLoS One. 2015;10(9):e0136267.
162. Heidbreder CA, Newman AH. Current perspectives on selective dopamine D(3) receptor antagonists as pharmacotherapeutics for addictions and related disorders. Ann N Y Acad Sci. 2010;1187:4–34.
163. Le Foll B, Goldberg SR, Sokoloff P. The dopamine D3 receptor and drug dependence: effects on reward or beyond? Neuropharmacology. 2005;49(4):525–41.

164. Xi ZX, et al. Blockade of mesolimbic dopamine D3 receptors inhibits stress-induced rein-statement of cocaine-seeking in rats. Psychopharmacology. 2004;176(1):57–65.
165. Higley AE, et al. Dopamine D(3) receptor antagonist SB-277011A inhibits methamphet-amine self-administration and methamphetamine-induced reinstatement of drug-seeking in rats. Eur J Pharmacol. 2011;659(2–3):187–92.
166. Berridge KC, Robinson TE. What is the role of dopamine in reward: hedonic impact, reward learning, or incentive salience? Brain Res Brain Res Rev. 1998;28(3):309–69.
167. Flagel SB, et al. Individual differences in the propensity to approach signals vs goals promote different adaptations in the dopamine system of rats. Psychopharmacology. 2007;191(3):599–607.
168. Flagel SB, et al. A selective role for dopamine in stimulus-reward learning. Nature. 2011;469(7328):53–7.
169. Di Ciano P, et al. Differential involvement of NMDA, AMPA/kainate, and dopamine recep-tors in the nucleus accumbens core in the acquisition and performance of pavlovian approach behavior. J Neurosci. 2001;21(23):9471–7.
170. Berridge KC, Robinson TE. Parsing reward. Trends Neurosci. 2003;26(9):507–13.
171. Dickinson A, Smith J, Mirenowicz J. Dissociation of Pavlovian and instrumental incentive learning under dopamine antagonists. Behav Neurosci. 2000;114(3):468–83.
172. Wolterink G, et al. Relative roles of ventral striatal D1 and D2 dopamine receptors in respond-ing with conditioned reinforcement. Psychopharmacology. 1993;110(3):355–64.
173. Beninger RJ, Ranaldi R. The effects of amphetamine, apomorphine, Skf-38393, quin-pirole and bromocriptine on responding for conditioned reward in rats. Behav Pharmacol. 1992;3(2):155–63.
174. Beninger RJ, Phillips AG. The effects of pimozide during pairing on the transfer of classical conditioning to an operant discrimination. Pharmacol Biochem Behav. 1981;14(1):101–5.
175. Fletcher PJ, Higgins GA. Differential effects of ondansetron and alpha-flupenthixol on responding for conditioned reward. Psychopharmacology. 1997;134(1):64–72.
176. Sutton MA, Rolfe NG, Beninger RJ. Biphasic effects of 7-OH-DPAT on the acquisition of responding for conditioned reward in rats. Pharmacol Biochem Behav. 2001;69(1–2):195–200.
177. Day JJ, et al. Nucleus accumbens neurons encode Pavlovian approach behaviors: evidence from an autoshaping paradigm. Eur J Neurosci. 2006;23(5):1341–51.
178. Hall J, et al. Involvement of the central nucleus of the amygdala and nucleus accum-bens core in mediating Pavlovian influences on instrumental behaviour. Eur J Neurosci. 2001;13(10):1984–92.
179. Taylor JR, Robbins TW. Enhanced behavioural control by conditioned reinforcers follow-ing microinjections of d-amphetamine into the nucleus accumbens. Psychopharmacology. 1984;84(3):405–12.
180. Everitt BJ, Wolf ME. Psychomotor stimulant addiction: a neural systems perspective. J Neurosci. 2002;22(9):3312–20.
181. Cocker PJ, Vonder Haar C, Winstanley CA. Elucidating the role of D4 receptors in mediating attributions of salience to incentive stimuli on Pavlovian conditioned approach and condi-tioned reinforcement paradigms. Behav Brain Res. 2016;312:55–63.
182. Fraser KM, et al. Examining the role of dopamine D2 and D3 receptors in Pavlovian condi-tioned approach behaviors. Behav Brain Res. 2016;305:87–99.
183. Zeeb FD, et al. Low impulsive action, but not impulsive choice, predicts greater con-ditioned reinforcer salience and augmented nucleus accumbens dopamine release. Neuropsychopharmacology. 2016;41(8):2091–100.
184. Yang Y, et al. Positive association between trait impulsivity and high gambling-related cogni-tive biases among college students. Psychiatry Res. 2016;243:71–4.
185. Marsden CA. Dopamine: the rewarding years. Br J Pharmacol. 2006;147(Suppl 1):S136–44.
186. Jaber M, et al. Dopamine receptors and brain function. Neuropharmacology. 1996;35(11):1503–19.

The Neurobiology of Gambling Disorder: Neuroscientific Studies and Computational Perspectives

7

Alexander Genauck and Nina Romanczuk-Seiferth

At a Glance This chapter gives an overview on neurobehavioral findings concerning gambling disorder (GD) [1–3]. We classify studies into classical and computational psychiatry studies and into three categories related to different symptom clusters: loss of control, craving, and neglect of other areas in life [3]. Studies using classical analyses are those that set into relationship measured random variables by estimating their respective means, variances, and covariances. Computational psychiatry studies and computational analyses are those that explicitly assume one or several cognitive-computational processes responsible for generating the data [4]. Analyses could involve reinforcement learning models fit to behavioral choice data [5, 6] or neural network models fit to brain data [7]. Computational psychiatry aims at taking a closer look at processes underlying psychological disorders. Note that we will also use a computational psychiatry perspective when reporting on the classical neurobiological GD studies here. This means we will review primary research articles with respect to computationally relevant processes such as cue reactivity, response inhibition, gain and loss processing, uncertainty, and delay processing as well as learning from reward and punishment.

A. Genauck (✉)
Department of Psychiatry and Psychotherapy, Charité—Universitätsmedizin Berlin, Berlin, Germany

Bernstein Center for Computational Neuroscience Berlin, Berlin, Germany
e-mail: alexander.genauck@charite.de

N. Romanczuk-Seiferth
Department of Psychiatry and Psychotherapy, Charité—Universitätsmedizin Berlin, Berlin, Germany
e-mail: nina.seiferth@charite.de

© Springer Nature Switzerland AG 2019
A. Heinz et al. (eds.), *Gambling Disorder*, https://doi.org/10.1007/978-3-030-03060-5_7

7.1 Introduction

7.1.1 General

Gambling disorder (GD) is characterized by continued gambling for money despite severe negative consequences. Here gambling is defined as "placing something of value at risk in the hopes of gaining something" [1]. GD has been a growing health concern [8–11]. Burdens of GD patients include loss of social structures, developing psychiatric comorbidities, as well as financial ruin [12, 13]. Recently, GD has been classified as an addiction alongside substance-use disorders (SUDs), such as alcohol or cocaine dependence [14]. This new classification was indicated because GD and SUDs are characterized by similar core symptoms (including craving, withdrawal, tolerance) and because both GD and SUDs show similar neurobehavioral signatures [3, 15–19]. Specifically in SUDs and GD, relevant core functions such as cue reactivity, response inhibition, and reward-based decision-making have been associated with changes in the dopaminergic reward network including the striatum and prefrontal cortex [2, 20–32]. Note that GD studies concerning these functional alterations in addiction allow conclusions regarding the biopsychological core features of addictive disorders in general. This is because GD is an addictive disorder itself but may develop without the influence of an external psychotropic substance. Thus, investigating GD allows us to understand better how addictive disorders can develop through the interactions of bio-psycho-social vulnerabilities with learning processes. The mentioned studies have mostly been based on qualitative or statistical models of neural functioning leading to valuable but flashlight evidence of changes in the neural system of people suffering from GD. As a response, computational psychiatry has pushed toward applying quantitative behavioral models to characterize more comprehensively deviations in neural functioning in psychological disorders [5, 33–37]. Computational models of behavior and brain functioning try to mathematically formulate a supposed mechanism and often make more precise and more quantitative predictions than classical statistical approaches in psychiatric research [38, 39].

This chapter aims at summarizing the neurobehavioral findings regarding GD from a computational psychiatry perspective and presents recent studies which already use computational models (CMs) of GD behavior. This text would like to argue that computational modeling of behavioral and neural data may enhance the sensitivity, specificity, and interpretability of GD studies and as such is a valuable addition to the toolbox of GD researchers.

7.1.2 Neurobiological Research in GD

Neurobiological research in GD has been greatly influenced by neurobiological research of SUDs. The Impaired Response Inhibition and Salience Attribution (I-RISA) model [40] connects two core features of SUDs which have striking parallels in GD [18]. Impaired salience attribution (the "I-SA" in I-RISA) relates to the influential incentive sensitization theory [41]. The theory states that in addiction the meso-cortico-limbic reward network is sensitized to stimuli (cues) that are associated with the drug or addictive behavior and desensitized to cues that signal other rewards. In other words, drug-related cues (e.g., pictures of alcoholic beverages, a certain smell) get special salience and thus grab attention. According to the theory, cues, when attended to, produce or amplify craving. In a state of withdrawal, the effect of attention grabbing and amplification of craving is enhanced. Impaired response inhibition (the "I-RI" in I-RISA) refers to the fact that SUD and GD subjects show heightened impulsivity—in the widest sense of the word as it is to note that there is a variability of definitions used for "impulsivity" [42, 43]. This could include a difficulty to suppress automatic stimulus-induced responses or a tendency to opt for riskier activities. Response inhibition refers mainly to the former and is thus defined as the process of inhibiting a prepotent, initiated, or automatic response [40]. Impaired decision-making is a hallmark of SUDs and GD [14, 16, 44–46]. Although impaired decision-making may be partly explained or influenced by impaired response inhibition, there are still processes in risky decision-making (namely, the process of deliberation and weighing of alternatives) that are qualitatively different from response inhibition [47]. In that sense the I-RISA framework should be expanded and called the I-RISADM (Impaired Response Inhibition, Salience Attribution and Decision Making) framework.

7.1.3   Computational Models

Computational models are used to model the mechanics of complex systems such as the brain. Psychologists and psychiatrists are interested in studying psychiatric phenomena such as anhedonia, hallucinations, or addiction. These ailments are constructs but eventually product of multiple layers of substrate, such as proteins, neurotransmitters, neurons, neural networks, as well as social networks. Computational models help us to connect those different layers of abstraction by formulating data-driven or strictly theory-driven models [38]. Importantly, computational models model the mechanisms and dynamics of processes leading to a certain phenomenon. This means researchers applying computational models essentially do this by building complex simulations of the brain or parts of it in order to generate predictions concerning the dependent variable and concerning the data generating process. In addiction research, computational models have mainly been reinforcement learning models simulating impaired learning from reward and punishment [48] or impaired decision-making [49].

7.2   Classical Studies on the Neurobiology of Gambling Disorder

7.2.1   Loss of Control

The symptom cluster "loss of control" mainly describes problems such as escalation of gambling, gambling more than planned, as well as experiencing difficulty to stop or inhibit gambling [14]. Loss of control on clinical level has been associated with impaired response inhibition in laboratory experiments [3]. GD subjects show increased levels of impulsiveness and low self-control using both questionnaires and response inhibition tasks [18, 50, 51]. GD relapse seems to be predictable using performance scores from response inhibition tasks [52].

7.2.1.1 Stopping a Primed Action

Loss of control may be grounded in the ability to inhibit actions, such as demanded in a go/no-go task. It has been observed that GD subjects show diminished response inhibition on the go/no-go task [53, 54]. van Holst et al. [55] have observed that problem gamblers (PRGs) are overall slower in this task but that they profit more from gamble pictures being associated with the go response than HC subjects (making less errors at inhibiting the no-go response). On neural level, this has been associated with stronger activity in VS, DLPFC, and anterior cingulate cortex (ACC) in PRG subjects during gamble pictures (go trials) present and lower activation of the DLPFC and ACC during no-go trials (neutral pictures). During neutral inhibition trials (go and no-go coupled with neutral pictures), PRGs were slower but performed similarly accurate as HCs. During these trials, PRGs showed more DLPFC and ACC activity. Gambling-related stimuli hence seem to be more salient for PRGs than for HCs. PRGs seem to rely on compensatory brain activity to achieve similar performance during response inhibition in a neutral context. However, gambling-related pictures (during go trials) appear to facilitate neutrally contextualized response inhibition as indicated by lower brain activity and fewer behavioral errors in PRGs during no-go trials. Note that this means that cue reactivity has an influence on performance of a response inhibition task. A computational model could capture, e.g., the pre-activation of certain brain areas by certain cues—brain areas that are needed for response inhibition or initiation [56].

7.2.1.2 Stopping a Primed Action and Choosing Another

Several studies using the Stroop task have shown increased problems for GD subjects to inhibit a prepotent response and choosing another [50, 57–59], although the predictive power of the Stroop task for GD relapse is being questioned [52]. Stroop tasks work by creating interference between a fast automatic response and a more difficult to produce but needed response. In the classical case, subjects need to name the color of the ink of a word which itself is the name of a color. Other versions use an emotional Stroop, where the words may be gambling related or neutral and subjects have to name the color of the word. A study by Potenza et al. (2013) [60] suggests that GD subjects in response to infrequent incongruent stimuli showed decreased activity in the left ventromedial prefrontal cortex (VMPFC) in comparison to HC subjects. It has further been shown that this VS activity is inversely correlated with gambling severity and also more positively correlated with treatment outcome. In other words, the more similar the neural activity related to Stroop performance is to the activity in healthy controls, the more it is associated with reduced symptom severity and increased propensity for successful treatment outcome. Hence, intact cognitive control, as indicated by specific functional magnetic resonance imaging (fMRI) activity in VS and VMPFC, may be a decisive component for successful therapy.

7.2.1.3 Stopping an Initiated Action

The ability to stop an already initiated action seems to be impaired in GD subjects [50]. Interestingly, the size of this effect has been predictive of relapse, while impulsivity questionnaire scores have not [52]. However, another study has not found diminished performance in GD in a similar task to test for the ability to stop an already initiated action, but a general decreased activity of the DMPFC during both successful and failed response inhibition [61].

7.2.1.4 Summary

GD subjects consistently show diminished response inhibition. This seems to be related to different functioning of DLPFC, ACC, VS, and MPFC. Response inhibition scores and associated neural signatures seem relevant in predicting treatment outcome, relapse, and symptom severity.

7.2.2   Craving

In addiction research, craving and withdrawal symptoms have been mostly explained by the incentive sensitization theory [41]. Two neurobehavioral paradigms have thus received special attention: attentional bias and cue reactivity. A meta-analysis has shown across various SUDs a modest but significant correlation of $r = 0.19$ between attentional bias for drug-related stimuli and craving [62]. This underlines the relationship between the two concepts. Also cue reactivity has repeatedly been linked to subjective craving [63].

Cue reactivity as a neurobehavioral paradigm tests for the effect of addiction-related stimuli on brain activity and behavior [21]. In SUDs, there is a rather consistent picture of enhanced activity increase in ventral striatum (VS), ventral medial prefrontal cortex (VMPFC), precuneus, temporal pole, cingulum, and other regions toward drug cues compared to HC subjects [64, 65]. The picture in GD is similar albeit a little less consistent.

Self-reported craving has been reported to be correlated with activations in the temporal pole in GD subjects [66]. Interestingly, unlike in SUD subject, GD compared to HC subjects have shown *diminished* activation of VMPFC, VS, cingulate, insula, inferior frontal gyrus (IFG), and other regions during exposure to gambling cues [67]. However, another study found *increased* activation of bilateral occipital cortex (visual processing) and subcortical (amygdala, parahippocampus) regions in problem-gambling subjects during cue exposure compared to HC subjects [68]. Exposed to video cues, GD subjects responded with increased craving and increased dorsolateral prefrontal (DLPFC), parahippocampal, and fusiform gyrus responses [69]. Further, GD subjects rated gambling cues more positively arousing than HC subjects and showed a larger late positivity component in the electroencephalogram (EEG) in response to gambling cues which is indicative of more emotional processing [70]. A recent study observed that gambling but not food cues lead to changes/correlation with subjective craving with respect to brain activity and functional connectivity in a reward-related circuitry (including ACC, VS, MPFC) [71]. Findings like this suggest enhanced cue reactivity in GD subjects that may be the result of learned motivated attention inducing subjective craving and relapse [70]. Indeed, GD subjects accompanied to real-life gambling situations reported higher craving when in the casino. However, this cue reactivity ceased with time spent in the casino and when subjects engaged in a negative mood induction task [72].

Gambling cues indeed increase craving as measured with subjective scales in GD subjects. Cue reactivity neural response patterns are complex and show some inconsistency across studies. Investigating cue reactivity in the context of specific gambling tasks may make neural cue reactivity signatures more specific. Cue reactivity may alter gain and loss sensitivity of the striatum, as well as response inhibition processes [73–75]. It may also modulate other decision-making processes [76].

7.2.3 Neglect of Other Areas in Life

Neglect of other areas in life may be regarded as the symptom cluster reflecting impaired decision-making in patients suffering from addictive disorders [3]. GD subjects engage in high-risk gambles instead of naturally rewarding activities. Further, they pursue these activities with relentless energy and vigor, showing great motivation (against literally all odds). Impaired decision-making may be due to impaired anticipation of rewards, punishments, delays, and probabilities, as well as altered processing of decision outcomes.

7.2.3.1 Gain Processing

Decisions to gamble are essentially value-based decisions. The investigation of gain or reward processing in the context of value-based decision-making is of great importance because it directly relates to the reward deficiency hypothesis (RDH) and the incentive salience hypothesis (ISH) of addiction [40, 77]. The RDH of addiction states that people suffering from addiction keep engaging in the addictive behavior to avoid a hypo-dopaminergic state. Natural rewards lead to too little subjective reward or dopamine (DA) transmission, so that a DA promoting substance has to be ingested [77]. The RDH has been challenged in the field of GD research [78]. The incentive salience hypothesis of addiction sees impaired gain processing as the result of increased salience for addiction-related stimuli and decreased salience of stimuli signaling natural rewards [41].

Gain processing needs to be dealt with at no less than two stages of the decision-making process. This is during the anticipatory and the outcome phase of any value-based decision [79]. During the anticipation, the subject needs to assess possible gains and process their magnitude, probability, and delay. During the outcome phase, the subject actually receives the gain and may use it. In that sense, the anticipation phase elicits motivation to approach ("wanting"), while the outcome phase elicits pleasure ("liking"). Comparing the expected with the actual gain received during the outcome phase constitutes the so-called prediction error which is essential to any learning process [80–83].

Anticipation

GD is related to strong feelings of wanting with respect to gambling for monetary wins [3]. This lets us suppose that gamblers should show a stronger DA signal in the VS region when anticipating uncertain rewards compared to HC [84]. The monetary incentive delay (MID) task measures affect and action vigor (response speed) related to anticipation of monetary gains [79]. Studies using this task have shown that GD subjects rather show decreased gain anticipatory activation in VS [85–87] or that there is no difference in gain anticipation between GD and HC subjects [30]. Within GD subjects, the abstinence and duration of illness correlated with insula activity [87]. It is important to note that the four mentioned studies did not use gambling stimuli in the MID task while it has been suggested that monetary gain anticipation in GD might only be altered if contextual stimuli are gambling related [73, 75]. Sescousse et al. [78] investigated gain anticipation under different contexts using different reward types: subjects could work for monetary rewards or erotic stimulus rewards. The authors used a modified MID task and observed that GD subjects profit from monetary reward (in comparison to erotic stimuli as rewards) because it decreased their reaction times. HC subjects did not show a difference in reaction times between the two reward types. Importantly, this behavioral effect seemed to be driven by a blunted reactivity in the VS toward erotic stimuli rather than an enhanced reactivity toward anticipated monetary rewards.

In some tasks we can distinguish a second kind of anticipation phase, i.e., the anticipation phase after response, but before the outcome is presented. We can call this waiting anticipation. Since the outcome is probabilistic and a bit delayed, an expectation is built up, what will come. This is especially visible in single-line slot machines with three wheels: here, if two wheels have settled and show two with identical pictures, the third wheel will be of utmost interest: an anticipation of a win will be generated, without the subject having to respond or making a decision, but simply having to wait.

In the MID task, there is such a waiting period after the response has been made but before the outcome is presented. In this period, the subject has a feeling of how well they performed on the fast-response task and they have a feeling about how certain a positive outcome is given that they were fast enough. This generates a prediction of the outcome. We could assume GD subjects to be overly optimistic and have stronger anticipatory affect during waiting gain anticipation. Indeed, a study by Worhunsky et al. [88] has observed that GD subjects show stronger activity in mesolimbic and ventro-cortical regions (especially VS) than HC during third-wheel reward anticipation. However, the study by Balodis et al. [85] has observed reduced activation in VMPFC and VS in GD during MID waiting gain anticipation. Hence, more studies are needed to understand the reactivity in GD subjects during waiting for the outcome phase.

Decision-making

So far we have talked about how GD subjects process gain in anticipation of a possible outcome and when they have to show a predetermined speedy response to achieve it or even just have to wait for it. But what about gain anticipation during more complex value-based decision-making? What if the subject does not only have to press a button fast enough and in the right moment but has to choose between various options with different uncertain outcomes? After all, many gambles, such as black jack, poker, and roulette, ask the gambler to pick the option which he or she thinks is most favorable. Importantly, also the decision to go to a gambling place (e.g., a casino) or do something else (meet friends) is a value-based decision in itself. However, perhaps contrary to intuition, there are only two studies which report altered (neural) gain processing during decision phases [74, 89].

The loss aversion (LA) paradigm allows us to disentangle gain and loss sensitivity during value-based decision-making [90]. In a study in our own group [89], we have found that GD subjects in a LA task show reduced loss aversion, however, only due to decreased loss sensitivity but not decreased gain sensitivity. This means GD subjects did not respond more strongly with ever more gamble acceptance if gains increased compared to HC subjects. However, GD subjects showed faster reaction times with gains increasing, contrary to HC subjects. This may be an indicator for faster evidence gathering in GD subjects, when gains are increasing [7]. GD subjects also showed a stronger gain-related functional connectivity from amygdala to bilateral posterior OFC compared to HC, which may mean that amygdala enhances the representation of gain values in the posterior OFC. This may lead to decreased loss aversion because losses are becoming less salient with gains increasing. In line with this, another study has found enhanced dorsal striatal activation with increasing gains during the decision phase in a guessing task [74].

Outcome

So far we have asked if gain anticipation or "wanting" is different in GD subjects. But do GD subjects also show differing "liking" processes? Do they like monetary gains more than HC subjects? Or do they, as the RDH would suggest, like them less and that is why they have to accumulate more to reach the same level of satisfaction? The study by Sescousse et al. [78] looked at the processing of cued outcomes. There were no differences in liking ratings both with respect to monetary and erotic stimuli. However, the authors observed in GD compared to HC subjects that monetary rewards elicited a response more in the posterior (as opposed to expected anterior) regions of the orbitofrontal cortex (OFC). This region is known to represent more primary reinforcers (e.g., sex and food). Further, during the outcome phase, the liking ratings of subjects correlated with the VS signal in response to monetary outcomes in both groups but in the case of erotic stimuli only in HC subjects. The authors interpreted that erotic stimuli in GD subjects, i.e., a natural reinforcer, cannot reliably be translated into a neural signal of motivation, perhaps explaining why erotic stimuli, i.e., a natural reinforcer, do not enhance approach motivation anymore. These results show us that money for GD subjects may not be more or less pleasurable but work more as primary reinforcers than actual primary reinforcers.

In contrast, another study [91] observed no differences between GD and HC subjects in neural representation of reward outcome during an MID task. Yet, looking more closely at the GD group, it became apparent that the insula signal during gain outcome presentation was higher in depressed subjects than in non-depressed GD subjects. This result highlights the need for subclassifications within the category of GD according to comorbid symptomatology and reminds us that GD samples often are very heterogeneous. Another study using a single-line slot machine task also did not find differences between GD and HC subjects during reward receipt [88].

In contrast, Reuter et al. [92] in a simple card-guessing task with gain and loss outcomes and illusionary choice observed reduced activity in response to reward receipt in VS and VMPFC in GD subjects, which was inversely correlated with GD severity. This means, in line with the RDH, that the stronger the activity in VS and VMPFC during reward receipt, the lower the GD severity.

In a seminal study by Miedl et al. [93], researchers let GD subjects play blackjack and compared them to occasional gamblers (OG). Subjects had to choose whether to hit or stand and received an outcome on every trial. During wins compared to losses, OG and GD subjects both showed similar activity in VS and posterior cingulate. However, GD subjects showed stronger activation than OG in right superior frontal and parietal areas, which the authors of this study interpreted as an activation of gambling-related action sequences stored in memory, perhaps to already prepare subsequent gambling.

Habib and Dixon [94] found that GD subjects in a slot machine task had no overlap with OG in their network of activated brain regions after winning outcomes. This network included bilateral temporal, parietal, and cingulate areas, bilateral cuneus, postcentral gyrus, the uncus extending into the amygdala bilaterally, cerebellum, brainstem, and inferior frontal gyrus.

Using a gambling task simulating real-life risky decision-making (the Iowa Gambling Task, IGT), another study has observed differences in gain outcome processing [95]. In this study, GD subjects decreased their heart rate after losses and wins, whereas the HC group showed a decrease in heart rate after losses but an increase in HR after wins. Absence of a HR increase after wins may imply that reward sensitivity is decreased in GD, the authors suggested. However, another study found no differences in neural responses to gain outcomes in the IGT [96].

We have seen that with respect to gain outcome processing, GD subjects show more pervasive brain networks coding for gain outcome and different peripheral physiological outcomes. In addition, it seems that gain outcome signal from classical reward-associated brain areas (VS, VMPFC, and VLPFC) is reduced. These results may interact with comorbid symptoms such as depression.

Summary

Monetary and natural gain anticipation seems to be blunted in the VS in GD subjects. In decision-making, increasing possible gains seem to lead to faster decisions and altered reactivity in parietal and dorsal striatal areas during the decision phase. There is ample evidence for altered neural processing in GD subjects during reward receipt.

7.2.3.2 Loss Processing

Loss processing in the context of gambling disorder is manifold just like gain processing. On the one hand, studies have investigated whether GD subjects anticipate losses in a different way than HC subjects. Researchers have asked whether GD subjects are more or less motivated when losses are at stake. On the other hand, studies have investigated how GD subjects react differently toward actual loss outcomes than HC subjects. Do they care less about losses or are losses even rewarding to them? Finally, researchers have also asked whether GD subjects learn differently from loss and punishments than HC subjects.

Anticipation

VS activity in the MID task has been observed increased compared to HC subjects during loss avoidance trials [30]. This may support the idea that losses at stake have a positive motivational impact on GD subject. Note that in real life avoiding losses means not being more vigorous but usually means to refrain from gambling all together—especially at slot machines. However, Balodis et al. [85] and Choi et al. [86] have seen decreased activation during loss anticipation in the same MID task in VS and in the ventro-medial caudate, respectively. In gain anticipation, we also introduced waiting anticipation. Note that in a slot machine task, there is no loss-related waiting period. In the MID task, Balodis et al. [85] report no group differences during waiting anticipation of losses.

Decision-making

Loss processing in static (one-shot) value-based decisions boils down to loss sensitivity or in other words anticipation of possible negative outcomes. This feature of the decision-making process can be well studied using the aforementioned LA task [90]. In the LA task, subjects are offered coin flip gambles with gain and loss outcomes of different magnitude. Subjects decide how much they feel motivated to take each gamble. By many gamble offerings and thus many answers by the participants, it is possible to compute their decision-related gain and loss sensitivity. We may define LA as the ratio of these sensitivities (sensitivity to loss/sensitivity to gain). LA has been observed reduced in GD subjects [25, 89, 97–100] and correlated with increased cognitive gambling-related distortions [89]. The reduction of LA is mainly seen in nonstrategic gamblers who have not yet received therapy. On neural level, LA is driven by brain areas such as the VS, the MPFC, insula, and amygdala which code for both gain and loss [90, 101, 102]. The study by Gelskov et al. [25] comparing GD and HC subjects on a LA task observed that GD showed stronger activation than HC subjects to extreme gambles (very favorable and very unfavorable) in a cortico-striatal executive network. Genauck et al. [89] observed that GD subjects displayed a decreased loss-related amygdala-VMPFC connectivity which may disturb a proper cost-benefit evaluation in this group [7, 103]. Loss sensitivity and LA seem to be reduced in GD subjects. This may be reflective of altered task-related brain connectivity, cortico-striatal functioning, and related to increased cognitive gambling-related distortions.

Outcome

After anticipation of losses and evaluation of losses during decisions, how do GD subjects react differently from HC subjects when actually experiencing losses? In line with the idea of losses as a motivating factor, GD subjects have been observed to respond with faster reaction times after losses, unlike HC subjects [53]. The study by Worhunsky et al. [88] showed a generally reduced neural reactivity in GD subjects compared to HC subjects during loss outcomes. Habib and Dixon [94] found similar evidence, while another study found no differences [96]. Habib and Dixon [94] found reduced activity after loss outcomes in the midbrain, an area known to code for prediction errors [83]. Further, they found that the unique network activating for losses in HC subjects was extensive, while in PG subjects it only comprised the superior parietal lobule (SPL). Also reduced loss outcome activity in the middle frontal gyrus and VMPFC was negatively associated with a GD symptom severity score. The study by Romanczuk-Seiferth et al. [30] found diminished activity in GD subjects during successful loss avoidance pointing to the possibility that subjects may not feel positively or learn from the fact that they were successful in loss avoidance. Hence, there is ample evidence that GD subjects tend to respond with blunted neural activity when experiencing losses which may be associated with increased GD symptom severity and higher gambling motivation in subsequent trials.

In gambling not all losses are simply losses. Losses that were attained but were almost a win are called "near misses." A near miss is most commonly seen in multi-wheel slot machines where the wheels successively stop. In the case of three wheels, when the first two wheels are showing the same symbol (AA), then the gambler can win. When the third wheel then shows a different symbol (AAB), then the gambler almost won, i.e., had a near miss. Research has shown that these losses are qualitatively different from normal losses [104]. It also seems that some people are motivated by near misses to gamble more [105–107], perhaps because it is interpreted as a signal that they are getting better at the game.

The study by Clark et al. [108] found that in healthy participants, near misses were rated as less pleasant than full misses. Interestingly, near miss outcomes recruited insula and striatal areas which also responded to monetary wins. What was missing in the near misses win circuitry in comparison to the real win circuitry was the activation of the rostral ACC (rACC). Depending on whether the subjects could exert control over the gamble (arranging the gamble vs. watching the computer arranging the gamble), rACC was activated during near misses in the high-control trials, and the opposite was true during low-control trials. This study shows that losses, when they are near-misses in high-control situations, can neurally be very similar to wins. Further, near miss neural reactivity in the midbrain has been shown correlated with gambling severity in regular (but not all GD) gamblers [109].

In contrast, the study by Worhunsky et al. [88], reporting on high-severity GD subjects, found that GD subjects showed diminished reactivity in VS compared to HC subjects during near misses which was interpreted as lower salience of these incidences. Non-GD gamblers in turn showed increased reactivity toward near misses vs. full misses in the VS and related areas.

Habib and Dixon [94] recruited more low-severity GD subjects and found that this group uniquely activated the right inferior occipital gyrus, the right uncus extending into the amygdala, the midbrain, and the cerebellum in response to near misses. They thus showed an activation pattern closer to wins than to losses, while in non-GD subjects this was the other way around. It thus seems that especially regular gamblers or low-severity GD subjects on neural level display near misses as more win-like. High-severity GD subjects, in turn, seem to react with a generally blunted loss outcome signal, as we have seen already with normal losses.

Summary
Increased loss anticipation signal in VS plus decreased loss-related activity during successful loss avoidance may explain increased gambling. This is because GD subjects may feel increased motivation to avoid losses but not feel enough satisfaction when actually being successful in avoiding losses. We have also seen that GD subjects display reduced LA, i.e., a reduced inhibition to accept gambles despite high losses at stake. In addition, regular gamblers seem to be motivated from near misses as if they were gains, while GD subjects generally display a decreased reactivity in VS and other regions toward losses. The progression from regular gambling to GD may thus correlate with progressive loss outcome desensitization. Decreased sensitivity to negative reinforcement [30, 110] as well as decreased sensitivity to losses may be supporting factors for loss chasing (gambling more to make up for losses) which further abets GD symptoms.

7.2.3.3 Uncertainty
So far, we have looked at gain and loss sensitivity because gains and losses are the possible outcomes of any gamble. However, the fundamental feature of any gamble is uncertainty. Gambles are by definition "risky," i.e., associated with uncertain outcomes. If we are unsure about an outcome O of an action α, it means O may turn out to be A or B. This is only important if A and B have different values. For example, the value of A might be smaller than the value of B. If I do not know which outcome O will take effect, in case I choose action α, then I am uncertain about $O(\alpha)$. This uncertainty can come now in two different flavors: choosing α may be risky or ambiguous [111]. If it is risky, then the gambler knows the probabilities (P) of the outcomes and is, technically, able to compute the expected value (EV) of α.

$$EV(\alpha) = P(A) * value(A) + P(B) * value(B) \qquad (7.1)$$

The expected value is the average outcome of the action if I were to choose that action an infinite number of times under the same conditions. The risk can then be defined as [112]:

$$Risk(\alpha) = P(A) * (value(A) - EV(\alpha))^2 + P(B) * (value(B) - EV(\alpha))^2 \quad (7.2)$$

High risk thus means high variance in the outcome. The higher the risk, the less informative the EV. Note that this risk assessment is objective. This means that it is computable by a computer if all the variables are known, but it does not mean that it is computed necessarily by a human to base their decision on. Still the EV and the risk (i.e., of an action outcome $O(\alpha)$) may be used as experimental manipulations to check how subjects react to that.

Yet, there is another form of uncertainty, as already mentioned, which is ambiguity. The outcome of an action is ambiguous when the values but not the probabilities are known to the subject. This case is actually much more common in real gambling situations. Subjects have a vague idea or must learn the probabilities of certain outcomes. Subjects may have a general idea whether an action has higher or lower risk, but they cannot completely be sure of it.

Risk

As mentioned risky gambles are defined as gambles where the probabilities of all action outcomes are known. Researchers have asked how GD subjects react toward risky gambles. Is high risk exciting for them? Is it motivating? Are GD subjects less risk averse than HC subjects? Note that high risk often means high possible losses. In that sense, studies on risk processing are closely related to studies on loss sensitivity. It has been observed that PG subjects perform worse on gambles where the probabilities of the outcomes are known [113]. Thus, GD subjects are indeed less risk averse than HC subjects (but do note the comments on this study in the computational section of this chapter). The study by Miedl et al. [93] also used the risk scenario (i.e., probabilities of action outcomes were known to gamblers). The authors let GD subjects play blackjack in a high-risk vs. a low-risk scenario. Subjects had to choose whether to hit or stand and received an outcome on every trial. Here, GD and OG subjects did not differ in behavior. However, while GD subjects showed activation during high risk and deactivation during low risk in temporal and thalamic areas, as well as inferior frontal gyrus (IFG), OG showed the opposite pattern. This may be interpreted as higher task engagement in a high-risk situation for GD subjects, while the opposite is true for OG subjects. Similar to the findings in loss anticipation, these results could mean that high-risk gambles are more interesting and engaging to GD subjects than to OG subjects. In that vein, Power et al. [114] have found that before making high-risk choices, GD subjects in an Iowa Gambling Task (IGT) compared to HC subjects show increased frontal lobe, basal ganglia, OFC, caudate, and amygdala activation. Over time GD subjects made more disadvantageous choice than HC subjects. However, the IGT is complex and manipulates not only risk but also delay of the wins and losses. Further, the probabilities of action outcomes are not completely explicit but have to be learned by the gambler. So it may be that risk is not the decisive feature to explain the increased motivation to opt for the high-risk gambles.

Note that both mentioned studies by Miedl et al. [93] and by Power et al. [114] used complex ecologically valid tasks. But no computational models were used to explicitly model the decision-making process of the subjects. The question is what information do the subjects incorporate into decision-making and what do they learn from the experienced outcomes? How do experienced losses or wins affect their risk sensitivity from trial to trial? The used analyses (comparing "high risk" vs. "low risk" trials) may be rather rough. We will see later that especially complex tasks which involve learning profit from analyses which are based on a computational model.

We have seen that risk seems to engage GD subjects more than OG and HC subjects. It may even lead to more disadvantageous decision-making. Risk ultimately means that possible gains and losses become more and more uncertain. As we have seen with LA (classically tested under circumstances of steady maximal risk, i.e., 50:50 coin flip gambles), HC subjects tend to overweight losses. This may be a heuristic to deal with the risk, i.e., the uncertainty. GD subjects perhaps do this less or even overweight gains in these situations [73].

Ambiguity
Ambiguous gambling situations (i.e., the probabilities of the action outcomes are unknown to the gambler) are more common in real-life gambling situations. GD subjects perform also worse on these kinds of gambles compared to HC subjects [113]. It further seems that performance on these kinds of gambles is a better predictor for GD symptom severity than performance on risk tasks [113].

The Balloon Analogue Risk-Taking Task (BART) tests the behavior of gamblers in response to an ambiguous gamble [115, 116]. On a computer screen, the gambler has to fill up a balloon with air. The more the gambler fills air into the balloon, the more they can win. However, the more air they fill into the balloon, the higher the probability that the balloon will pop and all the money accrued gets lost. Krmpotich et al. [117] observed no significant difference between GD subjects compared to HC subjects in risk-taking assessed with the BART.

The Iowa Gambling Task (IGT) is an extensively studied task where subjects have to learn probabilistically about four decks of cards by drawing a card on every trial. Over time subjects are able to learn through trial and error which decks are more advantageous and which are less. As mentioned earlier, the task is better classified as a task testing for reaction to ambiguous rather than risky gambles [113]. It has consistently been shown that GD subjects on average perform worse on the IGT [53, 113, 118], although there are exceptions [96]. Goudriaan et al. [95] investigated GD vs. HC subjects in an IGT task gathering peripheral-physiological data. During anticipation of disadvantageous decks, GD subjects showed less reduction of heart rate and lower skin conductance responses than HC subjects. Together with the altered neural signatures in response to high-risk gambles discussed earlier, this may mean that GD subjects fail to properly assess or anticipate high-risk gambles.

We have seen that GD subjects indeed react differently to risky and ambiguous gambles compared to HC subjects. Response to ambiguous gambles may even be a useful predictor for GD symptom severity. However, as we have also seen, risk is a higher-order gamble feature, already on mathematical level. Altered risk sensitivity in GD subjects is ultimately the product of altered gain, loss, as well as altered probability sensitivity [49, 119]. Computational models incorporating these basic processes may thus disentangle the neural disturbances leading to altered risk processing [112].

7.2.3.4 Delay
After discussing different magnitude sensitivities for gains and losses, as well as altered risk and probability sensitivity in GD subjects compared to HC subjects, we will now turn to delay as the final feature which needs to be incorporated in any

subjective value computation. The question whether a reward or a punishment will take effect immediately or, let us say, in a month, can be of vital importance and confers distinctive neural signatures [120]. Increased delay discounting (DD) of rewards has repeatedly been associated with addictive disorders [121]. Researchers have asked if also GD subjects show increased DD for rewards.

Indeed GD subjects show increased DD of rewards, and it has been associated with GD severity [93, 97, 122, 123]. Patients suffering from both GD and at least one SUD show even higher DD of rewards [124], although this finding has been challenged as a possible artifact due to differences in intelligence levels between GD and HC subjects [117]. Also casino environments seem to increase DD of rewards in GD subjects [125]. We are not aware of any neurobehavioral studies on DD of rewards in GD which use a non-computational approach to investigate the neural bases of GD subjects' increased DD of rewards. Note also that lower performance on the IGT may be due to increased DD to rewards. We will discuss this in a later section.

7.2.3.5 Learning from Reward and Punishment

When we talk about decision-making, we eventually have to talk about learning. People can only make decisions based on learned values and policies. We have seen so far that the value of an action outcome is subjective and draws upon experience and knowledge as to the possible gain, loss, associated probabilities, and delays. A policy is a decision-making style or more formally speaking the probability of choosing a certain option in a given situation, and given the learning history (whatever has been learned about the value, the probability, and the delay of the outcomes of the option in question).

Learning from punishment, according to reinforcement learning theory, should mean decreasing the likelihood of displaying the behavior which has been associated with punishment. In gambling, punishment means losing money. People should stop gambling when they are losing money. Through learning from punishment, the subjective value of the gamble should plummet, and so should the estimated probability of winning. However, GD subjects have been observed to stick with the same option despite received punishment (perseveration) [53]. This points to a learning impairment in GD subjects.

The so-called dopaminergic (DA) prediction error signal in the midbrain and in the VS has been brought into correlation with the prediction error (PE), the decisive learning signal from reinforcement learning [6, 126]. When an outcome is larger than the subjective value of an option, then it should be positive and we should see a burst in DA in the VS (positive prediction error). However, when it is smaller, then we should see a short silencing in comparison to tonic DA activity, indicative of a negative prediction error [83, 126]. In other words losing money should reduce DA activity and winning money increase DA activity.

In studying GD subjects, researchers often use probabilistic learning tasks to model the kind of learning that is pertinent to real-life gambling situations. Specifically, probabilistic learning means that the feedback is not deterministic when learning about a certain action outcomes. A bad option will mostly confer bad outcomes but *sometimes* also good outcomes or no outcomes.

Probabilistic Learning

Iowa Gambling Task

As we have discussed above, GD subjects generally perform worse on the Iowa Gambling Task (IGT) than HC subjects. Studies have used a sum score to assess performance in the IGT [99]. We have argued that impaired performance in the IGT may be due to differences in gain, loss, or probability sensitivity, or increased DD to rewards. However, it may also indicate a learning impairment. Perhaps PE DA signals are attenuated in GD subjects, and hence, they experience diminished learning signals from which to correctly compute a proper value estimate.

Linnet et al. [127] used an IGT in a positron emission tomography (PET) setting to measure DA release during IGT gambling. Note that PET is sluggish, and therefore we can only measure a mean DA release during gambling. The authors compared GD vs. HC subjects and observed that HC subjects ($n = 10$) and GD subjects ($n = 8$) who won money on the IGT showed comparable DA release. However, when comparing GD ($n = 8$) who lost money on the task and HC subjects ($n = 5$) who also lost money on the task, GD subjects showed more DA release in the striatum than HC subjects. In other words, GD subjects that lost money had DA release levels as if they were HC subjects that were winning. It thus seemed they experienced too many or too big positive PEs. Further, the authors found that DA receptor availability or overall DA release was not different between HC and GD subjects [128]. However, in GD subjects DA release was correlated with worse performance in the IGT and in HC vice versa [128]. This points to an impaired or—more precisely—inverse functioning of the DA system in GD subjects, where on the one hand objectively negative PEs seem to get "rewarded" with DA boosts and hence might reinforce risky choices. On the other hand, positive PEs lead to no DA shoot or a too small one, so that GD subjects learn too little about what the good decks are. In fact, a study by van Eimeren et al. [129] using DA agonists in Parkinson's disease patients suggested that the tonic stimulation of DA receptors specifically desensitizes the DA reward system by preventing decreases in DA transmission that occurs with negative PEs. The authors propose that in GD subjects lack of pauses in DA transmission impairs the extinction effect that losing should have on gambling.

Tanabe et al. [96] have also used the IGT in GD subjects with SUD (GD/SUD) and without SUD to test whether impaired decision-making in these cohorts is due to dysfunctions in MPFC and lateral prefrontal areas (Fig. 7.1). They found decreased activity during decision-making in both SUD and GD/SUD subjects, with least activity in GD/SUD subjects. As mentioned earlier the authors did not find differences with respect to gain or loss outcomes. The IGT is a complex decision-making task incorporating gain, loss, delay, and probability sensitivities. Decreased activity in certain brain areas during the decision-making period is thus hard to interpret. Below we will discuss a reanalysis of the aforementioned study where the authors used a computational model of the IGT significantly increasing interpretability of the results [130].

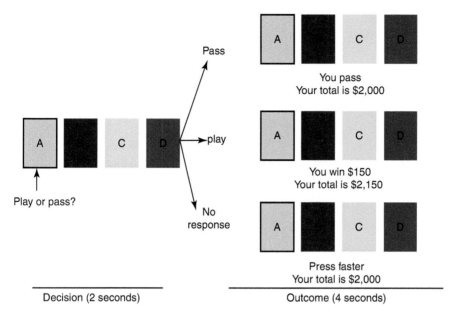

Fig. 7.1 The Iowa Gambling Task as adapted by Tanabe et al. [130]. In every trial, subjects are presented with four stacks of cards. Subjects have two options: pass or play. When playing then subjects have to draw a card from one of the stacks. Cards are associated with rewards and punishments. Through trial and error, subjects have to learn from which stacks to choose to accumulate wins. Two stacks are associated with occasional large wins but also large losses. The other two stacks are associated with small wins and small losses and will in the end lead to higher net gains. From: [130]: Figure 3 (Supp.). Reprinted with permission from the American Journal of Psychiatry, (Copyright ©2013). American Psychiatric Association. All Rights Reserved

We have seen that IGT performance is reduced in GD subjects. This may be related to impaired learning based on disturbances in PE signal generation in the striatum. Due to its complex nature, computational modeling of IGT data may prove particularly relevant.

Reversal Learning

A special challenge in learning from probabilistic feedback are reversals. This means the environment can change, such that what used to be good is now bad and what used to be bad is now good. This problem lies at the heart of addictive disorders because the challenge is to learn that a behavior which used to bring *mostly* pleasure now brings *mostly* pain [14, 131]. However, inferring from *probabilistic* feedback whether or not the environment has changed is a special challenge. After all a negative feedback may be indicative of a reversal or may be just noise. Addictive disorders have been repeatedly related to increased response perseveration in reversal learning tasks [29, 48, 132–134]. This may be a reflection of failure to learn from punishment or devaluation, as it may happen in real life. Despite the fact that the addicted patient gets negative feedback for a formerly pleasurable behavior (e.g., drinking alcohol), they will continue the behavior. Note that the reversal task lends itself for behavioral computational modeling and hence for model-based fMRI [48]. However, the task may also be analyzed in classical statistical ways. It has been found that the ability to adapt to reversals in the probabilistic reward feedback is predictive for relapse in GD subjects [52]. However, results from a reversal task in GD subjects using deterministic feedback (Wisconsin Card Sorting Task) has been observed not to be different from HC subjects [118]. Hence, reversal in probabilistic environments seems more relevant to studying GD.

de Ruiter et al. [135] have used the reversal learning task in GD subjects in an fMRI setting. They found that GD subjects performed worse than HC subjects and smokers (i.e., won less money). The authors concluded that this was due to response perseveration (sticking too long with an option that is no longer rewarded). Further, they correlated the win outcomes with fMRI data. They observed that GD subjects showed less responsiveness of the VLPFC to monetary gain. Hypo-responsiveness in the ventral (lateral) prefrontal cortex seems common in addictive disorders and related to impaired functioning of ventral striatal functioning [136]. However, the results of the study remain a bit unspecific. The gain trials lumped together are actually not all of the same kind, because they may constitute positive or negative PEs (which seem to be encoded in lateral prefrontal areas [137, 138]). Thus, the results are hard to interpret. Also the behavioral analysis is rough, even for a statistical analysis, because money won is the only variable analyzed. A computational approach modeling how subjects learn from positive and negative prediction errors in the reversal task would have probably been more informative (please see discussion below).

We have seen that GD subjects perform worse in probabilistic reversal learning tasks and that their performance may be predictive for relapse. However, without a computational model which explains the generation of reversal task behavior, it is difficult to explain the causes for this response perseveration. To our knowledge, there exist so far no reversal task studies in GD subjects using computational models. Reduced sensitivity to loss outcomes, in combination with steady high anticipatory motivation in response to high risk, may be explanatory factors.

Loss Chasing

The only diagnostic criterion of GD that is specific to the disorder compared to SUD is loss chasing. Loss chasing is the phenomenon that patients, after losses, rather than stopping gambling, feel an urge to gamble more, in order to make up for their losses [14]. In that sense, losses, paradoxically, seem to have a reinforcing effect for gambling behavior. In GD, it has been observed that they show increased speed after losses compared to HC subjects in the IGT, a card playing task, and in the go/no-go task [53]. This may be a reflection of the reinforcing or invigorating effect of losses for GD subjects. From a reinforcement learning perspective, where losses should yield demotivation of gambling behavior, this phenomenon cannot be so easily explained. A study by Campbell-Meiklejohn et al. [139] investigated the neural basis of loss chasing in HC subjects using fMRI. Subjects started with fictive 20,000 British Pounds. The task consisted of different kinds of blocks where subjects would start with losing amounts of 10, 20, 40, …, 160 pounds. After losing, subjects could choose to stick with the loss and start a new round or choose to chase the loss, i.e.,

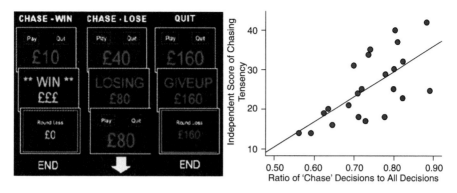

Fig. 7.2 Loss chasing game [139]. Left panel: Three different trials are displayed (from left to right). In the first trial, the subject started with losing 10 pounds, chooses to gamble (winning back 10 or losing 20) to get the money back, and wins. In the second trial, the person starts with losing 40 pounds, chooses to gamble, and loses 80 pounds. The person is then asked if they want to chase again or quit. In the third trial, the person starts with losing 160 pounds and immediately chooses to quit gambling. Right panel: Correlation of the loss chasing game score with an independent self-report gambling measure asking about chasing tendencies. The correlation highlights the validity of the task. Reprinted from [139], Figure 1. With permission from Elsevier

choose to gamble, where they could either win the money lost back or lose the same amount again. In case of losing, they would be able to choose again whether they would want to chase the complete loss or give up and accept the loss. In case of winning, subjects "won back" the loss and the block ended (Fig. 7.2). Chasing could only be done until an amount of 640 British Pounds was accrued (i.e., maximally six rounds of chasing). Probabilities of winning and losing were unknown to the subjects, so this was an ambiguous gambling task.

Subjects chased on 73% of the trials and stopped chasing after on average two chases. This indicates that subjects do not evaluate every trial independently. If that were the case, they should keep chasing. Subjectively, losses rather seem to "add up." Decisions to quit were associated with increased activity in dorsal anterior cingulate cortex (dACC), posterior cingulate, anterior insula, and parietal cortex and decreased activity in the VMPFC and subgenual ACC (sgACC). Decisions to chase were associated with decrease in activity in dACC and anterior insula and inferior frontal gyrus. In general, decisions to quit lead to more activity than decisions to chase. Further, subjects with high interpretive bias ("When I win, it is a sign that I mastered the game"; "When I lose, then it is bad luck") showed reduced activity in quitting associated areas (dACC, posterior cingulate, anterior insula).

The authors also took a reinforcement learning perspective of the task. They compared wins after chases against losses after chases (i.e., PE+ > PE−). This revealed stronger activity in VMPFC and posterior cingulate. This indicates that positive PEs yield to activation and negative PEs to deactivation in these areas. Both good and bad outcomes after chase decisions against decisions to quit (PE in general) were associated with activity in VS, putamen. Checking how negative outcomes after a chase followed by a decision to chase are different from negative outcomes after a chase followed by a decision to quit revealed increased activity in dACC, a known conflict monitoring area, and indicated earlier in being associated with increased propensity to quit.

The authors argue that their results are in line with previous studies, which have associated VMPFC and sgACC with appetitive states and dACC as well as anterior insula with the experience of disgust and anxiety. The presented study provides a valuable framework for the analysis of the neural basis of loss chasing. A recent study has used the task to compare GD and HC subjects in loss chasing [140]. GD subjects showed stronger activity during quitting in a medial frontal executive-processing network, including ACC. This may be interpreted as stronger activity need to successfully quit chasing in GD subjects compared to HC.

Near Misses

Near misses, as discussed earlier, seem to have a powerful affective effect [108]. In the mentioned study, it was found that near misses are unpleasant to HC subjects but they increase the desire to play, anyway. This is the case when the subjects have some control over the gamble. In other words, subjects learn falsely from feedback. This is perhaps the case because the slight control over the gamble lets them conclude that a near miss means that they almost made it and they only have to increase their effort. This is noteworthy because GD subjects tend to display bigger illusions of control [141]. Worhunsky et al. [88], as noted earlier, have found no effect of a near miss "as-if-win" circuit like Clark et al. [108] have in HC subjects. However, they found an increased anticipatory affect in GD subjects. It thus seems that near-miss effects are important in healthy gambling and, as mentioned earlier, early problem gambling [109]. Later, in GD subject, near misses are desensitized just like all loss outcomes. So they cannot have an effect on learning anymore. However, anticipation of gambling still invokes heightened motivation.

We have seen that GD subjects seem to learn worse from negative feedback and thus persevere in their gambling behavior. This may be due to impaired processing of probabilistic feedback, loss chasing, as well as increased motivation to gamble in response to near misses. Computational models of learning from rewards and punishments in GD subjects are needed to disentangle disturbances in the many subprocesses contributing to impaired learning.

7.3   Changes in the Neural Substrate

Since computational models in psychiatry are often used to relate clinically relevant behavior more distinctively to the underlying neural processes [38], we have to understand which neural "hardware" GD subjects are working with. In particular, it is important to understand in what way the GD brain is different from the HC brain, and we may then wonder how these differences in the "hardware" may influence the "software," i.e., the functions or behavior of GD subjects. Structural and physiological differences may be predisposing factors or may be results of repeated behavior and learning [142–144]. From extensive research on brain plasticity, we know that the brain may undergo substantial structural changes simply by training and practicing, without the application of any drug [145]. Essentially the very process of learning is reflected in structural changes, such as strengthening of synapses, building of new synapses, and the creation of new neural dendrites. Further, addictive disorders are known to influence and be influenced by alterations in neurotransmitter systems [146, 147]. Even without a computational model relating neural substrate, neural function, and clinically relevant behavior, researchers may ask whether changes in neural substrates are correlated with GD severity.

7.3.1   Gray Matter

Gray matter is comprised chiefly of neuronal somas, their dendrites, synapses, and unmyelinated axons [148]. Two studies investigating whole brain differences in gray matter have found no differences in gray matter volume between GD and HC subjects [149, 150]. Region of interest (ROI)-based studies have found in GD subjects reduced volume in the left hippocampus and right amygdala compared to HC subjects and a positive correlation between impulsivity self-report scores and left hippocampal and left amygdalar volumes in the GD group [151]. In a study by our own group [28], we used the prefrontal cortex (PFC) and VS as ROIs because of the importance of these brain regions with respect to reward processing and inhibitory control [84, 152]. We observed higher volume in the right prefrontal cortex and right VS in GD subjects compared with HC subjects. Hypertrophy was seen in bilateral putamen which was correlated with GD severity. Increased gray matter volume and/ or density may be due to increased number of synapses due to learning [153]. However, in neocortical areas, it may also point to an increased number of actual neurons, as has been observed in macaque monkeys [154]. More synapses and more neurons may lead to better signal-to-noise ratio in neural computations [155]. Hence, gray matter volume/density as putative proxies for computational efficiency should be taken into account when designing computational models of GD subjects' behavior.

7.3.2   White Matter

White matter is comprised mainly of myelinated axons and very few neuronal somas [148]. White matter integrity in GD compared to HC subjects has been investigated in only few GD studies. Joutsa et al. [150] have found no differences in white matter integrity, but the structural connectivity between several regions was reduced in GD subjects. Those were in the corpus callosum, the cingulum, the superior longitudinal fascicle, the inferior fronto-occipital fascicle, the anterior limb of internal capsule, the anterior thalamic radiation, the inferior longitudinal fascicle, and the uncinate/inferior fronto-occipital fascicle. Yip et al. [156] have found reduced genual corpus callosal white matter integrity in GD subjects which was correlated with a sensation seeking self-report measure. In a study by our group [157], we have observed increased functional connectivity during resting state between limbic regions and prefrontal regions, as well as reduced functional connectivity (correlation of fMRI time series between two regions) between prefrontal regions. Similar findings were reported by Tschernegg et al. [158]. The latter authors also applied a graph-theoretical approach to resting-state data from GD subjects to examine network properties on the global and nodal levels. GD subjects demonstrated no alterations in global network properties. At the nodal level, however, they showed alterations in network properties in the paracingulate cortex and the supplementary motor area (SMA). At an uncorrected threshold level, alterations also were observed in the inferior frontal gyrus and caudate.

We have seen that structural and functional connectivity alterations may be present in GD subjects. This should be taken into account when designing computational models of task-related neural functioning in GD subjects. Free parameters modeling connectivity strength between specific areas may be included in such models.

7.3.3　Neurotransmitters

7.3.3.1 Dopamine

Dopamine (DA) is arguably the most studied and most prominent neurotransmitter associated with addictive disorders. DA is so popular with addiction researchers because it seems to code for prediction errors and thus has major implications in learning, motivation, and action selection [83, 126]. Both the reward deficiency hypothesis and the incentive salience hypothesis of addiction are based in the mechanisms of the meso-cortico-limbic DA system [40, 41, 77]. Despite its prominence in addiction research, there is yet no DA medication for the treatment of addictive disorders [159]. DA medication studies using DA antagonists in GD subjects have yielded conflicting results [159]. However, a study by Zack and Poulos [160] has observed that high-impulsivity GD subjects profit from modafinil (a DA transporter inhibitor raising tonic extracellular DA levels), while low-impulsivity GD subjects rather become more pathological in relevant measures. This indicates the importance of defining subgroups of GD to understand the disorder and devise proper treatments.

Further, it is well-documented that some Parkinson's disease (PD) patients receiving DA agonist therapy (to counter atrophy of DA neurons) develop GD [159, 161]. A study by Steeves et al. [162] has investigated DA reactivity during a gambling task in PD patients under DA agonist therapy. One group of these patients had developed GD (PDGD); the other group had not (PD). The authors observed that PDGD subjects had a stronger increase in DA release in the VS during gambling vs. neutral trials in comparison to PD subjects. Further, the general binding of the DA receptor ligand in VS was reduced in PDGD subjects during both conditions. This hints at reduced VS D2/D3 receptor availability in PDGD patients. It is a common finding that VS D2/D3 receptors are reduced in SUD populations [163–165] and perhaps a predisposing factor for the development of addiction, in line with the reward deficiency hypothesis [166–169].

However, as already mentioned, Sescousse et al. [78] observed that the reward deficiency hypothesis does not seem to be valid in GD. Moreover, there is recurrent evidence that D2/D3 receptor density is not reduced in GD subjects but only correlated with GD symptom severity and subjective gambling high [23, 27, 127, 165]. This indicates that PDGD is etiologically different from GD in non-PD populations [161]. Further, in the pursuit of pharmacological treatments for GD, other DA receptors may need to be taken into consideration [170].

We have seen that DA receptor density and functioning are informative within GD subjects since they relate to gambling high and behavior and putatively cue reactivity [171]. However, DA variables seem not so informative to differ between HC and GD subjects. Computational models trying to explain behavior in GD should incorporate free parameters for tonic and phasic DA signaling, since these variables can have effects on the relative importance of the striatal prediction error.

7.3.3.2 Other Neurotransmitters

Norepinephrine or noradrenaline (NA) is a neurotransmitter that renders the body and brain ready for action. It is lowest during sleep and rises during wakefulness and is even more increased during stress [172, 173]. GD studies using blood and urine samples, as well as drug challenges and fMRI, have noted heightened levels of NA, suggesting increase in arousal and excitement associated to GD [174]. Another study [175] suggested that increased sensitivity to or increased release of NA elicits a stronger stress response in GD than in HC in the amygdala. Hence, GD subjects might be more easily triggered into action mode via noradrenergic processes. This might also facilitate risky and rash choices as seen in gambling.

Serotonin is a neurotransmitter implicated in a wide array of behaviors including sleep, sex, memory, and social behavior [176]. Most notably, serotonin has been linked to the computation and processing of negative prediction errors and to the behavioral changes ensuing [177, 178]. As a consequence, serotonergic signal has been suggested as the basis of LA in a computational neural network model [103]. Serotonin levels may be reduced in GD subjects [179]. However, studies investigating the effects of serotonergic agonists on GD severity have yielded mixed results [174].

Endorphins or opiodergic peptides have been associated especially with pleasure, pain reduction, and reward receipt processing. In other words, endorphins are integral in outcome processing and "liking" [180]. Notably, stimulation of opioid receptors in the ventral tegmentum (midbrain) and nucleus accumbens (VS) modulate the release of midbrain DA [181, 182]. Further, in detoxified alcohol-dependent patients, μ-opiate receptor density in the VS has been observed increased and correlated with subjective craving [183]. Endorphin release has been associated with gambling anticipation and winning during gambling [184]. Opioid antagonist therapy in GD subjects has yielded mixed results so far [174].

Neurotransmitter systems such as the NA or DA system are likely changed in GD subjects. Such changes should be considered in computational models based on neural architecture and neural mechanisms. However, studies on neurotransmitter system changes in GD are still anything but conclusive. For a detailed review on these studies and related pharmacological treatments studies, please refer to Bullock and Potenza [174].

7.4 Computational Studies on Gambling Disorder

In this section, we will review studies, which used computational modeling (CM) to discern the bases of neurobehavioral disturbances in GD. We will review studies which used computational models to analyze behavioral data from GD subjects and studies which used computational models to link mechanistically neural data to behavioral data. The latter studies will be limited to model-based fMRI studies [4]. Note that all studies reported in this section relate to the symptom cluster "neglect of other areas in life" [3]. Computational studies on loss of control (response inhibition) and craving (cue reactivity), to our knowledge, are yet non-existent in GD literature.

Research using computational modeling (CM) in GD has largely focused on explaining impaired decision-making. The models used are based on prospect theory [185] and reinforcement learning (RL) theory [6] (Fig. 7.3). Bayesian extensions of RL are also considered [186]. Prospect theory emphasizes the fact that the EV (Eq. (7.1) see above under Sect. 7.2.3.3) of a gamble is always subjective. It

$$Q(s_t, a_t) \leftarrow Q(s_t, a_t) + \alpha \left[r_{t+1} + \gamma \max_a Q(s_{t+1}, a) - Q(s_t, a_t) \right]$$

Initialize $Q(s, a)$ arbitrarily

Repeat (for each episode):

   Initialize s

   Repeat (for each step of episode):

      Choose a from s using policy derived from Q (e.g., ε-greedy)
      Take action a, observe r, s'
      $Q(s, a) \leftarrow Q(s, a) + \alpha[r + \gamma \max_{a'} Q(s', a') - Q(s, a)]$
      $s \leftarrow s'$;

   until s is terminal

Fig. 7.3 Temporal difference learning or Q-learning [6]. Depicted is a form of temporal difference learning, namely, Q-learning. The agent has to learn which action best to pick in any given state. The agent solves this task by caching and updating Q-values for every state-action pair. Q-values get updated on every trial by adding to the old respective Q-value (i.e., the predicted Q-value) a discounted prediction error. The discount parameter (learning rate) is α, which is assumed between 0 and 1. Note that if α is 1, then the experienced reward (reward plus estimated value of next state) completely replaces the old Q-value within one trial. The box below displays a program that simulates the behavior of an agent given a set of states and actions associated with certain reinforcement schedules. The program will converge to the agent picking the best action in all states given enough trials and a stationary environment. Note that this learning algorithm does not split updating values and preferences (critic vs. actor), as discussed later. Everything is only learned in Q-values. A policy is a set of rules governing how to choose from n actions available in a given state which are associated with n Q's. An ε-greedy policy picks always the action with the highest cached Q-value except sometimes (with a probability of ε) it picks randomly. Other policies exist, such as the softmax rule using a consistency parameter. r, reward; t, trial or time step; γ, discount rate for future state-action Q-values; s, state; s', new state after performing chosen action a; a', action in next state

depends on the current state of the agent, on their gain and loss sensitivity, on their probability sensitivity, and on their delay discounting of rewards and punishments. Note that we will use these parameters to structure this section, just as we have done when reporting on classical studies. RL theory is based in behaviorism and on Thorndike's law of effect [187]. The law of effect is the observation that agents repeat behaviors which are rewarded, i.e. reinforced. Bayesian RL incorporates the online estimation of probability distributions of reward returns to allow for an optimal trade-off between exploration and exploitation on every choice [186, 188]. Other (knowledge-based) decision-making models have been suggested to explain risky choices but not yet applied to GD subjects [189].

7.4.1   Gain and Loss Processing

A computational framework of gain processing eventually tries to answer how the objective values presented to a human (i.e., the anticipation of 10 € or the receipt of 10 €) are transformed into a subjective value. Using a CM on IGT data, Lorains et al. [99] have found heightened outcome-related gain and loss sensitivity in strategic problem gamblers but reduced outcome-related loss sensitivity in non-strategic gamblers. The ANDREA (Affective Neuroscience of Decision through Reward-based Evaluation of Alternatives) model presents a complete neurobehavioral spiking neuron model synthesizing how a brain could do this, also explaining phenomena such as loss aversion and the framing effect [103]. The model by Basten et al. [7] uses a similar approach and further relates the neural predictions to concrete fMRI signal hypotheses. Both models emphasize the co-working of multiple brain areas connected in a network. The models have been used to generate explorative hypotheses on neural data collected during a LA task performed by GD subjects [89]. The authors found that GD subjects showed stronger connectivity from amygdala to bilateral posterior OFC with rising monetary gains at stake. The posterior OFC has been associated with processing of more primary rewards [78]. Further the connectivity from amygdala to VMPFC with rising losses was stronger in HC than GD subjects, which may be indicative of an impaired cost-benefit computation [7].

The study by van Holst et al. [74] has already been discussed. Interestingly the authors performed both a linear correlation analysis with BOLD response in the striatum with the objective value (no computation assumed) and with the positive expected values, i.e. EV+ = objective gain value * P(objective gain value). This formula assumes a trial-by-trial transformation of the gain value based on the objective probability of winning known to the subject. Both variables lead to a significant group difference with PG subjects showing stronger dorsal stiatum (DS) signal, but using the computational value lead to a stronger group difference effect. Further, the EV+ signal in amygdala was negatively related to a GD symptom severity scale. This speaks in favor of computational values (based on specific assumptions of computed values represented by certain neural populations) which may lead to more apt descriptions of group differences in studies comparing GD and HC subjects. Also note that this result may be in line with the model by Piray et al. [131], which predicts growing action preferences in DS compared to reduced action values in VS.

We have seen that subjective gain values may be differently represented in OFC in GD compared to HC subjects. Further, neural network models of gain and loss anticipation suggest that the amygdala—a structure putatively assigning salience to represented values [190, 191]—may bias wins over losses during the assessment of offered gambles.

7.4.2 Learning from Reward and Punishment

When reporting on classical studies, computational modeling is particularly useful when dealing with learning paradigms. During gambling, GD subjects experience reward and punishments in response to their choices and hence are exposed to specific reinforcement schedules [187]. Computational modeling of choice behavior is particularly apt to investigate how GD subjects respond to such reinforcement schedules. In this context we will firstly focus on the findings of computational models capturing differences between GD and HC subjects in responding to rewards and punishments. In the classical studies section, we have seen that increasing gains at stake may lead to faster reaction times in GD subjects but not HC subjects. Other than that behavioral results on gain processing were inconclusive, and we have pointed out that computational models could discern better the contribution of gain sensitivity in explaining GD subjects' choice behavior. We have noted that especially the IGT is used to investigate GD subjects' gambling behavior but that its overall performance score falls short in explaining the exact structure of disadvantageous choice behavior in GD subjects.

Power et al. [114] have found decreased learning in the IGT task by computing an IGT summary score for every quartile of trials. Tanabe et al. [130] followed up on a previous IGT study [96] and demonstrated how computational modeling can increase the interpretability of neural and behavioral differences between a clinical group with SUDs and HC subjects on this task. The expectancy valence model (EVM) of the IGT assumes three free parameters: the sensitivity to gain outcome vs. loss outcome (ω), the learning rate (α), and the choice consistency growing over trials ($t^c/10$). SUD subjects showed reduced choice consistency over trials and a trend of reduced sensitivity to loss outcomes. There was no difference in the learning rate (α). Importantly the EVM, like any RL model, allows the modeling of prediction errors on every trial. There is ample evidence that the VS (but not the dorsal striatum) and ventral medial prefrontal (but not lateral) areas represent PEs which are used to update the action selection policy [192]. Tanabe et al. [130] observed that SUD subjects displayed a weaker PE signal in these areas than HC subjects. It tells us that people suffering from addiction generate less of a teaching signal to update their behavioral policy leading to greater losses when gambling. Krmpotich et al. [117] used the same analysis approach with GD subjects who also suffered from an SUD (SDGD) and subjects who only suffered from an SUD (SD subjects). They found again no reduced learning rate, but reduced consistency and reduced loss outcome sensitivity, with SDPG showing always the steepest reductions compared to both SD and HC subjects. The question would now be whether also GD subjects without SD show the same differences in the behavioral parameters and whether they also suffer from a reduced BOLD representation of the PE signal.

Lorains et al. [99] used the IGT in strategic (e.g., poker gamblers) (SPG) and non-strategic problem gamblers (e.g., slot machine gamblers) (NSPG) and acquired behavioral data. Only NSPG performed worse than HC subjects according to the sum score of the task. The authors also applied a CM to analyze the behavioral data. The prospect valence model (PVL) is an extension to the EVM. It includes a LA parameter for received outcomes (λ_{out}), a learning rate (α), a utility shape exponent (β), and a consistency parameter (c). SPG showed greater sensitivity to gains, higher outcome-related loss aversion, but lower consistency (more erratic, random behavior). There was no difference on the learning parameter α. NSPG showed similar PVL parameters as controls. They only showed lower outcome-related LA. Hence, GD subjects may differ not only in their net score but also on the structure of their choice behavior. Strategic gamblers actually show higher loss aversion than HC but more exploration behavior (random behavior) which may indicate more openness to explore against the odds. Non-strategic gamblers on the other hand seem to suffer mainly from reduced loss outcome sensitivity which in the end really hampers their learning. As mentioned earlier in the same study, Lorains et al. [99] also found a reduced anticipatory LA in NSG but not SG. The CM and the split of the gamblers group into NSG and SG have shown us what the target for therapy, at least for non-strategic gamblers, could be: increasing LA on anticipation and outcome level. We thus see that CMs can also help make neurobiological studies more translational with respect to devising new therapy methods and targets. Further, the results by Lorains et al. [99] are quite in line with the SDPG study by Krmpotich et al. [117]. However, the comparison of the PVL [99] and the EVM [117] also shows us that RL models are somewhat arbitrary. We can introduce always slightly different parameters in slightly different equations to account for new cognitive-affective theoretical ideas as to how the subjects may solve the task. This makes parameter comparisons across studies difficult. Computational models should thus be replicated in many studies. Further, multiple models should be tried and compared using established model comparison tools like cross-validation or Bayesian Information Criterion (BIC). Another approach is to devise RL models in a more principled way.

In fact, Piray et al. [131] have suggested a neutrally informed RL framework to explain the addictive learning behavior in GD subjects. For this, it is worthwhile to note that certain RL frameworks may be split into two components: the actor and the critic. The actor stores state-action-dependent preferences or in other words a policy, which returns a preference for each possible action in a given state. The critic, on the other hand, stores state-dependent values and computes prediction errors comparing adjacent states, especially with respect to actually chosen actions [131]. In a range of studies, the actor has been associated with functional behavior of the dorsal striatum, while the critic has been associated with the VS [131]. The authors suggest that addiction in general and GD may develop due to reduced levels of D1/D2 receptors in the VS. The dopaminergic efferents from posteromedial VTA to these receptors are needed to code for positive PEs. If D1/D2 receptors are low in VS, then the critic cannot produce adequate PEs. The authors show that this leads to an imbalance between preference updates in the DS and value updates in the VS. This, in turn, leads to an exaggerated preference for appetitive stimuli (gambling/drugs). Additional exposure to unnaturally high DA signal in combination with already reduced D1/D2 receptor availability leads to further reduction of this receptor availability. Consequently, even if the addictive behavior is now paired with punishment (e.g., electric shock, money loss), the preference for the behavior stays much higher than for the alternative action (refraining from gambling). This prediction of the model is reflective of the symptom "engaging in the addictive behavior despite negative consequences (Fig. 7.4)."

We have reported earlier that D2/D3 receptors do not seem to be reduced in striatum in GD subjects, but their density seems related to GD symptom severity. An initial or even progressed downregulation of D2 receptors as proposed by Piray et al. [131] as precondition for the development and maintenance for GD seems thus questionable. However, we do not know of studies which looked at D1 receptor density in

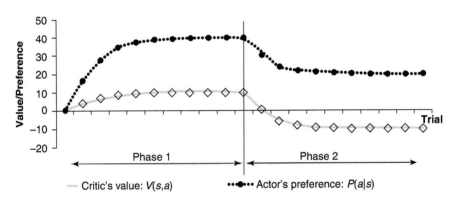

Fig. 7.4 The progression of addictive behavior. Temporal differences learning may neurally be implemented by an actor-critic model [131, 6]. Here, Q-learning is split in a seemingly redundant way: VS (the critic) is learning about action values and DS (the actor) is learning about action preferences. Note, that only preference values determine action selection. Value learning is important for generating prediction errors for learning both values and preferences. Hence, values and preferences should mirror each other. However, in the development of an addiction, this might change. The model by Piray et al. [131] suggests that an agent with a reduced D1/D2 receptor density (as an innate vulnerability) may develop addiction because the continuous onslaught of DA surges in the VS (by a drug or through gambling) in phase 1 leads to an escalation of action preference for the addictive behavior because the action value is insufficiently updated. Through successive DA surges the patient loses more DA receptors which exacerbates the divergence of value and preference cached by the critic and the actor, respectively. In the graph we see that the addictive behavior is preferred more and more by the actor, although the critic's valuation of the behavior is much lower. During phase 2, the addictive behavior is no longer rewarded but punished. Even though value and preference updating are now again coupled, the preference is so high that it cannot become negative. Hence, the addictive behavior is still chosen despite its negative value. Reprinted from [131]. Figure 1, p. 2349. © 2010 by the Massachusetts Institute of Technology. With permission from MIT Press Journals

VS, which might show the proposed reduction. Further, the PET studies reported on earlier focused on the striatum as a whole or on dorsal striatum and substantia nigra [23]. However, Piray et al. [131] argue that the DS may respond with higher and higher metabolism due to the increased preference for addiction-related actions, but receptor downregulation in these areas is not part of their computational model. It is further interesting to note that the model by Piray et al. [131] works solely on a disturbance in positive PEs in VS. The authors' model may even explain that long-time exposure to high DA surges may start the cascade of reduced DA receptor density, decreased VS PE's and increased preference for the addictive behavior. In fact a PET study reported earlier has shown reduced striatal DA signal putatively related to positive PEs in GD subjects [128]. Note that the model by Piray et al. [131] essentially proposes a lower and lower learning rate in the critic (VS) compared to the actor (DS). Giving some support to this model prediction, a study by Lim et al. [193] in a community sample of regular gamblers found that in a reward learning task, learning rates were negatively correlated with an impulsivity self-reporting scale. The result must be interpreted with care, since the authors did not use a RL model strictly splitting actor and critic. Sensitivity to objective reward magnitudes in that study was not correlated with impulsivity. Interestingly, the authors also found that high-impulsivity gamblers tended to be more response perseverant after large wins. This could be a reflection of an increasingly biased preference in the actor due to DA surges.

We have seen that there are still few studies using computational models to investigate GD subjects' response to reinforcement schedules and probabilistic learning tasks. However, first results and modeling efforts highlight the importance of focusing on PEs, associated learning rates, and loss aversion. There is some evidence that GD subjects show reduced generation of PEs in ventral prefrontal areas. This may also lead to a reduced sensitivity to loss outcomes and response perseveration.

7.4.3 Uncertainty

Reinforcement schedules in gambling situations are probabilistic by definition. Subjects have to deal with uncertainty and probabilistic feedback. Any outcome will only take effect with some probability. Shead and Hodgins [194] found that HC subjects do not perceive probabilities objectively but discount or magnify probabilities, especially when they are very large. Using the objective EV as baseline and a hyperbolic probability discounting function, it has been found that college students magnify the probability of gains, when the probability of winning is high [194]. In other words, when the probability of winning is around 0.7 or higher, college students tend to overestimate the probability of winning [194]. However, when probability of winning is low, their estimation of winning (i.e., their subjective value estimation) lines up with the mathematically optimal model, i.e., the EV [194]. In losses, it is the same picture. College students tend to overestimate the probability of losses when the probability of losing is at about 0.7 or higher. In other words, with respect to gains, HC subjects are risk seeking, while with respect to losses subjects are risk averse.

Shead et al. [195] did not find among problem gamblers that more problematic gambling is associated with stronger overestimation of winning probability or stronger underestimation of losing probability. However, the authors found that problem gamblers who expect gambling to enhance positive mood overestimate winning probabilities and underestimate losing probabilities compared to those who think of gambling as good for alleviating bad mood and those who think of gambling having no effect on mood. Miedl et al. [49] tested GD subjects against HC subjects in winning probability discounting using the same probability discounting model as Shead et al. [195]. They found a trend in GD subjects overestimating winning probabilities compared to HC subjects. On brain level, subjective value derived from the probability-discounting model was overall not differently distributed in GD compared to HC subjects. An exception was the OFC, where GD subjects seemed to inversely represent value. Note that in the last two studies the objective probabilities were known to the subjects at all times. We have already mentioned in the classical studies that GD subjects tend to be more risk seeking, when probabilities are known [113]. However, the computational studies presented here challenge this conclusion.

With respect to ambiguity, we saw in the classical studies section that subjects performed mostly worse. However, the summary task scores used did not allow deciding whether this was due to probability discounting differences. Lim et al. [193] used a two-armed bandit task in a community sample of regular gamblers. Each arm (i.e., option) in the task was associated with some reward magnitude. Unknown to the subject were the winning probabilities. Those were stable for 120 trials for both options and later changed and swapped regularly (reversal). In that sense, the game was a probability tracking game. The authors used a Bayesian learning model [188] and a RL model. They observed that the Bayesian optimal probability estimate was used more if subjects scored low on the non-planning facet of the Barrat Impulsiveness Scale (BIS) [196] and also if they scored low on a self-report scale measuring illusions of predictive control over gambles. Using RL modeling incorporating the learning about and the sensitivity to probabilities, the authors observed that high-impulsivity (non-planning scale in BIS) gamblers tend to underestimate high probabilities and overestimate low probabilities, while low-impulsivity gamblers displayed almost correct probability estimation. However, this must be the product of both decreased learning about probabilities and distorted probability sensitivities, because the learning rate also negatively correlated with non-planning impulsivity.

Hence, there is only a trend that GD subjects show different probability sensitivities compared to HC subjects. The OFC, as mentioned in the context of gain representation and delayed values [49, 78], perhaps also here is a brain area showing distorted value representation in GD subjects. In situations of ambiguity, learning about probabilities may be distorted especially in high-impulsive gamblers. Hence, we need more studies that focus on GD subjects' processing of uncertainty.

7.4.4 Delay

Note that the IGT, which is very often used, only implicitly measures delay discounting because card decks with small steady rewards combined with small punishments are set against card decks giving intermittent large rewards with inter-mittent large punishments. Choosing high-risk card desks may be interpreted as a decreased sensitivity to variance of outcomes but also as an increased delay dis-counting with respect to the possible small rewards in the future and/or the big punishments in the past. Power et al. [114] found that before high-risk choices, GD subjects compared to HC subjects show larger increased frontal lobe, basal ganglia, OFC, caudate, and amygdala activation. The authors interpreted this as increased salience of risky bets, perhaps similar to a cue reactivity contrast, but it may also be interpreted as increased delay discounting in GD subjects. This is a shortcoming of the complexity of the IGT and its lack of orthogonalization of delay and risk.

Miedl et al. [49] used a pure DD-of-rewards task and, based on a hyperbolic discounting function, computed subject- and trial-specific values of the money value in the future for GD and HC subjects. DD was increased in GD subjects. Across all subjects the subjective values correlated positively with activity in the VS, MPFC, and lateral parietal and posterior cingulate. This may indicate that these areas are involved in the anticipation of the future reward. In GD subjects, the sub-jective value was more correlated with activity in the DS. Furthermore, the better the subjective value correlated with OFC, VS, and SN/VTA, the lower the GD severity. This is in line with the Piray et al. model [131], which predicts a shift of value representation from VS to DS as indicative of addiction progression [131]. Piray et al. [131] note that DS represents all options (in this case the delayed and the immediate choice), while the VS represents mainly the to-be-chosen option. Since GD subjects tend to prefer choosing the immediate reward, it makes sense that the value of the future reward is rather found in the DS in the GD cohort. Miedl et al. [76] have further investigated how GD subjects are influenced by gambling-related cues when evaluating delayed rewards (Fig. 7.5).

Gambling pictures were sorted according to subjective craving induced. During high-craving trials, subjects tended to increase their delay discounting. Further, while in low-craving trials, there was a positive correlation with subjective value of the delayed reward in VS and midbrain, this correlation faltered or reversed during high-craving pictures (Fig. 7.6). According to the Piray et al. [131] model, this may mean that under high-craving conditions delayed rewards become less considered as a viable option.

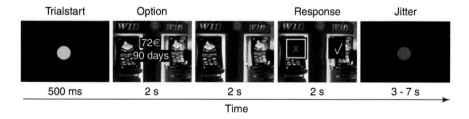

Fig. 7.5 Delay discounting task from the Miedl et al. [76] study. Participants had to always choose between an immediate reward of 20 € and a larger delayed reward. Gambling scenes were shown in the background. Reprinted from [76], Figure 1. With permission from The Society for Neuroscience

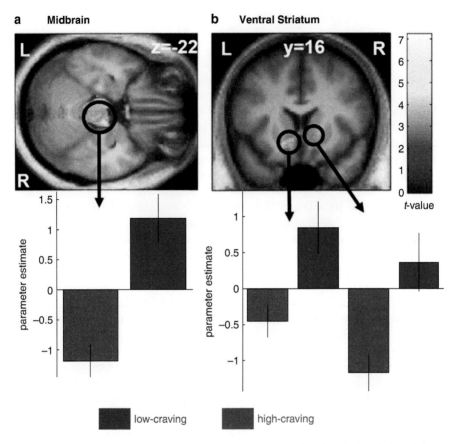

Fig. 7.6 Delay discounting and cue reactivity. Results from Miedl et al. [76]. Correlation of signal with the subjective value of the delayed reward gets inversed when high-craving pictures are presented in the background of the delay-discounting task. Reprinted from [76], Figure 3. With permission from The Society for Neuroscience

In addition to the well-established finding that GD subjects tend to discount future rewards more than HC subjects, we have seen that GD subjects also represent future rewards less in VS but more in DS, indicative of addiction progression. Craving-inducing cues might exacerbate this effect. More studies on the interaction of processes associated with symptom clusters (response inhibition, craving, decision-making) should be conducted to increase ecological validity of tasks and understand the co-working of these processes [55]. Computational models lend themselves well to deal with the ensuing increase in task complexity.

7.5   Discussion

In this chapter, we have reviewed classical studies investigating the neurobiological bases of GD. While doing this, we have taken a computational psychiatry perspective by trying to focus on relevant disturbances of neurocognitive processes, which may constitute the basis for specific GD symptoms. We have further presented several GD studies, which used computational modeling (CM), and have argued that such an approach is to be favored. This is because CM often allows for better mapping of the neural substrate's functions to clinically relevant behavior. Throughout this chapter, we have focused on the three main symptom clusters: loss of control, craving, and neglect of other areas in life. Thus, we use this structure again to summarize and discuss the findings presented in this chapter.

7.5.1   Loss of Control

Loss of control has mainly been associated with impaired response inhibition. GD subjects consistently show diminished response inhibition. This seems to relate to altered functioning of DLPFC, ACC, VS, and MPFC. Response inhibition scores and associated neural signatures seem relevant in predicting treatment outcome, relapse, and symptom severity. To our knowledge, there are no computational models yet trying to capture reduced response inhibition in GD subjects. Reinforcement learning models do not seem adequate for this, but rather real-time neural network models predicting exact reaction time differences [155].

7.5.2   Craving

Gambling cues increase craving as measured with subjective reporting scales in GD subjects. Neural response patterns of cue reactivity are complex and show some inconsistency across studies. Investigating cue reactivity in the context of specific gambling tasks may make neural cue reactivity signatures more specific. Cue reactivity may alter gain and loss sensitivity of the striatum, as well as response inhibition and decision-making processes.

7.5.3   Neglect of Other Areas in Life

7.5.3.1   Gain and Loss Processing

Monetary and natural gain anticipation seems to be blunted in the VS in GD subjects. In decision-making increasing possible gains seem to lead to faster decisions and altered reactivity in parietal and dorsal striatal areas during the decision phase. We have seen that subjective gain values may be differently represented in OFC in GD compared to HC subjects. Further, neural network models of gain and loss anticipation suggest that amygdala—a structure putatively assigning salience to represented values [7, 103] —may bias wins over losses during the assessment of offered gambles.

Increased loss anticipation signal in VS plus decreased loss-related activity during successful loss avoidance may explain increased gambling. This is because GD subjects may feel increased motivation to do away with losses but not feel enough satisfaction when actually being successful in avoiding losses. We have also seen that GD subjects display reduced loss aversion both during gamble anticipation and during gamble outcomes. In addition, regular gamblers seem to be motivated from near misses as if they were gains, while GD subjects display a generally decreased reactivity in VS and other regions toward losses. The progression from regular gambling to GD may thus correlate with progressive loss outcome desensitization. Decreased sensitivity to negative reinforcement as well as decreased sensitivity to losses may be supporting factors for loss chasing which further abets GD symptoms.

7.5.3.2 Uncertainty and Delay

We have seen that risk seems to engage GD subjects more than regular gamblers and HC subjects. It may even lead to more disadvantageous decision-making. Risk ultimately means that possible gains and losses become more and more uncertain. As we have seen with LA (classically tested under circumstances of steady maximal risk, i.e., 50:50 coin flip gambles), HC subjects tend to overweight losses. This may be a heuristic to deal with the risk, i.e., the uncertainty. GD subjects perhaps do this less or even overweight gains in these situations. We have seen that GD subjects also react differently to ambiguous gambles compared to HC subjects. Response to ambiguous gambles but not risky gambles may be a useful predictor for GD symptom severity. However, as we have also seen, risk is a higher-order gamble feature, already on mathematical level. Computational modeling studies have shown only trends for GD subjects showing different probability sensitivities compared to HC subjects. The OFC, as mentioned in the context of representation of gain and delayed values, may be again a brain area showing distorted value representation in GD subjects. In situations of ambiguity, learning about probabilities may be distorted especially in high-impulsive gamblers.

Delay discounting of rewards is increased in GD subjects and correlates with severity. In addition, a computational modeling study has observed that delayed values are represented more in DS which may be indicative of addiction progression.

7.5.3.3 Learning from Reward and Punishments

There is ample evidence for altered neural processing in GD subjects during reward receipt. We have seen that IGT performance is reduced in GD subjects. This may be related to impaired learning based on disturbances in PE signal generation in the striatum. We have also seen that GD subjects perform worse in probabilistic reversal learning tasks and that their performance may be predictive for relapse. GD subjects seem to learn worse from negative feedback and thus persevere in their gambling behavior. Reduced sensitivity to loss outcomes, in combination with steady high anticipatory motivation in response to high risk, may be explanatory factors. Computational models have supported these ideas. First results and modeling efforts highlight the importance of focusing on PEs, associated learning rates, and loss sensitivity. There is some evidence that GD subjects show reduced generation of PEs in ventral prefrontal areas. This may also lead to a reduced sensitivity to loss outcomes and response perseveration. Different set-up of RL models may yield different conclusions. Principled model comparisons and model consistency across studies are thus needed.

Loss chasing is of particular interest for understanding GD since it is the only diagnostic criterion not shared with SUDs. Reduced loss aversion on outcome and anticipation level may fuel loss chasing. There is evidence that GD subjects need to activate a medial-prefrontal executive control network more strongly when deciding to quit than HC subjects.

Near misses in the context of learning seem especially dangerous for regular gamblers who may develop GD. Later, in GD subjects, near misses seem desensitized just like all other loss outcomes. So they cannot have an effect on learning anymore. However, motivation for gambling stays high and is easily evoked by relevant cues.

7.5.4   Changes in Neural Substrate

Unlike, e.g., alcohol-dependent subjects [21], GD subjects show only very circumscribed gray matter reductions. These are seen in hippocampus and amygdala and may correlate with impulsivity. GD subjects show increased volume in DS which seems to correlate with GD severity. According to the model by Piray et al. [131], this may be indicative of addiction progression. With respect to white matter, structural and functional connectivity alterations may be present in GD subjects. We have seen that DA receptor density and functioning are informative within GD subjects since they relate to gambling high and severity and putatively cue reactivity. Future computational modeling studies in GD subjects should incorporate information on gray matter, white matter, and neurotransmitter differences between GD and HC subjects For instance, the model by Piray et al. [131] offers parameters for DA receptor density and DA receptor sensitivity.

References

1. Potenza MN. Neurobiology of gambling behaviors. Curr Opin Neurobiol. 2013a;23:660–7.
2. Quester S, Romanczuk-Seiferth N. Brain imaging in gambling disorder. Curr Addict Rep. 2015;2:220–9.
3. Romanczuk-Seiferth N, van den Brink W, Goudriaan AE. From symptoms to neurobiology: pathological gambling in the light of the new classification in DSM-5. Neuropsychobiology. 2014;70:95–102.
4. Stephan KE, Iglesias S, Heinzle J, Diaconescu AO. Translational perspectives for computational neuroimaging. Neuron. 2015;87:716–32.
5. Sebold M, Deserno L, Nebe S, Schad DJ, Garbusow M, Hägele C, et al. Model-based and model-free decisions in alcohol dependence. Neuropsychobiology. 2014;70:122–31.
6. Sutton RS. Introduction to reinforcement learning. Cambridge, MA: MIT Press; 1998.
7. Basten U, Biele G, Heekeren HR, Fiebach CJ. How the brain integrates costs and benefits during decision making. Proc Natl Acad Sci. 2010;107:21767–72.
8. Bischof A, Meyer C, Bischof G, John U, Wurst FM, Thon N, et al. Suicidal events among pathological gamblers: the role of comorbidity of axis I and axis II disorders. Psychiatry Res. 2015;225:413–9.
9. Bundeszentrale für gesundheitliche Aufklärung. Glücksspielverhalten und Glücksspielsucht in Deutschland. Ergebnisse des Surveys 2013 und Trends. Bundeszentrale Für Gesundheitliche Aufklär. 2014.

10. Meyer C, Bischof A, Westram A, Jeske C, de Brito S, Glorius S, et al. The "Pathological Gambling and Epidemiology" (PAGE) study program: design and fieldwork. Int J Methods Psychiatr Res. 2015;24:11–31.
11. Raylu N, Oei TPS. Pathological gambling: a comprehensive review. Clin Psychol Rev. 2002;22:1009–61.
12. Grinols EL, Mustard DB. Business profitability versus social profitability: evaluating industries with externalities, the case of casinos. Manag Decis Econ. 2001;22:143–62.
13. Ladouceur R, Boisvert J-M, Pépin M, Loranger M, Sylvain C. Social cost of pathological gambling. J Gambl Stud. 1994;10:399–409.
14. American Psychiatric Association. Diagnostic and statistical manual of mental disorders: DSM-5. American Psychiatric Association, DSM-5 task force. Arlington, VA: American Psychiatric Association; 2013.
15. Clark L. Disordered gambling: the evolving concept of behavioral addiction. Ann N Y Acad Sci. 2014;1327:46–61.
16. Clark L, Averbeck B, Payer D, Sescousse G, Winstanley CA, Xue G. Pathological choice: the neuroscience of gambling and gambling addiction. J Neurosci. 2013;33:17617–23.
17. Fauth-Bühler M, Mann K, Potenza MN. Pathological gambling: a review of the neurobiological evidence relevant for its classification as an addictive disorder. Addict Biol. 2017;22:885–97.
18. Leeman RF, Potenza MN. Similarities and differences between pathological gambling and substance use disorders: a focus on impulsivity and compulsivity. Psychopharmacology. 2012;219:469–90.
19. Petry NM, Blanco C, Auriacombe M, Borges G, Bucholz K, Crowley TJ, et al. An overview of and rationale for changes proposed for pathological gambling in DSM-5. J Gambl Stud. 2014;30:493–502.
20. Beck A, Schlagenhauf F, Wüstenberg T, Hein J, Kienast T, Kahnt T, et al. Ventral striatal activation during reward anticipation correlates with impulsivity in alcoholics. Biol Psychiatry. 2009;66:734–42.
21. Beck A, Wüstenberg T, Genauck A, Wrase J, Schlagenhauf F, Smolka MN, et al. Effect of brain structure, brain function, and brain connectivity on relapse in alcohol-dependent patients relapse in alcohol-dependent patients. Arch Gen Psychiatry. 2012;69:842–52.
22. Bickel WK, Miller ML, Yi R, Kowal BP, Lindquist DM, Pitcock JA. Behavioral and neuroeconomics of drug addiction: competing neural systems and temporal discounting processes. Drug Alcohol Depend. 2007;90(Suppl 1):S85–91.
23. Boileau I, Payer D, Chugani B, Lobo D, Behzadi A, Rusjan PM, et al. The D2/3 dopamine receptor in pathological gambling: a positron emission tomography study with [11C]-(+)-propyl-hexahydro-naphtho-oxazin and [11C] raclopride. Addiction. 2013;108:953–63.
24. Garbusow M, Schad DJ, Sebold M, Friedel E, Bernhardt N, Koch SP, et al. Pavlovian-to-instrumental transfer effects in the nucleus accumbens relate to relapse in alcohol dependence. Addict Biol. 2016;21:719–31.
25. Gelskov SV, Madsen KH, Ramsøy TZ, Siebner HR. Aberrant neural signatures of decision-making: pathological gamblers display cortico-striatal hypersensitivity to extreme gambles. Neuroimage. 2016;128:342–52.
26. Heinz A, Siessmeier T, Wrase J, Buchholz HG, Gründer G, Kumakura Y, et al. Correlation of alcohol craving with striatal dopamine synthesis capacity and D2/3 receptor availability: a combined [18F]DOPA and [18F]DMFP PET study in detoxified alcoholic patients. Am J Psychiatry. 2005b;162:1515–20.
27. Joutsa J, Johansson J, Niemelä S, Ollikainen A, Hirvonen MM, Piepponen P, et al. Mesolimbic dopamine release is linked to symptom severity in pathological gambling. Neuroimage. 2012;60:1992–9.
28. Koehler S, Hasselmann E, Wüstenberg T, Heinz A, Romanczuk-Seiferth N. Higher volume of ventral striatum and right prefrontal cortex in pathological gambling. Brain Struct Funct. 2015;220:469–77.

29. Park SQ, Kahnt T, Beck A, Cohen MX, Dolan RJ, Wrase J, et al. Prefrontal cortex fails to learn from reward prediction errors in alcohol dependence. J Neurosci. 2010;30:7749–53.
30. Romanczuk-Seiferth N, Koehler S, Dreesen C, Wüstenberg T, Heinz A. Pathological gambling and alcohol dependence: neural disturbances in reward and loss avoidance processing. Addict Biol. 2015;20:557–69.
31. Schott BH, Minuzzi L, Krebs RM, Elmenhorst D, Lang M, Winz OH, et al. Mesolimbic functional magnetic resonance imaging activations during reward anticipation correlate with reward-related ventral striatal dopamine release. J Neurosci. 2008;28:14311–9.
32. Wrase J, Schlagenhauf F, Kienast T, Wustenberg T, Bermpohl F, Kahnt T, et al. Dysfunction of reward processing correlates with alcohol craving in detoxified alcoholics. Neuroimage. 2007;35:787–94.
33. Genauck A, Huys QJ, Heinz A, Rapp MA. Pawlowsch-Instrumentelle Transfereffekte bei Alkoholabhängigkeit. SUCHT. 2013;59:215–23.
34. Huys QJM, Cools R, Gölzer M, Friedel E, Heinz A, Dolan RJ, et al. Disentangling the roles of approach, activation and valence in instrumental and Pavlovian responding. PLoS Comput Biol. 2011;7:e1002028.
35. Huys QJM, Deserno L, Obermayer K, Schlagenhauf F, Heinz A. Model-free temporal-difference learning and dopamine in alcohol dependence: examining concepts from theory and animals in human imaging. Biol Psychiatry Cogn Neurosci Neuroimaging. 2016a;1:401–10.
36. Schad DJ, Jünger E, Sebold M, Garbusow M, Bernhardt N, Javadi A-H, et al. Processing speed enhances model-based over model-free reinforcement learning in the presence of high working memory functioning. Decis Neurosci. 2014;5:1450.
37. Sebold M, Schad DJ, Nebe S, Garbusow M, Jünger E, Kroemer NB, et al. Don't think, just feel the music: individuals with strong Pavlovian-to-instrumental transfer effects rely less on model-based reinforcement learning. J Cogn Neurosci. 2016;28:985–95.
38. Huys QJM, Maia TV, Frank MJ. Computational psychiatry as a bridge from neuroscience to clinical applications. Nat Neurosci. 2016b;19:404–13.
39. Paulus MP, Huys QJM, Maia TV. A roadmap for the development of applied computational psychiatry. Biol Psychiatry Cogn Neurosci Neuroimaging. 2016;1:386–92.
40. Goldstein RZ, Volkow ND. Drug addiction and its underlying neurobiological basis: neuroimaging evidence for the involvement of the frontal cortex. Am J Psychiatry. 2002;159:1642–52.
41. Robinson TE, Berridge KC. Incentive-sensitization and addiction. Addiction. 2001;96:103–14.
42. Reynolds B, Ortengren A, Richards JB, de Wit H. Dimensions of impulsive behavior: Personality and behavioral measures. Personal Individ Differ. 2006;40:305–15.
43. Whiteside SP, Lynam DR. The Five Factor Model and impulsivity: using a structural model of personality to understand impulsivity. Personal Individ Differ. 2001;30:669–89.
44. Bechara A, Damasio H. Decision-making and addiction (part I): impaired activation of somatic states in substance dependent individuals when pondering decisions with negative future consequences. Neuropsychologia. 2002;40:1675–89.
45. Bechara A, Dolan S, Hindes A. Decision-making and addiction (part II): myopia for the future or hypersensitivity to reward? Neuropsychologia. 2002;40:1690–705.
46. Clark L. Decision-making during gambling: an integration of cognitive and psychobiological approaches. Philos Trans R Soc Lond Ser B Biol Sci. 2010;365:319–30.
47. Rangel A, Camerer C, Montague PR. A framework for studying the neurobiology of value-based decision making. Nat Rev Neurosci. 2008;9:545–56.
48. Reiter AM, Heinze H-J, Schlagenhauf F, Deserno L. Impaired flexible reward-based decision-making in binge eating disorder: evidence from computational modeling and functional neuroimaging. Neuropsychopharmacology. 2017;42:628–37.
49. Miedl SF, Peters J, Büchel C. Altered neural reward representations in pathological gamblers revealed by delay and probability discounting. Arch Gen Psychiatry. 2012;69:177–86.
50. Goudriaan AE, Oosterlaan J, De Beurs E, Van Den Brink W. Neurocognitive functions in pathological gambling: a comparison with alcohol dependence, Tourette syndrome and normal controls. Addiction. 2006b;101:534–47.

51. Moccia L, Pettorruso M, De Crescenzo F, De Risio L, di Nuzzo L, Martinotti G, et al. Neural correlates of cognitive control in gambling disorder: a systematic review of fMRI studies. Neurosci Biobehav Rev. 2017;78:104–16.
52. Goudriaan AE, Oosterlaan J, Beurs ED, Brink WVD. The role of self-reported impulsivity and reward sensitivity versus neurocognitive measures of disinhibition and decision-making in the prediction of relapse in pathological gamblers. Psychol Med. 2008;38:41–50.
53. Goudriaan AE, Oosterlaan J, de Beurs E, van den Brink W. Decision making in pathological gambling: a comparison between pathological gamblers, alcohol dependents, persons with Tourette syndrome, and normal controls. Cogn Brain Res. 2005;23:137–51.
54. Kertzman S, Lowengrub K, Aizer A, Vainder M, Kotler M, Dannon PN. Go–no-go performance in pathological gamblers. Psychiatry Res. 2008;161:1–10.
55. van Holst RJ, van Holstein M, van den Brink W, Veltman DJ, Goudriaan AE. Response inhibition during cue reactivity in problem gamblers: an fMRI study. PLoS One. 2012a;7:e30909.
56. Zhang J, Berridge KC, Tindell AJ, Smith KS, Aldridge JW. A neural computational model of incentive salience. PLoS Comput Biol. 2009;5:e1000437.
57. Kertzman S, Lowengrub K, Aizer A, Nahum ZB, Kotler M, Dannon PN. Stroop performance in pathological gamblers. Psychiatry Res. 2006;142:1–10.
58. McCusker CG. Cognitive biases and addiction: an evolution in theory and method. Addiction. 2001;96:47–56.
59. McCusker CG, Gettings B. Automaticity of cognitive biases in addictive behaviours: further evidence with gamblers. Br J Clin Psychol. 1997;36:543–54.
60. Potenza MN, Steinberg MA, Skudlarski P, et al. Gambling urges in pathological gambling: a functional magnetic resonance imaging study. Arch Gen Psychiatry. 2003;60:828–36.
61. de Ruiter MB, Oosterlaan J, Veltman DJ, van den Brink W, Goudriaan AE. Similar hyporesponsiveness of the dorsomedial prefrontal cortex in problem gamblers and heavy smokers during an inhibitory control task. Drug Alcohol Depend. 2012;121:81–9.
62. Field M, Munafò MR, Franken IHA. A meta-analytic investigation of the relationship between attentional bias and subjective craving in substance abuse. Psychol Bull. 2009;135:589–607.
63. Carter BL, Tiffany ST. Meta-analysis of cue-reactivity in addiction research. Addiction. 1999;94:327–40.
64. Chase HW, Eickhoff SB, Laird AR, Hogarth L. The neural basis of drug stimulus processing and craving: an activation likelihood estimation meta-analysis. Biol Psychiatry. 2011;70:785–93.
65. Schacht JP, Anton RF, Myrick H. Functional neuroimaging studies of alcohol cue reactivity: a quantitative meta-analysis and systematic review. Addict Biol. 2013;18:121–33.
66. Balodis IM, Lacadie CM, Potenza MN. A preliminary study of the neural correlates of the intensities of self-reported gambling urges and emotions in men with pathological gambling. J Gambl Stud. 2012b;28:493–513.
67. Potenza MN. The neurobiology of pathological gambling and drug addiction: an overview and new findings. Philos Trans R Soc B Biol Sci. 2008;363:3181–9.
68. Goudriaan AE, de Ruiter MB, van den Brink W, Oosterlaan J, Veltman DJ. Brain activation patterns associated with cue reactivity and craving in abstinent problem gamblers, heavy smokers and healthy controls: an fMRI study. Addict Biol. 2010;15:491–503.
69. Crockford DN, Goodyear B, Edwards J, Quickfall J, el-Guebaly N. Cue-induced brain activity in pathological gamblers. Biol Psychiatry. 2005;58:787–95.
70. Wölfling K, Mörsen CP, Duven E, Albrecht U, Grüsser SM, Flor H. To gamble or not to gamble: at risk for craving and relapse--learned motivated attention in pathological gambling. Biol Psychol. 2011;87:275–81.
71. Limbrick-Oldfield EH, Mick I, Cocks RE, McGonigle J, Sharman SP, Goldstone AP, et al. Neural substrates of cue reactivity and craving in gambling disorder. Transl Psychiatry. 2017;7:e992.
72. Kushner MG, Abrams K, Donahue C, Thuras P, Frost R, Kim SW. Urge to gamble in problem gamblers exposed to a casino environment. J Gambl Stud Co-Spons Natl Counc Probl Gambl Inst Study Gambl Commer Gaming. 2007;23:121–32.

73. van Holst RJ, Veltman DJ, van den Brink W, Goudriaan AE. Right on cue? Striatal reactivity in problem gamblers. Biol Psychiatry. 2012c;72:e23–4.
74. van Holst RJ, Veltman DJ, Büchel C, van den Brink W, Goudriaan AE. Distorted expectancy coding in problem gambling: is the addictive in the anticipation? Biol Psychiatry. 2012d;71:741–8.
75. Leyton M, Vezina P. On cue: striatal ups and downs in addictions. Biol Psychiatry. 2012;72:e21–2.
76. Miedl SF, Büchel C, Peters J. Cue-induced craving increases impulsivity via changes in striatal value signals in problem gamblers. J Neurosci. 2014;34:4750–5.
77. Blum K, Braverman ER, Holder JM, Lubar JF, Monastra VJ, Miller D, et al. The reward deficiency syndrome: a biogenetic model for the diagnosis and treatment of impulsive, addictive and compulsive behaviors. J Psychoactive Drugs. 2000;32:1–112.
78. Sescousse G, Barbalat G, Domenech P, Dreher J-C. Imbalance in the sensitivity to different types of rewards in pathological gambling. Brain. 2013;136:2527–38.
79. Knutson B, Westdorp A, Kaiser E, Hommer D. FMRI visualization of brain activity during a monetary incentive delay task. Neuroimage. 2000;12:20–7.
80. Berridge KC. Food reward: brain substrates of wanting and liking. Neurosci Biobehav Rev. 1996;20:1–25.
81. Berridge KC, Robinson TE. The mind of an addicted brain: neural sensitization of wanting versus liking. Curr Dir Psychol Sci. 1995;4:71–6.
82. Berridge KC, Robinson TE, Aldridge JW. Dissecting components of reward: 'liking', 'wanting', and learning. Curr Opin Pharmacol. 2009;9:65–73.
83. Schultz W, Dayan P, Montague PR. A neural substrate of prediction and reward. Science. 1997;275:1593–9.
84. Knutson B, Adams CM, Fong GW, Hommer D, et al. Anticipation of increasing monetary reward selectively recruits nucleus accumbens. J Neurosci. 2001;21:1–5.
85. Balodis IM, Kober H, Worhunsky PD, Stevens MC, Pearlson GD, Potenza MN. Diminished frontostriatal activity during processing of monetary rewards and losses in pathological gambling. Biol Psychiatry. 2012a;71:749–57.
86. Choi J-S, Shin Y-C, Jung WH, Jang JH, Kang D-H, Choi C-H, et al. Altered brain activity during reward anticipation in pathological gambling and obsessive-compulsive disorder. PLoS One. 2012;7:e45938.
87. Tsurumi K, Kawada R, Yokoyama N, Sugihara G, Sawamoto N, Aso T, et al. Insular activation during reward anticipation reflects duration of illness in abstinent pathological gamblers. Front Psychol. 2014;5:1013.
88. Worhunsky PD, Malison RT, Rogers RD, Potenza MN. Altered neural correlates of reward and loss processing during simulated slot-machine fMRI in pathological gambling and cocaine dependence. Drug Alcohol Depend. 2014;145:77–86.
89. Genauck A, Quester S, Wüstenberg T, Mörsen C, Heinz A, Romanczuk-Seiferth N. Reduced loss aversion in pathological gambling and alcohol dependence is associated with differential alterations in amygdala and prefrontal functioning. Sci Rep. 2017;7:16306.
90. Tom SM, Fox CR, Trepel C, Poldrack RA. The neural basis of loss aversion in decision-making under risk. Science. 2007;315:515–8.
91. Fauth-Bühler M, Zois E, Vollstädt-Klein S, Lemenager T, Beutel M, Mann K. Insula and striatum activity in effort-related monetary reward processing in gambling disorder: The role of depressive symptomatology. Neuroimage Clin. 2014;6:243–51.
92. Reuter J, Raedler T, Rose M, Hand I, Gläscher J, Büchel C. Pathological gambling is linked to reduced activation of the mesolimbic reward system. Nat Neurosci. 2005;8:147–8.
93. Miedl SF, Fehr T, Meyer G, Herrmann M. Neurobiological correlates of problem gambling in a quasi-realistic blackjack scenario as revealed by fMRI. Psychiatry Res Neuroimaging. 2010;181:165–73.
94. Habib R, Dixon MR. Neurobehavioral evidence for the "Near-Miss" effect in pathological gamblers. J Exp Anal Behav. 2010;93:313–28.

95. Goudriaan AE, Oosterlaan J, de Beurs E, van den Brink W. Psychophysiological determinants and concomitants of deficient decision making in pathological gamblers. Drug Alcohol Depend. 2006a;84:231–9.
96. Tanabe J, Thompson L, Claus E, Dalwani M, Hutchison K, Banich MT. Prefrontal cortex activity is reduced in gambling and nongambling substance users during decision-making. Hum Brain Mapp. 2007;28:1276–86.
97. Brevers D, Cleeremans A, Verbruggen F, Bechara A, Kornreich C, Verbanck P, et al. Impulsive action but not impulsive choice determines problem gambling severity. PLoS One. 2012b;7:e50647.
98. Giorgetta C, Grecucci A, Rattin A, Guerreschi C, Sanfey AG, Bonini N. To play or not to play: a personal dilemma in pathological gambling. Psychiatry Res. 2014;219:562–9.
99. Lorains FK, Dowling NA, Enticott PG, Bradshaw JL, Trueblood JS, Stout JC. Strategic and non-strategic problem gamblers differ on decision-making under risk and ambiguity. Addiction. 2014;109:1128–37.
100. Takeuchi H, Kawada R, Tsurumi K, Yokoyama N, Takemura A, Murao T, et al. Heterogeneity of loss aversion in pathological gambling. J Gambl Stud. 2016;32:1143–54.
101. Barkley-Levenson EE, Van Leijenhorst L, Galván A. Behavioral and neural correlates of loss aversion and risk avoidance in adolescents and adults. Dev Cogn Neurosci. 2013;3:72–83.
102. Canessa N, Crespi C, Motterlini M, Baud-Bovy G, Chierchia G, Pantaleo G, et al. The functional and structural neural basis of individual differences in loss aversion. J Neurosci. 2013;33:14307–17.
103. Litt A, Eliasmith C, Thagard P. Neural affective decision theory: choices, brains, and emotions. Cogn Syst Res. 2008;9:252–73.
104. Clark L, Bechara A, Damasio H, Aitken MRF, Sahakian BJ, Robbins TW. Differential effects of insular and ventromedial prefrontal cortex lesions on risky decision-making. Brain. 2008;131:1311–22.
105. Kassinove JI, Schare ML. Effects of the "near miss" and the "big win" on persistence at slot machine gambling. Psychol Addict Behav. 2001;15:155–8.
106. Parke J, Griffiths M. Gambling addiction and the evolution of the "near miss". Addict Res Theory. 2004;12:407–11.
107. Reid RL. The psychology of the near miss. J Gambl Behav. 1986;2:32–9.
108. Clark L, Lawrence AJ, Astley-Jones F, Gray N. Gambling near-misses enhance motivation to gamble and recruit win-related brain circuitry. Neuron. 2009;61:481–90.
109. Chase HW, Clark L. Gambling severity predicts midbrain response to near-miss outcomes. J Neurosci. 2010;30:6180–7.
110. Solomon RL, Kamin LJ, Wynne LC. Traumatic avoidance learning: the outcomes of several extinction procedures with dogs. J Abnorm Psychol. 1953;48:291–302.
111. Platt ML, Huettel SA. Risky business: the neuroeconomics of decision making under uncertainty. Nat Neurosci. 2008;11:398–403.
112. Minati L, Grisoli M, Franceschetti S, Epifani F, Granvillano A, Medford N, et al. Neural signatures of economic parameters during decision-making: a functional MRI (fMRI), electroencephalography (EEG) and autonomic monitoring study. Brain Topogr. 2012;25:73–96.
113. Brevers D, Cleeremans A, Goudriaan AE, Bechara A, Kornreich C, Verbanck P, et al. Decision making under ambiguity but not under risk is related to problem gambling severity. Psychiatry Res. 2012a;200:568–74.
114. Power Y, Goodyear B, Crockford D. Neural correlates of pathological gamblers preference for immediate rewards during the Iowa Gambling Task: An fMRI Study. J Gambl Stud. 2011;28:623–36.
115. Lejuez CW, Magidson JF, Mitchell SH, Sinha R, Stevens MC, De Wit H. Behavioral and biological indicators of impulsivity in the development of alcohol use, problems, and disorders. Alcohol Clin Exp Res. 2010;34:1334–45.
116. White TL, Lejuez CW, de Wit H. Test-retest characteristics of the Balloon Analogue Risk Task (BART). Exp Clin Psychopharmacol. 2008;16:565–70.

117. Krmpotich T, Mikulich-Gilbertson S, Sakai J, Thompson L, Banich MT, Tanabe J. Impaired decision-making, higher impulsivity, and drug severity in substance dependence and pathological gambling. J Addict Med. 2015;9:273–80.
118. Cavedini P, Riboldi G, Keller R, D'Annucci A, Bellodi L. Frontal lobe dysfunction in pathological gambling patients. Biol Psychiatry. 2002;51:334–41.
119. Petry NM. Discounting of probabilistic rewards is associated with gambling abstinence in treatment-seeking pathological gamblers. J Abnorm Psychol. 2012;121:151–9.
120. Ballard K, Knutson B. Dissociable neural representations of future reward magnitude and delay during temporal discounting. Neuroimage. 2009;45:143–50.
121. MacKillop J, Amlung MT, Few LR, Ray LA, Sweet LH, Munafò MR. Delayed reward discounting and addictive behavior: a meta-analysis. Psychopharmacology. 2011;216:305–21.
122. Alessi SM, Petry NM. Pathological gambling severity is associated with impulsivity in a delay discounting procedure. Behav Process. 2003;64:345–54.
123. Dixon MR, Marley J, Jacobs EA. Delay discounting by pathological gamblers. J Appl Behav Anal. 2003;36:449–58.
124. Petry NM, Casarella T. Excessive discounting of delayed rewards in substance abusers with gambling problems. Drug Alcohol Depend. 1999;56:25–32.
125. Dixon MR, Jacobs EA, Sanders S. Contextual control of delay discounting by pathological gamblers. J Appl Behav Anal. 2006;39:413–22.
126. Schultz W. Predictive reward signal of dopamine neurons. J Neurophysiol. 1998;80:1–27.
127. Linnet J, Peterson E, Doudet DJ, Gjedde A, Møller A. Dopamine release in ventral striatum of pathological gamblers losing money. Acta Psychiatr Scand. 2010;122:326–33.
128. Linnet J, Møller A, Peterson E, Gjedde A, Doudet D. Inverse association between dopaminergic neurotransmission and Iowa Gambling Task performance in pathological gamblers and healthy controls. Scand J Psychol. 2011;52:28–34.
129. van Eimeren T, Ballanger B, Pellecchia G, Miyasaki JM, Lang AE, Strafella AP. Dopamine agonists diminish value sensitivity of the orbitofrontal cortex: a trigger for pathological gambling in Parkinson's disease? Neuropsychopharmacology. 2009;34:2758–66.
130. Tanabe J, Reynolds J, Krmpotich T, Claus E, Thompson LL, Du YP, et al. Reduced neural tracking of prediction error in substance-dependent individuals. Am J Psychiatry. 2013;170:1356–63.
131. Piray P, Keramati MM, Dezfouli A, Lucas C, Mokri A. Individual differences in nucleus accumbens dopamine receptors predict development of addiction-like behavior: a computational approach. Neural Comput. 2010;22:2334–68.
132. Calu DJ, Stalnaker TA, Franz TM, Singh T, Shaham Y, Schoenbaum G. Withdrawal from cocaine self-administration produces long-lasting deficits in orbitofrontal-dependent reversal learning in rats. Learn Mem. 2007;14:325–8.
133. Deserno L, Beck A, Huys QJM, Lorenz RC, Buchert R, Buchholz H-G, et al. Chronic alcohol intake abolishes the relationship between dopamine synthesis capacity and learning signals in the ventral striatum. Eur J Neurosci. 2015;41:477–86.
134. Jentsch JD, Olausson P, Garza RDL, Taylor JR. Impairments of reversal learning and response perseveration after repeated, intermittent cocaine administrations to monkeys. Neuropsychopharmacology. 2002;26:183–90.
135. de Ruiter MB, Veltman DJ, Goudriaan AE, Oosterlaan J, Sjoerds Z, van den Brink W. Response perseveration and ventral prefrontal sensitivity to reward and punishment in male problem gamblers and smokers. Neuropsychopharmacology. 2008;34:1027–38.
136. Goldstein RZ, Volkow ND. Dysfunction of the prefrontal cortex in addiction: neuroimaging findings and clinical implications. Nat Rev Neurosci. 2011;12:652–69.
137. Gläscher J, Daw N, Dayan P, O'Doherty JP. States versus rewards: dissociable neural prediction error signals underlying model-based and model-free reinforcement learning. Neuron. 2010;66:585–95.
138. Schultz W, Dickinson A. Neuronal coding of prediction errors. Annu Rev Neurosci. 2000;23:473–500.

139. Campbell-Meiklejohn DK, Woolrich MW, Passingham RE, Rogers RD. Knowing when to stop: the brain mechanisms of chasing losses. Biol Psychiatry. 2008;63:293–300.
140. Worhunsky PD, Potenza MN, Rogers RD. Alterations in functional brain networks associated with loss-chasing in gambling disorder and cocaine-use disorder. Drug Alcohol Depend. 2017;178:363–71.
141. MacKillop J, Anderson EJ, Castelda BA, Mattson RE, Donovick PJ. Convergent validity of measures of cognitive distortions, impulsivity, and time perspective with pathological gambling. Psychol Addict Behav. 2006;20:75.
142. Hyman SE, Malenka RC, Nestler EJ. Neural mechanisms of addiction: the role of reward-related learning and memory. Annu Rev Neurosci. 2006;29:565–98.
143. Kauer JA, Malenka RC. Synaptic plasticity and addiction. Nat Rev Neurosci. 2007;8:844–58.
144. Nestler EJ. Molecular basis of long-term plasticity underlying addiction. Nat Rev Neurosci. 2001;2:119–28.
145. Draganski B, Gaser C, Busch V, Schuierer G, Bogdahn U, May A. Neuroplasticity: changes in grey matter induced by training. Nature. 2004;427:311–2.
146. Lüscher C, Malenka RC. Drug-evoked synaptic plasticity in addiction: from molecular changes to circuit remodeling. Neuron. 2011;69:650–63.
147. Russo SJ, Dietz DM, Dumitriu D, Morrison JH, Malenka RC, Nestler EJ. The addicted synapse: mechanisms of synaptic and structural plasticity in nucleus accumbens. Trends Neurosci. 2010;33:267–76.
148. Purves D. Neuroscience. 4th ed. Sunderland, MA: Sinauer Associates, Inc.; 2008.
149. van Holst RJ, de Ruiter MB, van den Brink W, Veltman DJ, Goudriaan AE. A voxel-based morphometry study comparing problem gamblers, alcohol abusers, and healthy controls. Drug Alcohol Depend. 2012b;124:142–8.
150. Joutsa J, Saunavaara J, Parkkola R, Niemelä S, Kaasinen V. Extensive abnormality of brain white matter integrity in pathological gambling. Psychiatry Res Neuroimaging. 2011;194:340–6.
151. Rahman AS, Xu J, Potenza MN. Hippocampal and amygdalar volumetric differences in pathological gambling: a preliminary study of the associations with the behavioral inhibition system. Neuropsychopharmacology. 2014;39:738–45.
152. Aron AR, Robbins TW, Poldrack RA. Inhibition and the right inferior frontal cortex: one decade on. Trends Cogn Sci. 2014;18:177–85.
153. Kleim JA, Lussnig E, Schwarz ER, Comery TA, Greenough WT. Synaptogenesis and Fos expression in the motor cortex of the adult rat after motor skill learning. J Neurosci. 1996;16:4529–35.
154. Gould E, Reeves AJ, Graziano MS, Gross CG. Neurogenesis in the neocortex of adult primates. Science. 1999;286:548–52.
155. Eliasmith C. How to build a brain: a neural architecture for biological cognition. Oxford: Oxford University Press; 2013.
156. Yip SW, Lacadie C, Xu J, Worhunsky PD, Fulbright RK, Constable RT, et al. Reduced genual corpus callosal white matter integrity in pathological gambling and its relationship to alcohol abuse or dependence. World J Biol Psychiatry. 2013;14:129–38.
157. Koehler S, Ovadia-Caro S, van der ME, Villringer A, Heinz A, Romanczuk-Seiferth N, et al. Increased functional connectivity between prefrontal cortex and reward system in pathological gambling. PLoS One. 2013;8:e84565.
158. Tschernegg M, Crone JS, Eigenberger T, Schwartenbeck P, Fauth-Bühler M, Lemènager T, et al. Abnormalities of functional brain networks in pathological gambling: a graph-theoretical approach. Front Hum Neurosci. 2013;7:625.
159. Potenza MN. How central is dopamine to pathological gambling or gambling disorder? Front Behav Neurosci. 2013b;7:206.
160. Zack M, Poulos CX. Effects of the atypical stimulant modafinil on a brief gambling episode in pathological gamblers with high vs. low impulsivity. J Psychopharmacol (Oxf). 2009;23:660–71.

161. Heiden P, Heinz A, Romanczuk-Seiferth N. Pathological gambling in Parkinson's disease: what are the risk factors and what is the role of impulsivity? Eur J Neurosci. 2017;45:67–72.
162. Steeves TDL, Miyasaki J, Zurowski M, Lang AE, Pellecchia G, Eimeren TV, et al. Increased striatal dopamine release in Parkinsonian patients with pathological gambling: a [11C] raclopride PET study. Brain. 2009;132:1376–85.
163. Dalley JW, Fryer TD, Brichard L, Robinson ESJ, Theobald DEH, Lääne K, et al. Nucleus accumbens D2/3 receptors predict trait impulsivity and cocaine reinforcement. Science. 2007;315:1267–70.
164. Heidbreder CA, Gardner EL, Xi Z-X, Thanos PK, Mugnaini M, Hagan JJ, et al. The role of central dopamine D3 receptors in drug addiction: a review of pharmacological evidence. Brain Res Rev. 2005;49:77–105.
165. Volkow ND, Wang GJ, Fowler JS, Logan J, Hitzemann R, Ding YS, et al. Decreases in dopamine receptors but not in dopamine transporters in alcoholics. Alcohol Clin Exp Res. 1996;20:1594–8.
166. Gelernter J, Goldman D, Risch N. The A1 allele at the D2 dopamine receptor gene and alcoholism: a reappraisal. JAMA. 1993;269:1673–7.
167. Gelernter J, Kranzler H. D2 dopamine receptor gene (DRD2) allele and haplotype frequencies in alcohol dependent and control subjects: no association with phenotype or severity of phenotype. Neuropsychopharmacology. 1999;20:640–9.
168. Klein TA, Neumann J, Reuter M, Hennig J, von Cramon DY, Ullsperger M. Genetically determined differences in learning from errors. Science. 2007;318:1642–5.
169. Uhl G, Blum K, Noble E, Smith S. Substance abuse vulnerability and D2 receptor genes. Trends Neurosci. 1993;16:83–8.
170. Cocker PJ, Le Foll B, Rogers RD, Winstanley CA. A selective role for dopamine D_4 receptors in modulating reward expectancy in a rodent slot machine task. Biol Psychiatry. 2014;75:817–24.
171. van Holst RJ, van den Brink W, Veltman DJ, Goudriaan AE. Brain imaging studies in pathological gambling. Curr Psychiatry Rep. 2010;12:418–25.
172. Aston-Jones G, Bloom FE. Activity of norepinephrine-containing locus coeruleus neurons in behaving rats anticipates fluctuations in the sleep-waking cycle. J Neurosci. 1981;1:876–86.
173. Skosnik PD, Chatterton RT Jr, Swisher T, Park S. Modulation of attentional inhibition by norepinephrine and cortisol after psychological stress. Int J Psychophysiol. 2000;36:59–68.
174. Bullock SA, Potenza MN. Pathological gambling: neuropsychopharmacology and treatment. Curr Psychopharmacol. 2012;1:67–85.
175. Elman I, Becerra L, Tschibelu E, Yamamoto R, George E, Borsook D. Yohimbine-induced amygdala activation in pathological gamblers: a pilot study. PLoS One. 2012;7:e31118.
176. Muller CP, Jacobs B. Handbook of the behavioral neurobiology of serotonin, vol. 21. London: Academic Press; 2009.
177. Daw ND, Kakade S, Dayan P. Opponent interactions between serotonin and dopamine. Neural Netw. 2002;15:603–16.
178. Dayan P, Huys QJM. Serotonin, inhibition, and negative mood. PLoS Comput Biol. 2008;4:e4.
179. Nordin C, Eklundh T. Altered CSF 5-HIAA disposition in pathologic male gamblers. CNS Spectr. 1999;4:25–33.
180. Esch T, Stefano GB. The neurobiology of pleasure, reward processes, addiction and their health implications. Neuroendocrinol Lett. 2004;25:235–51.
181. Chiara GD, Imperato A. Drugs abused by humans preferentially increase synaptic dopamine concentrations in the mesolimbic system of freely moving rats. Proc Natl Acad Sci U S A. 1988;85:5274–8.
182. Spanagel R, Herz A, Shippenberg TS. Opposing tonically active endogenous opioid systems modulate the mesolimbic dopaminergic pathway. Proc Natl Acad Sci U S A. 1992;89:2046–50.
183. Heinz A, Reimold M, Wrase J, Hermann D, Croissant B, Mundle G, et al. Correlation of stable elevations in striatal μ-opioid receptor availability in detoxified alcoholic patients with

alcohol craving: a positron emission tomography study using carbon 11-labeled carfentanil. Arch Gen Psychiatry. 2005a;62:57–64.

184. Shinohara K, Yanagisawa A, Kagota Y, Gomi A, Nemoto K, Moriya E, et al. Physiological changes in Pachinko players; beta-endorphin, catecholamines, immune system substances and heart rate. Appl Hum Sci. 1999;18:37–42.

185. Kahneman D, Tversky A. Prospect theory: an analysis of decision under risk. Econom J Econom Soc. 1979;47:263–91.

186. Strens M. A Bayesian framework for reinforcement learning. ICML. 2000:943–950. At http://web.eecs.utk.edu/~itamar/courses/ECE-692/paper1c.pdf.

187. Herrnstein RJ. On the law of effect. J Exp Anal Behav. 1970;13:243–66.

188. Behrens TEJ, Woolrich MW, Walton ME, Rushworth MFS. Learning the value of information in an uncertain world. Nat Neurosci. 2007;10:1214–21.

189. Iglesias A, del Castillo MD, Serrano JI, Oliva J. A computational knowledge-based model for emulating human performance in the Iowa Gambling Task. Neural Netw. 2012;33:168–80.

190. Anderson AK, Phelps EA. Lesions of the human amygdala impair enhanced perception of emotionally salient events. Nature. 2001;411:305–9.

191. Gottfried JA, O'Doherty J, Dolan RJ. Encoding predictive reward value in human amygdala and orbitofrontal cortex. Science. 2003;301:1104–7.

192. Joel D, Niv Y, Ruppin E. Actor–critic models of the basal ganglia: new anatomical and computational perspectives. Neural Netw. 2002;15:535–47.

193. Lim MSM, Jocham G, Hunt LT, Behrens TEJ, Rogers RD. Impulsivity and predictive control are associated with suboptimal action-selection and action-value learning in regular gamblers. Int Gambl Stud. 2015;15:489–505.

194. Shead NW, Hodgins DC. Probability discounting of gains and losses: implications for risk attitudes and impulsivity. J Exp Anal Behav. 2009;92:1–16.

195. Shead NW, Callan MJ, Hodgins DC. Probability discounting among gamblers: differences across problem gambling severity and affect-regulation expectancies. Personal Individ Differ. 2008;45:536–41.

196. Patton JH, Stanford MS, Barratt ES. Factor structure of the Barratt impulsiveness scale. J Clin Psychol. 1995;51:768–74.

Pharmacological Interventions in Gambling Disorder

8

Gustavo C. Medeiros and Jon E. Grant

8.1 Introduction

Gambling disorder (GD) is associated with a wide range of negative consequences such as familial, occupational, legal, and financial difficulties as well as suicidality and lower quality of life [1–3]. Despite the significant personal and social impact, the number of clinical trials in GD is relatively small.

With respect to the management of GD, the most established therapeutic approaches are either psychotherapy (particularly cognitive behavioral therapy) or pharmacological interventions. Although psychotherapeutic treatments have shown significant benefits [4, 5], there are some difficulties in providing psychological treatment on a large scale given the insufficient number of trained therapists [5]. Consequently, pharmacological interventions are an important tool in the therapeutic arsenal.

Pharmacotherapy in GD has some important aims. First, psychotropic drugs are important to effectively treat co-occurring psychiatric disorders, which are highly prevalent in GD [3]. Alcohol-use disorder, substance-use disorder, major depression, and anxiety disorders are particularly common in subjects with GD. Second, some medications appear to reduce urges to gamble and gambling behavior independent of any underlying co-occurring psychiatric disorder. Therefore, there are medications that appear to target the pathophysiology of GD. In this chapter, we will review the evidence regarding the different pharmacotherapies that have been investigated in GD.

G. C. Medeiros (✉)
Department of Psychiatry, University of Texas, Southwestern Medical Center, Dallas, TX, USA

J. E. Grant
Department of Psychiatry and Behavioral Neuroscience, University of Chicago, Chicago, IL, USA
e-mail: jongrant@uchicago.edu

© Springer Nature Switzerland AG 2019
A. Heinz et al. (eds.), *Gambling Disorder*, https://doi.org/10.1007/978-3-030-03060-5_8

8.2   Classification and Clinical Approaches

GD, previously called pathological gambling, has been theoretically associated with different categories of mental disorders. Understanding the diverse approaches to the categorization of GD provides important insight into the different strategies used in clinical trials.

GD was originally thought to belong to the obsessive-compulsive disorder spectrum. This parallel was established due to the repetitive thoughts and behaviors associated with gambling in disordered gamblers. There was also a theory that GD was a bipolar spectrum disorder, i.e., the inappropriate gambling behavior would be a consequence of underlying hypomanic/cyclothymic states. The assumptions that GD was an obsessive-compulsive spectrum disorder incentivized trials focused on selective serotonin reuptake inhibitors—SSRIs [6]. Similarly, the affective theory of GD led to clinical studies with mood stabilizers and antipsychotics.

Phenomenological, genetic, epidemiological, and neurobiological research over the ensuing years has suggested that GD actually has much more in common with addictions, especially alcohol-use disorders [7–10]. This understanding of GD as a type of behavioral addiction has led to a stronger interest in medications that directly or indirectly might modulate the reward system and/or the prefrontal cortex to improve inhibition. Based on this conceptualization of GD, trials using opioid antagonists (naltrexone, nalmefene) or glutamate modulators (N-acetylcysteine, memantine, topiramate) have been conducted.

Although the number of clinical trials for GD in the last decade has increased, the available evidence available is still limited. There is no drug approved by the Food and Drug Administration (FDA) and no established treatment guidelines. Since there are still significant rates of relapse and chronicity in GD, the need for more and larger clinical trials is evident. Despite these limitations, clinical trials have provided important insights with respect to pharmacological interventions in GD.

8.3   The Reward System

The reward system comprises complex and interconnected neurocircuits affiliated with pleasure, reward-seeking, and motivation. A basic understanding of its structures and neurotransmitters gives important insights regarding pharmacological interventions in GD. The reward system consists of evolutionary old circuits located deep in the brain. Natural behaviors such as food and sex classically activate the reward system, and this stimulation is essential to the repetition of these vital behaviors. Other behaviors such as gambling were found to stimulate the reward system as well. In other words, gambling "hijacks" a neurocircuitry naturally associated with reward and repetition of behaviors. This is a major process in the development of disordered gambling.

Two major structures of the reward system are the ventral tegmental area and the nucleus accumbens. They use dopamine as primary neurotransmitter. The strength by which substances or behaviors stimulate the reward system (thought to be largely via dopamine release) is roughly correlated with the addictive potential. In this context, dopaminergic agonists such as the drug pramipexole have been linked with the development of impulsive/addictive behaviors (such as disordered gambling) as a side effect.

It is important to note that the dopamine release is under control of secondary pathways that use diverse neurotransmitters. One of the major modulators of the reward system is the opioid system, i.e., endogenous opioids indirectly control the release of dopamine in the reward system. Hence, by modulation of dopamine activity, opioid drugs may modulate pleasure, excitement, and craving [11]. Thus, several clinical trials have investigated opioid antagonists such as naltrexone and nalmefene for GD.

Part of the complexity of the reward system comes from its connections with other brain regions such as the hippocampus (associated with memory) and the prefrontal cortex (associated with planning and decision-making). Glutamatergic neurocircuits seem to modulate the interaction between the prefrontal cortex and the nucleus accumbens, a main component of the reward system [12]. It is postulated that glutamate is implicated with the regulation of motivational responses and reward-seeking behaviors [12]. Consequently, medications that affect the glutamatergic neurotransmission may also benefit disordered gamblers.

8.4   Opioid Antagonists

Endogenous opioids indirectly modulate dopamine release in the reward system. Consequently, several trials investigated the efficacy of opioid antagonists in GD (main trials displayed in Table 8.1). Opioid antagonists are probably the class of medication with the strongest evidence for GD.

Table 8.1 Summary of clinical trials conducted with opioid antagonists for gambling disorder

Study	Drug	Sample	Study design	Duration	Result
Kim and Grant [13]	Naltrexone	n = 17	Open-label flexible dose trial	6 weeks	Positive
Kim et al. [14]	Naltrexone	n = 83	Double-blind, placebo-controlled	12 weeks	Positive
Grant et al. [15]	Nalmefene	n = 207	Double-blind, placebo-controlled	16 weeks	Positive
Grant et al. [16]	Naltrexone	n = 73	Double-blind, placebo-controlled	18 weeks	Positive
Toneatto et al. [17]	Naltrexone	n = 52	Double-blind, placebo-controlled	11 weeks	Negative
Grant et al. [18]	Nalmefene	n = 233	Double-blind, placebo-controlled	16 weeks	Positive
Kovanen et al. [19]	Naltrexone	n = 101	Double-blind, placebo-controlled as needed design + psychological support	20 weeks	Negative

Naltrexone and nalmefene have been the opioid antagonists investigated. Naltrexone is available orally and intramuscularly (long-acting formulation). Nalmefene presents less hepatotoxicity and has a longer half-life than naltrexone. Nalmefene is available in oral and intravenous preparations, but only the intravenous form is available in the United States.

The results of opioid antagonists in the treatment of GD are encouraging. The clinical trials also suggest that the majority of the responders tend to show improvement within 4 weeks of treatment [13]. Although individual responses vary, some additional research suggests that they may be preferentially effective in gambling disordered individuals with urges to gamble, comorbid alcohol-use disorder, or a family history of alcohol-use disorders [16, 18].

Regarding the side effect profile, the most common adverse reaction is nausea [13, 19]. Regular checking of liver enzymes is suggested. Opioid antagonists are contraindicated in opioid-use disorders as they may precipitate a withdrawal syndrome.

8.5   Glutamatergic Drugs

As seen in the section reward system (see above), glutamate has been implicated in neurocircuits important for the regulation of motivational responses and reward-seeking behaviors [12]. There have been trials assessing the efficacy of glutamatergic drugs in GD. The main glutamatergic agents investigated are N-acetylcysteine (NAC), memantine, topiramate, and amantadine. The mechanism of action of these drugs is complex and includes modulation of different neurotransmitters, i.e., they do not have an exclusive action on glutamate receptions.

NAC

NAC has been used for decades in the treatment of paracetamol intoxication and respiratory conditions. Due to its modulation of glutamatergic neurotransmission, NAC has been increasingly investigated for the treatment of a range of addictive behaviors [20]. NAC has shown efficacy in some clinical trials on cocaine-use disorders and cannabis-use disorders.

One clinical trial assessed the efficacy of NAC in GD, and the reduction in gambling symptoms was promising [21]. Additionally, the fact that NAC has been used for a long time and tends to be well tolerated (benign side effect profile) should encourage further investigations in GD. With respect to the dose used, research in addictions has tended to use doses higher than in other clinical indications. Studies have used doses ranging from 1.2 g/day to 3.6 g/day. The positive trial in GD used 1.8 g/day.

Memantine

Memantine is an antagonist of N-methyl-D-aspartate NMDA glutamate receptors. This medication has shown pro-cognitive effects in disorders such as Alzheimer's disease. It was also effective in treating alcohol-use disorder [22].

This medication is promising since it may modulate not only urges to gamble but also produce addition to cognitive enhancement via modulation of the prefrontal cortex. Regarding the cognitive effects of memantine, it is possible that this medication promotes cognitive flexibility and, therefore, improves cognitive distortions associated with continuous gambling despite negative consequences. An open-label trial showed that memantine was well tolerated and associated with improvement in measures of gambling behavior and neuropsychology [18]. However, this is, from the best of our knowledge, the only study investigating this medication in GD.

Topiramate

Topiramate has shown promise in the management of impulsive and addictive behaviors such as binge eating and alcohol-use disorder [23, 24]. The two double-blind, placebo-controlled trials conducted in GD with this medication demonstrated mixed results. Berlin et al. [25] found that topiramate was not superior to placebo, while de Brito et al. [26] had positive results for topiramate combined with cognitive restructuring.

Amantadine

Amantadine is a psychotropic drug classically used for Parkinson's disease. It has glutamatergic and NMDA-blocking activities and increases dopaminergic neurotransmission. One small double-blind, placebo-controlled clinical trial demonstrated that amantadine was effective for the treatment of GD in Parkinson's disease [27]. The dose used was 200 mg/day.

8.6 Antidepressants

SSRIs

SSRIs are probably the most investigated class of drugs in GD. There have been several clinical trials examining SSRIs including fluoxetine, fluvoxamine, paroxetine, citalopram, and escitalopram. They have shown mixed results and a tendency to have high rates of placebo effect. Due to the inconsistent results and the high comorbidity of GD and depression, there is some question whether the positive trials with SSRIs were largely due to alleviating depressive or anxiety symptoms rather than targeting GD symptoms specifically. There is evidence that SSRIs might be appropriate for gamblers with co-occurring anxiety disorder [28]. Open-label studies with citalopram and fluoxetine have shown positive results in non-depressed subjects [29, 30]; however, the lack of double-blind placebo-controlled trial significantly weakens the evidence. In light of this discussion, SSRIs may be particularly appropriate for GD comorbid with depression or anxiety disorders.

Bupropion

Bupropion is a dual antidepressant with noradrenergic and dopaminergic effects, and the medication has been used for impulsive/addictive disorders. Bupropion is indicated for smoking cessation and has demonstrated reduction in urges and symptoms of nicotine withdrawn [31]. It also has some efficiency in attention deficit hyperactivity disorder (ADHD)—[32]. Nonetheless, bupropion demonstrated mixed results in GD. A preliminary open-label clinical study showed efficacy [33], but a later double-blind, placebo-controlled trial was negative [34]. Consequently, there is no solid evidence that bupropion is efficient in GD.

8.7   Mood Stabilizers

There were some studies assessing the efficiency of mood stabilizers in GD. These clinical trials were mainly performed with subjects with bipolar disorder or bipolar spectrum disorder. The use of mood stabilizers is particularly interesting for the comorbidity GD and bipolar disorder.

Lithium and Valproate

A single-blind trial observed that lithium and valproate were associated with statistical improvement in gambling behavior [35]. A later double-blind placebo-controlled study showed that lithium was superior to placebo in subjects with a bipolar spectrum disorder and co-occurring GD [36].

Carbamazepine

The evidence for carbamazepine in GD is weak. There is only a small ($n = 8$) open-label trial with positive results [37].

8.8   Atypical Antipsychotics

The idea that antipsychotics could be effective in GD was based on the following: (1) GD appears to have clinical similarities to bipolar disorder and obsessive compulsive disorder, conditions in which antipsychotics have shown some efficacy; and (2) lithium, a mood stabilizer, has demonstrated effectiveness compared to placebo in subjects with bipolar spectrum disorders and GD.

Olanzapine

Olanzapine is the only antipsychotic medication formally investigated for the treatment of GD. Additionally to the dopamine antagonist action, this drug has some effect on neurocircuits rich in dopamine and serotonin, two neurotransmitters that have been implicated in the pathophysiology of GD. In spite of that, two double-blind, placebo-controlled clinical trials found that olanzapine did not differ from placebo in the treatment of GD [38, 39].

8.9 Other Drugs

Modafinil

Modafinil is a stimulant drug that increases dopaminergic and adrenergic tone in the central nervous system. It is classically used in patients with attention deficit hyperactivity disorder (ADHD) and has some evidence for the comorbidity of ADHD and cocaine-use disorder [40]. In a clinical trial with GD, modafinil reduced gambling behavior in highly impulsive gamblers but worsened gambling behavior in subjects with low impulsivity [41].

8.10 Future Directions

GD is a clinically heterogeneous disorder, and different subtypes of disordered gamblers have been identified [42, 43]. As a result of this, it is important to understand the effects of medications on different gambling domains and, therefore, which medications are more appropriated for specific subgroups of disordered gamblers. For example, there is evidence that opioid antagonists are particularly efficient for subjects with personal and/or family history of alcohol-use disorder/substance-use disorder. Similar insights are needed in order to develop customized pharmacological treatments. There is a need for larger clinical trials that give the opportunity of analysis of subtypes.

Another crucial point is to better elucidate how pharmacotherapy and psychotherapy interact. There are a few clinical trials where medications were used concomitantly with psychotherapeutic approaches [26, 44]. It is therefore possible that pharmacotherapy may have synergistic effects with psychotherapy.

As in other fields in psychiatry, the majority of clinical trials have examined only short-term outcomes. Hence, it is important to assess midterm and long-term effects of medication.

Finally, in many pharmacotherapy trials, there has been little information about optimal dose or duration of treatment needed for GD.

8.11 Conclusions

- Despite the significant personal and social impact, the number of pharmacotherapy clinical trials in GD is relatively small.
- Due to the high rates of co-occurring psychiatric disorders in individuals with GD, especially alcohol-use disorders, substance-use disorders, mood disorders,

and anxiety disorders, pharmacotherapy needs to address the potentially complex interaction of GD and these other disorders.

- Some evidence suggest that pharmacological interventions may have a synergistic effect on psychotherapeutic approaches. Psychotherapeutic treatments (especially cognitive behavioral therapy) have demonstrated efficacy in GD. Which medications may be most effective when used in combination with psychotherapy however remains unknown.
- Despite some promising results, pharmacological interventions for GD are currently used off-label, i.e., no drug is formally approved by the Food and Drug Administration. Therefore, it is necessary to inform patients about the nature of the treatment and discuss in detail risks and benefits.
- More double-blind, placebo-controlled trials are needed. There is a need for larger studies that might help develop customized pharmacological interventions.

References

1. Black DW, Moyer T, Schlosser S. Quality of life and family history in pathological gambling. J Nerv Ment Dis. 2003;191(2):124–6.
2. Grant JE, Kim SW. Quality of life in kleptomania and pathological gambling. Compr Psychiatry. 2005;46(1):34–7.
3. Petry NM, Stinson FS, Grant BF. Comorbidity of DSM-IV pathological gambling and other psychiatric disorders: results from the national epidemiologic survey on alcohol and related conditions [CME]. J Clin Psychiatry. 2005;66(5):564–74.
4. Pallesen S, Mitsem M, Kvale G, Johnsen BH, Molde H. Outcome of psychological treatments of pathological gambling: a review and meta-analysis. Addiction. 2005;100(10):1412–22.
5. Petry NM, Ammerman Y, Bohl J, Doersch A, Gay H, Kadden R, et al. Cognitive-behavioral therapy for pathological gamblers. J Consult Clin Psychol. 2006;74(3):555.
6. Lupi M, Martinotti G, Acciavatti T, Pettorruso M, Brunetti M, Santacroce R, et al. Pharmacological treatments in gambling disorder: a qualitative review. Biomed Res Int. 2014;2014:537306.
7. American Psychiatric Association. Diagnostic and statistical manual of mental disorders (DSM-5®). American Psychiatric Pub. 2013.
8. Blanco C, Moreyra P, Nunes EV, Saiz-Ruiz J, Ibanez A. Pathological gambling: addiction or compulsion? Semin Clin Neuropsychiatry. 2001;6(3):167–76.
9. Potenza MN. The neurobiology of pathological gambling. Semin Clin Neuropsychiatry. 2001;6(3):217–26.
10. Yip SW, Potenza MN. Treatment of gambling disorders. Curr Treat Options Psychiatry. 2014;1(2):189–203.
11. Kim SW. Opioid antagonists in the treatment of impulse-control disorders. J Clin Psychiatry. 1998;59(4):159–64.
12. Kalivas PW. The glutamate homeostasis hypothesis of addiction. Nat Rev Neurosci. 2009;10(8):561–72.
13. Kim SW, Grant JE. An open naltrexone treatment study in pathological gambling disorder. Int Clin Psychopharmacol. 2001;16(5):285–9.
14. Kim SW, Grant JE, Adson DE, Shin YC. Double-blind naltrexone and placebo comparison study in the treatment of pathological gambling. Biol Psychiatry. 2001;49(11):914–21.
15. Grant JE, Potenza MN, Hollander E, Cunningham-Williams R, Nurminen T, Smits G, Kallio A. Multicenter investigation of the opioid antagonist nalmefene in the treatment of pathological gambling. Am J Psychiatry. 2006;163(2):303–12.

16. Grant JE, Kim SW, Hollander E, Potenza MN. Predicting response to opiate antagonists and placebo in the treatment of pathological gambling. Psychopharmacology. 2008;200(4):521–7.
17. Toneatto T, Brands B, Selby P. A randomized, double-blind, placebo-controlled trial of naltrexone in the treatment of concurrent alcohol use disorder and pathological gambling. Am J Addict. 2009;18(3):219–25.
18. Grant JE, Chamberlain SR, Odlaug BL, Potenza MN, Kim SW. Memantine shows promise in reducing gambling severity and cognitive inflexibility in pathological gambling: a pilot study. Psychopharmacology. 2010;212(4):603–12.
19. Kovanen L, Basnet S, Castren S, Pankakoski M, Saarikoski ST, Partonen T, Alho H, Lahti T. A randomised, double-blind, placebo-controlled trial of as-needed naltrexone in the treatment of pathological gambling. Eur Addict Res. 2016;22(2):70–9.
20. Asevedo E, Mendes AC, Berk M, Brietzke E. Systematic review of N-acetylcysteine in the treatment of addictions. Rev Bras Psiquiatr. 2014;36(2):168–75.
21. Grant JE, Kim SW, Odlaug BL. N-acetyl cysteine, a glutamate-modulating agent, in the treatment of pathological gambling: a pilot study. Biol Psychiatry. 2007;62(6):652–7.
22. Evans SM, Levin FR, Brooks DJ, Garawi F. A pilot double-blind treatment trial of memantine for alcohol dependence. Alcohol Clin Exp Res. 2007;31(5):775–82.
23. Arbaizar B, Gómez-Acebo I, Llorca J. Efficacy of topiramate in bulimia nervosa and binge-eating disorder: a systematic review. Gen Hosp Psychiatry. 2008;30(5):471–5.
24. Shinn AK, Greenfield SF. Topiramate in the treatment of substance-related disorders: a critical review of the literature. J Clin Psychiatry. 2010;71(5):634–48.
25. Berlin HA, Braun A, Simeon D, Koran LM, Potenza MN, McElroy SL, et al. A double-blind, placebo-controlled trial of topiramate for pathological gambling. World J Biol Psychiatry. 2013;14(2):121–8.
26. de Brito AMC, de Almeida Pinto MG, Bronstein G, Carneiro E, Faertes D, Fukugawa V, et al. Topiramate combined with cognitive restructuring for the treatment of gambling disorder: a two-center, randomized, double-blind clinical trial. J Gambl Stud. 2016;33(1):249–63.
27. Thomas A, Bonanni L, Gambi F, Di Iorio A, Onofrj M. Pathological gambling in Parkinson disease is reduced by amantadine. Ann Neurol. 2010;68(3):400–4.
28. Grant JE, Potenza MN. Escitalopram treatment of pathological gambling with co-occurring anxiety: an open-label pilot study with double-blind discontinuation. Int Clin Psychopharmacol. 2006;21(4):203–9.
29. Gandara JJ, Sanz O, Gilaberte I. Fluoxetine: open-trial in pathological gambling. In Annual meeting of the American Psychiatric Association. 1999. p. 16–21.
30. Posternak MA. An open-label study of citalopram in the treatment of pathological gambling. J Clin Psychiatry. 2002;63(1):44–8.
31. Hughes JR, Stead LF, Hartmann-Boyce J, Cahill K, Lancaster T. Antidepressants for smoking cessation. Cochrane Database Syst Rev. 2014;(1):CD000031.
32. Moriyama TS, Polanczyk GV, Terzi FS, Faria KM, Rohde LA. Psychopharmacology and psychotherapy for the treatment of adults with ADHD—a systematic review of available meta-analyses. CNS Spectr. 2013;18(06):296–306.
33. Black DW. An open-label trial of bupropion in the treatment of pathologic gambling. J Clin Psychopharmacol. 2004;24(1):108–11.
34. Black DW, Arndt S, Coryell WH, Argo T, Forbush KT, Shaw MC, et al. Bupropion in the treatment of pathological gambling: a randomized, double-blind, placebo-controlled, flexible-dose study. J Clin Psychopharmacol. 2007;27(2):143–50.
35. Pallanti S, Quercioli L, Sood E, Hollander E. Lithium and valproate treatment of pathological gambling: a randomized single-blind study. J Clin Psychiatry. 2002;63(7):559–64.
36. Hollander E, Pallanti S, Allen A, Sood E, Rossi NB. Does sustained-release lithium reduce impulsive gambling and affective instability versus placebo in pathological gamblers with bipolar spectrum disorders? Am J Psychiatry. 2005;162(1):137–45.
37. Black DW, Shaw MC, Allen J. Extended release carbamazepine in the treatment of pathological gambling: an open-label study. Prog Neuropsychopharmacol Biol Psychiatry. 2008;32(5):1191–4.

38. McElroy SL, Nelson EB, Welge JA, Kaehler L, Keck PE Jr. Olanzapine in the, treatment of pathological gambling: a negative randomized placebo-controlled trial. J Clin Psychiatry. 2008;69(3):433–40.
39. Fong T, Kalechstein A, Bernhard B, Rosenthal R, Rugle L. A double-blind, placebo-controlled trial of olanzapine for the treatment of video poker pathological gamblers. Pharmacol Biochem Behav. 2008;89(3):298–303.
40. Dackis CA, Kampman KM, Lynch KG, Pettinati HM, O'brien CP. A double-blind, placebo-controlled trial of modafinil for cocaine dependence. Neuropsychopharmacology. 2005;30(1):205–11.
41. Zack M, Poulos CX. Effects of the atypical stimulant modafinil on a brief gambling episode in pathological gamblers with high vs. low impulsivity. J Psychopharmacol. 2008;23(6):660–71.
42. Blaszczynski A, Nower L. A pathways model of problem and pathological gambling. Addiction. 2002;97(5):487–99.
43. Ledgerwood DM, Petry NM. Psychological experience of gambling and subtypes of pathological gamblers. Psychiatry Res. 2006;144(1):17–27.
44. Grant JE, Odlaug BL, Chamberlain SR, Potenza MN, Schreiber LR, Donahue CB, Kim SW. A randomized, placebo-controlled trial of N-acetylcysteine plus imaginal desensitization for nicotine-dependent pathological gamblers. J Clin Psychiatry. 2013;75(1):39–45.

Psychological Interventions in Gambling Disorder

9

Meredith K. Ginley, Carla J. Rash, and Nancy M. Petry

Gambling disorder is characterized by clinical impairment from negative consequences of gambling [1]. Examples of problems include an inability to control or stop gambling behavior, preoccupation with gambling, and negative financial, relational, and work or educational consequences. In the United States, for example, gambling disorder affects about 0.4–2.0% of adults, with an additional 1.3–2.3% of adults considered problem gamblers [2–6]. Problem gamblers are individuals who experience some adverse effects related to their gambling but not to the extent that the diagnostic threshold is met.

Few persons with gambling problems access treatment, with only 7–12% of individuals with a lifetime diagnosis of gambling disorder reporting a history of professional treatment or mutual support group participation [7]. Despite low engagement in treatment, about 50% of people with lifetime gambling disorder do not have a current diagnosis, suggesting that natural recovery is common. Therefore, efficacious interventions for gambling disorder have to improve upon natural recovery rates.

A number of types of psychotherapies for gambling have been evaluated. Therapy modalities include full-length professionally delivered treatments, brief interventions, and self-directed workbooks. This chapter will review current empirical support for psychotherapy for gambling disorder, including different theoretical approaches, and other factors, such as intensity and format (i.e., group, individual, workbook, computer-facilitated). We will focus on moderate- to large-sized randomized controlled trials that include an average of at least 25–30 participants per

M. K. Ginley (✉)
Calhoun Cardiology Center—Behavioral Health, UConn Health, Farmington, CT, USA

Department of Psychology, East Tennessee State University, Johnson City, TN, USA
e-mail: ginleym@etsu.edu

C. J. Rash · N. M. Petry
Calhoun Cardiology Center—Behavioral Health, UConn Health, Farmington, CT, USA
e-mail: rashc@uchc.edu; npetry@uchc.edu

© Springer Nature Switzerland AG 2019
A. Heinz et al. (eds.), *Gambling Disorder*, https://doi.org/10.1007/978-3-030-03060-5_9

condition as recommended by Chambless and Hollon [8]. This chapter will highlight major gambling-related treatment outcomes and between treatment condition comparisons, with a focus on treatment dropout.

Treatment dropout is emphasized due to high rates of discontinuation among individuals in psychotherapy for gambling disorder, with rates that can commonly reach or even exceed 50% and a median dropout rate of 38% [9]. This rate is nearly double the average treatment dropout from psychotherapy in general, which is still high at 20% [10]. Dropout rates can greatly impact conclusions about treatment efficacy. Treatment discontinuation also has important clinical implications, with therapists unable to determine if patients do not return to subsequent therapy sessions because they have gotten better or they are failing to benefit. In the following sections, we discuss treatment completion and outcomes in full-length professionally delivered treatments and in self-guided or workbook-based interventions. We will also review motivational psychotherapy interventions developed specifically to address low engagement and retention in gambling treatment.

9.1 Professionally Delivered Behavior Therapy and Cognitive Therapy

Behavior therapies help patients change by focusing on eliminating unwanted behaviors and replacing them with more desirable actions. Cognitive therapies attempt to identify and challenge faulty thinking patterns, also called cognitive distortions (see [11]). Cognitive-behavioral treatments integrate both aspects. Table 9.1 provides an overview of the randomized controlled trials of these treatments.

Ladouceur et al. [12] randomly assigned 88 individuals with gambling disorder to cognitive therapy or a waitlist control condition. Treatment sessions continued until the patient stopped gambling completely. Thus, treatment was lengthy and lasted up to 20 sessions (average treatment time was 11 h). Treatment dropout was high at around 50%. Therapy completers showed significant posttreatment improvement on most gambling-related variables compared to participants on the waitlist. In a later study that explored the same therapy delivered in a group format [13], 71 participants with gambling disorder were randomized to either group cognitive therapy or a waitlist control. Treatment completion was higher relative to the individual format, with 74% of participants attending the 10 weekly, 2-h group sessions. At posttreatment, 88% of the gamblers who had completed treatment no longer met criteria for gambling disorder compared to 20% of waitlisted participants. Treatment gains were maintained through 6-, 12-, and 24-month follow-ups, although between-group comparisons were not possible due to the study design, and analyses in both these studies included only treatment completers.

Moving beyond a waitlist design, Smith et al. [14] compared cognitive therapy to a specific behavioral therapy—exposure therapy, in which patients were exposed to gambling situations without wagering, with cash restriction during exposure tasks gradually lessening over time. Eighty-seven problem gamblers were randomly assigned to one of the two conditions. Using intent-to-treat analyses that included

Table 9.1 Randomized trials of full-length professionally delivered treatments, self-directed workbook, and Internet-based interventions, and motivational interventions with or without cognitive-behavioral therapy

Authors, year	Population	Treatment conditions	N	Treatment duration (sessions)	Completed treatment	Summary treatment comparison (for gambling outcomes)
Professionally delivered behavior therapy and cognitive therapy						
Ladouceur et al. [12]	Gambling disorder	1. Waitlist	29	–	–	Cognitive tx: more symptom improvement
		2. Cognitive therapy	59	≤20 sessions	~50%	
Ladouceur et al. [13]	Gambling disorder	1. Waitlist	25	–	–	Cognitive tx: more symptom improvement
		2. Group cognitive therapy	46	10 weeks	74%	
Smith et al. [14]	Problem gamblers	1. Cognitive therapy	44	~12 weeks	68%	Both txs: symptom improvement; no significant condition differences
		2. Exposure therapy	43	(~12)	49%	
Professionally delivered CBT						
Petry et al. [15]	Gambling disorder	1. GA referral	63	–	–	Both CBT txs: greater abstinence
		2. CBT workbook	84	8 weeks (8)	37%	
		3. Individual CBT	84	8 weeks (8)	61%	
Oei et al. [16]	Problem gamblers	1. Waitlist	28	–	Not reported	Both CBT txs: more improvement than waitlist; no significant tx condition differences
		2. Group CBT	37	6 weeks (6)		
		3. Individual CBT	37	6 weeks (6)		
Self-directed CBT interventions						
Hodgins et al. [17]	Problem gamblers	1. CBT workbook mailed once	85	1	63% read materials	Both txs: correspond to symptom reduction; no significant condition differences
		2. CBT workbook in repeated mailings	84	11 months (8)	(not reported by group)	

(continued)

Table 9.1 (continued)

Authors, year	Population	Treatment conditions	N	Treatment duration (sessions)	Completed treatment	Summary treatment comparison (for gambling outcomes)
Campos et al. [18]	Problem gamblers	1. CBT workbook plus therapist guidance	47	20 weeks	~50% (not reported by group)	Workbook plus guidance condition: higher abstinence rates
		2. CBT workbook	40			
Luquiens et al. [19]	Problem gamblers	1. Waitlist	264	6 weeks	–	Some symptom improvement for all conditions; no significant condition differences
		2. Normative feedback via email	293		22%	
		3. Email with CBT workbook	264		17%	
		4. Email with CBT workbook plus therapist guidance	301		5%	
Motivational interventions and professionally delivered CBT						
Grant et al. [20]	Gambling disorder	1. GA referral	35	1 (1)	86%	MI + CBT: higher abstinence rates
		2. MI + CBT	33	8 (6)	76%	
Petry et al. [21]	Problem gamblers	1. Assessment only	48	–	–	Brief advice only tx to significantly decrease gambling behavior; MI + CBT decrease on one gambling outcome
		2. Brief advice/feedback	37	1 (1)	100%	
		3. MI	55	1(1)	94%	
		4. MI + CBT	40	4 weeks (4)	33%	
Petry et al. [22]	Problem gamblers	1. Brief psychoeducation	69	1 (1)	100%	At txs improved symptom outcomes; MI + CBT greater reduction $ spent and gambling problems
		2. Brief advice	66	1 (1)	100%	
		3. MI + CBT	82	4 weeks (4)	28%	
Carlbring et al. [23]	Problem gamblers	1. Waitlist	46	–	–	Both MET and CBT: more improvement than waitlist, no significant tx condition differences
		2. Individual MET	54	9 weeks (4)	43%	
		3. Group CBT	50	9 weeks (8)	29%	
Larimer et al. [24]	Problem gamblers	1. Assessment only	51	–	–	Both txs: significant symptom improvements; no significant tx condition differences
		2. MI	52	1 (1)	85%	
		3. Group CBT	44	6 weeks (4–6)	<41%	

Motivational interventions and self-directed treatments

Study	Population	Treatment	N	Follow-up	Completion %	Outcomes
Hodgins et al. [25]	Problem gamblers	1. Waitlist	35	–	–	Both workbook conditions: more improvement than waitlist, workbook + MI greater short-term improvements, no significant long-term tx condition differences
		2. CBT workbook	35	–	56% read workbook (not reported by group)	
		3. CBT workbook + MI phone call	32	1		
Hodgins et al. [26]	Problem gamblers	1. Waitlist	65	6 weeks	Not reported	Both MI conditions: greater short-term improvements, no significant long-term tx condition differences
		2. CBT workbook	82	6 weeks		
		3. CBT workbook + MI phone call	83	6 weeks (1)		
		4. CBT workbook + MI booster calls	84	36 weeks (7)		
LaBrie et al. [27]	Problem gamblers	1. Waitlist	102	–	Not reported	Both workbook conditions: greater improvements, no significant condition differences
		2. CBT workbook + MI in workbook	108	–		
		3. CBT workbook + MI in workbook + phone call	105	3 months (1)		
Diskin and Hodgins [28]	Problem gamblers	1. CBT workbook + control interview	39	1 (1)	50%	MI condition: greater improvements on some gambling-related outcomes
		2. CBT workbook + MI in person session	42	1 (1)	64%	
Cunningham et al. [29]	Problem gamblers	1. Waitlist	69	–	–	MI partial feedback condition: greater improvements on some gambling outcomes; no other significant condition differences
		2. MI partial feedback	70	1 (1)	100%	
		3. MI full feedback	70	1 (1)	100%	
Neighbors et al. [30]	Problem gamblers	1. Personalized normative feedback via computer	124	1 (1)	100%	Feedback condition: reduced $ lost and reduced symptoms short-term follow-up; no condition differences on symptoms long-term
		2. Attention control	128	1 (1)	100%	

Notes: *CBT* cognitive-behavioral therapy, *GA* Gamblers Anonymous, *MET* motivational enhancement therapy, *MI* motivational interviewing; tx(s), treatment(s). Summary treatment comparison includes only select major treatment outcomes with emphasis on between treatment condition comparisons all randomized participants, both treatments significantly reduced gambling at the 3-month follow-up with no significant differences between conditions. At the 6-month follow-up, 79.3% of cognitive therapy treatment participants and 82.6% of the exposure therapy treatment participants no longer met criteria for gambling disorder, rates which again did not differ. Exposure therapy had a higher dropout rate of 51% compared to 32% in the cognitive condition. However, treatment effects were achieved in a shorter time frame (average of one to three sessions) in the exposure condition relative to the cognitive therapy condition. The increased dropout in the exposure treatment may have been due to intervention-related factors (e.g., dislike of the treatment) or participants feeling better sooner and deciding they no longer needed treatment.

Overall, cognitive therapy, whether delivered in a group or individual format, appears to provide greater reductions in gambling symptoms than a waitlist control. Still, there is limited evidence that cognitive therapy is superior to other active therapies, such as behavioral therapy, or even to natural reductions in gambling that occur over time. Furthermore, attrition from cognitive therapy is fairly high, and research on this intervention remains limited. Many aspects of cognitive approaches have been incorporated into integrated treatment models such as cognitive-behavioral therapy (CBT), which has been more extensively studied.

9.2　Professionally Delivered Cognitive-Behavioral Therapy

Cognitive-behavioral therapy (CBT) merges cognitive and behavioral approaches. The first controlled trial [15] of CBT for gambling problems used the eight-session protocol developed by Petry [31]. Petry et al. [15] randomized 231 individuals with gambling disorder to one of three conditions: Gamblers Anonymous (GA) referral plus CBT workbook (one chapter to be completed each week over 8 weeks), GA referral plus therapist-directed CBT using the same workbook content in 8 weekly individual sessions delivered by a therapist, or referral to GA only. While gambling decreased overall for participants across all study conditions, participants in both CBT conditions had significantly larger reductions in gambling problems, with 69% of participants in therapist-delivered CBT condition and 51% of those in CBT workbook condition no longer meeting gambling disorder criteria at posttreatment, compared to 47% of those with the GA referral-only condition. Treatment completion data indicated that therapist-delivered content resulted in higher levels of engagement with the CBT (61% completed versus 37% in the workbook condition), and completion of the CBT, whether in a workbook or individual session format, was significantly related to outcomes. Results suggest therapist interaction can increase engagement in CBT, and CBT spurred greater behavior change than a GA referral alone.

With the initial success of CBT, Oei et al. [16] sought to determine whether group or individually delivered CBT was optimal. They randomized participants with problem gambling to individual CBT, group CBT, or a waitlist control. Participants in both CBT conditions reduced their gambling in comparison to the waitlist condition by the end of treatment. Treatment gains were maintained in the two active conditions, and no differences were reported at the 6-month follow-up. This study did not report upon treatment completion rates, limiting the ability to draw conclusions about differential engagement for group or individual CBT, but these data suggest both group and individual formats of CBT appear to reduce gambling.

9.3 Self-Directed CBT Interventions

Although the Petry et al. [15] study found that fewer patients with gambling disorder completed a CBT workbook than individual CBT sessions, gamblers with less severe problems may be more willing to utilize self-directed interventions than visit a therapist weekly. CBT workbook-based interventions may reduce some treatment barriers including treatment cost and transportation issues, and these options may also be associated with less stigma than seeking help from a mental health professional. Some studies have evaluated workbook and computer-facilitated versions of CBT in problem gamblers.

Hodgins et al. [17] randomized problem gamblers ($N = 169$) to receive a relapse prevention workbook based on CBT principles in its entirety immediately following study enrollment or to receive the workbook in sections eight times over an 11-month time frame. Just over 60% of participants reported completing the workbook, and spaced delivery did not improve completion rates or treatment outcomes. Regardless of delivery format, 23% reported recent abstinence from gambling at a 1-year follow-up, and 30–46% were no longer gambling problematically depending on assessment measure. These recovery rates, however, are similar to those noted for spontaneous improvement in epidemiological studies (33–36%; [7]) and are highlighted by the authors' study as mirroring recovery rates found in a previous study on the natural process of relapse [32]. Whether the workbook improved upon natural recovery could not be determined with this study design due to the lack of a control group.

In a similar study, Campos et al. [18] examined whether providing therapist guidance improved workbook utilization. Problem gamblers were randomly assigned to a CBT workbook plus therapist guidance or to a workbook-only condition where a research assistant checked in five times over 20 weeks to see if chapters had been completed. Therapist guidance improved abstinence rates at the end of treatment and 1 year later compared to those in the workbook-only condition. However, failure to complete the workbook was again high (>50%), and this study did not report completion rates by condition making it unclear if therapist guidance influenced workbook adherence and whether that related to improvements.

Subsequently, Linquiens et al. [19] explored therapist guidance for an Internet-based intervention, and they recruited non-treatment-seeking gamblers by offering an Internet-based gambling disorder screening to poker players on an online website. Players identified as problem gamblers ($N = 1122$) were randomized into four treatment conditions: waitlist control, normative feedback related to the results of their screening via single email, a CBT workbook emailed in a single downloadable file, or the same CBT program emailed weekly by a psychologist providing personalized email guidance associated with chapter content. Treatment dropout rate was high across all treatment conditions (83%), and the therapist-guided CBT condition had the highest dropout rate (95%). On average, participants showed some reductions in gambling at the 6-week follow-up with no significant differences observed between conditions. The particularly low treatment completion rates in this study are probably related to the fact that these gamblers were not seeking treatment. These data suggest when active gamblers are not seeking treatment, therapist facilitation may lead to increased treatment dropout relative to more "hands-off" approaches.

Across these studies, self-delivered CBT generally decreased gambling and gambling symptoms over time, but most studies did not include an attention control condition obviating the ability to determine the efficacy of CBT workbooks. Further, generally only about half the patients, even those who sought treatment, completed the workbook, and very few among the non-treatment seekers. Therapist facilitation, no matter how minimal, may improve outcomes, but only among those who are actively seeking treatment.

9.4 Motivational Interventions

As highlighted above, many individuals, even those who actively seek and start gambling treatment, do not receive the full recommended course of therapy. Going beyond general therapist guidance, motivational interviewing (MI) and motivational enhancement therapy (MET) were developed to facilitate increased treatment engagement for individuals with substance use disorders. The goal of both is to overcome barriers of treatment initiation and increase overall investment in therapy by supporting an individual's commitment to changing problem behavior. MI typically refers to a single-session intervention focused on the collaborative development of a change plan [33], while MET uses several sessions to comprehensively target internal motivation and includes personalized feedback related to a specific behavior targeted for change [34].

Motivational interventions have been widely adapted for use with problem gambling populations. Depending on the trial, MI has been delivered as a standalone intervention, integrated into a CBT intervention, or administered prior to a CBT intervention. Very brief motivational interventions, including single-session MI and personalized feedback only, have also been used to directly circumvent low treatment retention by ensuring the complete intervention occurs at a single point of contact.

9.5 Motivational Interventions and Professionally Delivered CBT

MI has been applied in an attempt to enhance completion of professionally delivered CBT. Grant et al. [20] compared 68 individuals with gambling disorder who were randomly assigned to MI plus CBT or to a GA referral condition. The MI plus

CBT (based on [31]) lasted 8 weeks. Participants in the MI plus CBT condition reported greater reduction in gambling at the posttreatment follow-up compared to participants in the GA referral condition, and 76% of participants completed the treatment. Interpretations about long-term effects were not possible as participants in the GA referral condition subsequently received the active treatment, and the specific impact of MI could not be isolated in this design.

Petry et al. [21] also explored the use of single-session interventions compared to an abbreviated multi-session MI/CBT intervention for non-gambling treatment seeking individuals who screened positive for gambling problems when assessed in waiting rooms of medical clinics and substance use clinics. Participants ($N = 180$) were randomly assigned into an assessment-only condition, 10 min of brief advice about gambling, a single MI session, or the same MI session plus three sessions of CBT. All randomized patients completed both single-session interventions, but only 33% of participants in the four-session condition completed treatment. When compared to the assessment-only condition, brief advice was the only condition that significantly decreased gambling behavior between baseline and the 6-week and 9-month follow-ups, but there were also no significant differences between the three active interventions. This study suggests that a very brief intervention may be useful in this population.

In a later study, Petry et al. [22] randomly assigned 217 substance abuse treatment patients who screened positive for gambling problems to 10–15 min of brief psycho-education about gambling; 10–15 min of brief advice on gambling-related norms, risk factors, and methods to prevent more gambling-related problems; or four sessions of MI plus CBT for gambling (as based on [31]). All participants also received standard substance abuse treatment. The single-session gambling interventions were provided immediately following the baseline evaluation ensuring all participants assigned to them received them, but only 28% of participants assigned to the MI plus CBT condition completed all four sessions. At a 5-month follow-up assessment, gambling-related symptoms reduced for participants across all conditions. Brief advice decreased gambling days between baseline and the 5-month follow-up to a greater degree than the brief psychoeducation condition. The MI plus CBT condition did not reduce days gambled compared to brief advice, but it did result in greater reductions in money spent gambling and gambling-related problems at the 5-month follow-up. At a 24-month follow-up, participants in all groups reported continued reductions in money spent and problems relative to baseline, with participants assigned to the MI plus CBT condition significantly more likely than those assigned to the brief interventions to be in long-term recovery from problem gambling. Overall, for individuals receiving concurrent substance use treatment, gambling-related symptoms significantly decreased over time, with the MI plus CBT condition resulting in the greatest clinical improvement, even though few participants completed all four sessions.

MET, with its more intensive content than MI, has also been evaluated as a stand-alone intervention for the treatment of gambling problems. Carlbring et al. [23] randomized 150 participants with problem gambling to four sessions of individual MET, eight sessions of group CBT (as based on [35]), or a waitlist control. Individuals in both active treatment conditions had significant declines in gambling-related symptomology compared to participants in the waitlist control group. No differences were found between active treatment conditions. Rates of engagement in both treatments were low and not significantly different, with 43% completing MET and 29% completing CBT. Given the different study designs, it remains unknown whether the addition of MET or MI to CBT is superior for reducing gambling-related symptoms compared to MET or CBT alone, but several studies have found benefits of one or both of these interventions combined.

Like MET, MI as an independent intervention has also been directly compared to CBT. In addition to the study by Petry et al. [21], Larimer et al. [24] explored the use of a single-session MI intervention for 147 university students with problem gambling. Participants were randomly assigned to either a single-session of MI or four to six sessions of group CBT (based on [31]) or an assessment-only control condition. Participants in both the CBT and the MI intervention conditions significantly reduced gambling frequency. The CBT intervention group had high attrition, with less than half of participants attending at least 50% of the sessions. Results suggest a single session of MI had a similar impact on gambling-related symptoms as a more extensive CBT intervention.

In sum, adding MI to CBT may improve retention rates in CBT, but no studies have been designed to isolate the impact of integrating MI with CBT in the context of professionally delivered therapy. Nevertheless, the two approaches combined appear to yield some benefits. Due to its brevity, MI on its own is more likely to be completed than more extensive CBT interventions, and MI on its own is useful for reducing gambling in some populations, although it has not been evaluated as a standalone treatment relative to an attention control condition.

9.6   Motivational Interventions and Self-Directed Treatments

Self-directed treatments require individuals to be internally motivated to complete them. MI has been evaluated as a method to increase completion of these types of interventions as well. Hodgins et al. [25] randomly assigned 102 problem gamblers to a waitlist control, a CBT workbook, or a CBT workbook enhanced by an MI phone session. Hodgins et al. [26] later varied whether MI was delivered in a single phone call or via six booster calls over a 9-month period. In both these studies, participants receiving any form of MI phone contact gambled less at posttreatment and 1-, 3-, 6-, and 9-month follow-ups than those who received the workbook-only conditions, with participants in the 2001 sample also gambling less at a 24-month follow-up. However, there was little evidence of benefit from repeated therapist contact [26]. As neither study reported workbook completion rates by condition, it is not possible to determine if MI phone calls increased treatment engagement directly, and more therapist contact was not associated with better outcomes than a single therapist contact.

LaBrie et al. [27] conducted a study similar to the treatment design of Hodgins et al. [25, 26], with the exception that MI was directly integrated into the CBT workbook and the phone call condition was simply a 5-min scripted phone call introducing the program and acting as a guide to the workbook. While not reaching statistical significance, participants in both active treatment conditions were 20% more likely to have achieved periods of abstinence when assessed at a 3-month follow-up than participants in the waitlist condition, but again no benefits were found for the addition of therapist contact. The researchers again did not note workbook completion rates. Rates of recent abstinence in the waitlist control group were also substantial, and the authors attributed the lack of statistically significant differences between treatment and control conditions to reductions in gambling for participants across all conditions.

Diskin and Hodgins [28] sought to examine if, instead of a phone call, a single face-to-face MI intervention could increase completion and impact of a CBT workbook. Eighty-one problem gamblers were randomized to either a MI plus CBT workbook condition or a structured psychiatric interview (to serve as a matched attention control) plus the CBT workbook. Workbooks were handed out at the conclusion of the in-person session or interview. Fifty percent of participants in the workbook-only condition and 64% in the MI plus workbook condition reported completing the workbook. At the 12-month follow-up, MI plus CBT workbook participants were spending less money gambling and wagering on fewer days than participants in the workbook-only condition. However, gambling severity did not differ by condition, suggesting benefits were not consistent across all gambling domains.

The impact of very brief motivational materials has also been explored by Cunningham et al. [29]. They randomized problem gamblers ($N = 209$) to one of the three conditions: waitlist control, MI with personalized feedback that included normative information about gambling, and MI with personalized feedback but no comparison of participant's gambling to population norms. Feedback for both conditions was imbedded within the MI materials. As the intervention occurred at the initial point of contact, all participants completed the treatment. Participants who received the partial feedback with no gambling norms, but not those who received the full personalized feedback, reported a reduction in days gambling compared to the waitlist condition. Given that feedback was incorporated within MI materials, it is not possible to determine the extent to which participants interacted with the personalized feedback, but these results suggest normative feedback information may not be particularly useful.

In contrast, another study found benefits of normative personalized feedback. Neighbors et al. [30] assigned 252 problem gambling college students to a single-session computer-delivered personalized feedback condition providing college student gambling norms or to an attention control condition. At 3-month post-intervention, the normative feedback condition participants had reduced gambling symptoms and money lost relative to the controls. At the 6-month follow-up, participants in the active intervention condition continued to report significantly less gambling loss than the attention control participants, with no between-condition differences for gambling symptoms. These findings suggest preliminary support for very brief interventions with college student problem gamblers as well as support for a computer-delivered intervention, but as in most studies, treatment effects were not consistent across all domains.

Together, these studies suggest that integrating minimal MI with CBT-based workbooks may be helpful, but benefits are not pronounced or consistent. Applying personalized feedback related to gambling norms has had mixed effects on improving outcomes.

9.7 Conclusion

Many interventions designed to treat gambling problems suffer from low rates of engagement and completion. Despite high dropout rates, some treatments have yielded benefits in reducing gambling problems, namely, CBT. CBT reduced gambling and related problems compared to waitlist and other control conditions in several studies, whether the CBT was delivered in an individual or group format. Adding MI to CBT certainly does not hurt, and may help enhance engagement and outcomes, but studies have yet to isolate benefits of including motivational interventions alongside professionally delivered CBT.

Self-directed treatments may also reduce gambling-related symptoms in some contexts. Workbooks and computer-facilitated programs have extended traditional CBT interventions beyond the mental health clinic. While minimal therapist contact appears to enhance initial engagement in these forms of self-directed treatment, at least for some populations of gamblers, therapist contact does not universally translate to measureable impacts on long-term gambling outcomes, and more therapist contact does not lead to additive benefits.

Motivational interventions have also been studied on their own. They outperform waitlist controls in some cases, and very brief motivational or personalized feedback interventions may be sufficient for creating behavior change, particularly in some groups of problem gamblers not actively seeking treatment. These single-session interventions may be as good at spurring change as some longer interventions, especially for less severe problem gamblers, and by their nature, they are not associated with the high rates of attrition found in longer-term interventions.

Overall, no treatment modality or format has resulted in markedly superior rates of treatment retention or outcomes compared to other active treatments, but the greatest support to date is for CBT, with or without MI/MET. Gambling problems tend to dissipate over time in most persons, so it is imperative that study designs include attention control conditions to assess efficacy. Regardless of the type of therapy provided, few persons with gambling problems remain engaged in lengthy treatments. Further development and evaluation of brief interventions may be most relevant in the context of treating gambling problems.

Acknowledgments Preparation of this manuscript was supported in part by NIH grants R21-DA031897, P50-DA09241, P60-AA03510, R01-HD075630, R01-AA021446, and R01-AA023502. Additional support was provided by the Connecticut Institute for Clinical and Translational Science (CICATS) at the University of Connecticut. The content is solely the responsibility of the authors and does not necessarily represent the official views of CICATS.

References

1. American Psychiatric Association. Diagnostic and statistical manual of mental disorders. 5th ed. Washington, DC: American Psychiatric Publishing; 2013.
2. Gerstein D, Volberg RA, et al. Gambling impact and behavior study: report to the national gambling impact study commission. Chicago: National Opinion Research Center; 1999.

3. Kessler RC, Hwang I, et al. DSM-IV pathological gambling in the National Comorbidity Survey Replication. Psychol Med. 2008;38(09):1351–60.

4. Petry NM, Stinson FS, et al. Comorbidity of DSM-IV pathological gambling and other psychiatric disorders: results from the National Epidemiologic Survey on Alcohol and Related Conditions [CME]. J Clin Psychiatry. 2005;66(5):564–74.

5. Welte J, Barnes G, et al. Alcohol and gambling pathology among US adults: prevalence, demographic patterns and comorbidity. J Stud Alcohol. 2001;62(5):706–12.

6. Welte JW, Barnes GM, et al. Gambling and problem gambling in the United States: changes between 1999 and 2013. J Gambl Stud. 2015;31(3):695–715.

7. Slutske WS. Natural recovery and treatment-seeking in pathological gambling: results of two US national surveys. Am J Psychiatry. 2006;163(2):297–302.

8. Chambless DL, Hollon SD. Defining empirically supported therapies. J Consult Clin Psychol. 1998;66(1):7.

9. Melville KM, Casey LM, et al. Psychological treatment dropout among pathological gamblers. Clin Psychol Rev. 2007;27(8):944–58.

10. Swift JK, Greenberg RP. Premature discontinuation in adult psychotherapy: a meta-analysis. J Consult Clin Psychol. 2012;80(4):547.

11. Fortune EE, Goodie AS. Cognitive distortions as a component and treatment focus of pathological gambling: a review. Psychol Addict Behav. 2012;26(2):298.

12. Ladouceur R, Sylvain C, et al. Cognitive treatment of pathological gambling. J Nerv Ment Dis. 2001;189(11):774–80.

13. Ladouceur R, Sylvain C, et al. Group therapy for pathological gamblers: a cognitive approach. Behav Res Ther. 2003;41(5):587–96.

14. Smith DP, Battersby MW, et al. Cognitive versus exposure therapy for problem gambling: randomised controlled trial. Behav Res Ther. 2015;69:100–10.

15. Petry NM, Ammerman Y, et al. Cognitive-behavioral therapy for pathological gamblers. J Consult Clin Psychol. 2006;74(3):555–67.

16. Oei TP, Raylu N, et al. Effectiveness of group and individual formats of a combined motivational interviewing and cognitive behavioral treatment program for problem gambling: a randomized controlled trial. Behav Cogn Psychother. 2010;38(2):233–8.

17. Hodgins DC, Currie SR, et al. Does providing extended relapse prevention bibliotherapy to problem gamblers improve outcome? J Gambl Stud. 2007;23(1):41–54.

18. Campos MD, Rosenthal RJ, et al. A self-help manual for problem gamblers: the impact of minimal therapist guidance on outcome. Int J Ment Health Addict. 2015;14:579–96.

19. Luquiens A, Tanguy ML, et al. The efficacy of three modalities of internet-based psychotherapy for non-treatment-seeking online problem gamblers: a randomized controlled trial. J Med Internet Res. 2016;18(2):e36.

20. Grant JE, Donahue CB, et al. Imaginal desensitization plus motivational interviewing for pathological gambling: randomized controlled trial. Br J Psychiatry. 2009;195(3):266–7.

21. Petry NM, Weinstock J, et al. A randomized trial of brief interventions for problem and pathological gamblers. J Consult Clin Psychol. 2008;76(2):318–28.

22. Petry NM, Rash CJ, et al. A randomized control trial of brief interventions for problem gambling in substance abuse treatment patients. J Consult Clin Psychol. 2016;84(10):874–86.

23. Carlbring P, Jonsson J, et al. Motivational interviewing versus cognitive behavioral group therapy in the treatment of problem and pathological gambling: a randomized controlled trial. Cogn Behav Ther. 2010;39(2):92–103.

24. Larimer ME, Neighbors C, et al. Brief motivational feedback and cognitive behavioral interventions for prevention of disordered gambling: a randomized clinical trial. Addiction. 2012;107(6):1148–58.

25. Hodgins DC, Currie SR, et al. Motivational enhancement and self-help treatments for problem gambling. J Consult Clin Psychol. 2001;69:50–7.

26. Hodgins DC, Currie SR, et al. Randomized trial of brief motivational treatments for pathological gamblers: more is not necessarily better. J Consult Clin Psychol. 2009;77(5):950–60.

27. LaBrie RA, Peller AJ, et al. A brief self-help toolkit intervention for gambling problems: a randomized multisite trial. Am J Orthopsychiatry. 2012;82(2):278–89.
28. Diskin KM, Hodgins DC. A randomized controlled trial of a single session motivational intervention for concerned gamblers. Behav Res Ther. 2009;47(5):382–8.
29. Cunningham JA, Hodgins DC, et al. A randomized controlled trial of a personalized feedback intervention for problem gamblers. PLoS One. 2012;7(2):e31586.
30. Neighbors C, Rodriguez LM, et al. Efficacy of personalized normative feedback as a brief intervention for college student gambling: a randomized controlled trial. J Consult Clin Psychol. 2015;83(3):500.
31. Petry NM. Pathological gambling: etiology, comorbidity, and treatment. Washington, DC: American Psychological Association Press; 2005.
32. Hodgins DC, el-Guebaly N. Retrospective and prospective reports of precipitants to relapse in pathological gambling. J Consult Clin Psychol. 2004;72(1):72.
33. Miller WR, Rollnick S. Motivational interviewing: helping people change. New York: Guilford Press; 2012.
34. Miller WR. Motivational enhancement therapy manual: a clinical research guide for therapists treating individuals with alcohol abuse and dependence. Rockville, MD: DIANE Publishing; 1995.
35. Ortiz L. Till spelfriheten! Kognitiv beteendeterapivid spelberoende [CBT for pathological gambling]. Stockholm: Natur & Kultur; 2006.

Innovative Treatment Approaches in Gambling Disorder

10

Leroy Snippe, Marilisa Boffo, Sherry H. Stewart, Geert Dom, and Reinout W. Wiers

10.1 Introduction

Treating disordered gambling can be challenging. There is ample empirical evidence suggesting a complex and dynamic interaction of genetic, developmental, cognitive, psychosocial, and environmental factors in the development and maintenance of excessive gambling behavior [1, 2]. There is also a growing recognition that gambling disorder (GD) and substance use disorders (SUDs) share clinical, endophenotypical and neurobiological similarities [3, 4], culminating in the inclusion of GD in the substance-related and addictive disorders category of the latest DSM-5 [5]. Furthermore, individuals suffering from GD are not a homogeneous group. Rather, disordered gamblers report distinct motivations for gambling [6], as well as a range of different intra- and interpersonal characteristics in the symptomatological expression of GD [7].

L. Snippe (✉)
University of Amsterdam, Amsterdam, Netherlands

University of Antwerp, Antwerpen, Belgium
e-mail: l.snippe@uva.nl

M. Boffo · R. W. Wiers
University of Amsterdam, Amsterdam, Netherlands
e-mail: R.W.H.J.Wiers@uva.nl

S. H. Stewart
Dalhousie University, Halifax, NS, Canada
e-mail: sstewart@dal.ca

G. Dom
University of Antwerp, Antwerpen, Belgium

Antwerp University Hospital, Edegem, Belgium
e-mail: geert.dom@uantwerpen.be

© Springer Nature Switzerland AG 2019
A. Heinz et al. (eds.), *Gambling Disorder*, https://doi.org/10.1007/978-3-030-03060-5_10

Designing effective interventions for GD is further challenged by the difficulty in reaching individuals suffering from gambling problems. Less than 10% of disordered gamblers ever seek help and enter treatment [8, 9]. This is partly related to most gamblers having difficulties to acknowledge they have a problem. Among those who do, the most frequently reported reasons for not seeking help include shame, stigma, and difficulties in disclosing personal issues, lack of motivation to stop gambling, desire for self-reliance, lack of awareness of treatment options, concerns about treatment content and quality, or issues with treatment attendance and costs [10, 11].

As local gambling opportunities continue to change and grow, with greater acceptability and accessibility and the progressive legalization of varieties of online gambling services, there is an urgent need for the development of effective prevention initiatives and support programs. Despite the surge of empirical studies on various therapeutic approaches (cf. Chap. 9 by Ginley, Rash, & Petry), the evidence on the differential and long-term effectiveness of these therapeutic approaches is still limited [12]. Thus, it is impossible to define "best practice" treatment standards for addressing disordered gambling at this time.

This chapter presents an overview of recent advances in research on innovative treatment approaches and modalities for gambling problems, ranging from training interventions based on addiction models, neuromodulation techniques, and employment of modern digital technology, to tailored interventions and integration of multiple methods. Altogether, these novel domains of research on gambling interventions share the goal of enhancing therapeutic effects and overcoming barriers and limitations to existing treatment programs by meeting the heterogeneous needs and demands of this particular clinical population.

10.2 Cognitive Training

10.2.1 Dual-Process Models of Addictive Behaviors

Dual-process models describe addiction as the result of an imbalance between two different types of neurocognitive processes: a bottom-up impulsive motivational processing network in which limbic structures such as the ventral striatum and amygdala play a crucial role, and top-down control processes representing inhibition of impulses based on long-term and goal-directed reflective considerations, associated with a network including the dorsolateral prefrontal cortex [13, 14]. However, dual-process models have theoretical problems and have been criticized for being neurologically implausible [15]. As a solution, neurocognitive models have been proposed emphasizing temporal dynamics dependent on the reinforcement of cognitive functions together with iterative reprocessing, in which the features of cognitive-motivational processes shift from impulsive to reflective with more reprocessing [16, 17]. It is important to be aware of these theoretical developments when considering recent advances in cognitive interventions in addiction [18, 19].

One crucial ingredient of interventions in addiction is to help people to develop a long-term perspective, including personal goals that conflict with continuation of the addictive behavior [20, 21]. This is directly compatible with the motivational interviewing approach, a therapeutic technique originally developed by William ("Bill") Miller in the context of addiction treatment and now applied more widely [22]. However, sometimes motivation alone is not enough for a successful quitting attempt. Theoretically, motivation may be present but not sufficient by itself or not readily enough activated to change the outcome of response selection processes, in particular in situations that advantage impulsive responding. In other words, the addicted person may know at some level that discontinuation of the addictive behavior would be better in view of long-term goals, but at the same time addiction-related cues may capture attention, may trigger memory associations and elicit trains of thought related to continuation, and in some cases even trigger action tendencies toward the addictive behavior [18, 23]. In recent years, several varieties of cognitive training have been developed, which may help motivated clients to bias their addiction-related decision-making toward a discontinuation of the addictive behavior. While these training programs have been rather successful as add-on to regular treatment of SUDs, especially when added to inpatient treatment for alcoholism [18, 24, 25], we do not know yet whether this approach works for problematic gambling as well. Further, a mechanism hypothesized to play a role in the disproportional influence of bottom-up, cue-elicited processes is neural sensitization resulting in sensitized responses to cues predicting the addictive behavior [14, 26], based on the work of Robinson and Berridge [27, 28], and we do not know whether this mechanism plays a similar role in gambling. However, there are indications that similar cognitive biases, such as attentional bias, also occur in gamblers (e.g., [29]; for a narrative review, see [30]), strengthening the case for cognitive training in gambling.

Cognitive training paradigms can be classified into two broad types: those aimed at modifying impulses and those aimed at increasing cognitive control in general [18]. The first type of training aims to modify cognitive biases automatically triggered by addiction-related stimuli (i.e., Cognitive Bias Modification paradigms). The training can focus on attentional processes (attentional bias retraining), action tendencies (approach bias retraining), or memory processes (e.g., evaluative conditioning). The second class of training typically involves many sessions of training general cognitive control functions such as working memory and has been applied with some success to addiction [31–33].

10.2.2 Cognitive Bias Modification

Cognitive bias modification (CBM) refers to a class of cognitive training paradigms that target specific automatic attentional, behavioral, or evaluative biases triggered by addiction-related cues. These biases have repeatedly been shown to play an important role in addiction, leading researchers to believe that finding a way to modify these biases could drastically advance the treatment of addiction [18]. Encouraged by results in the domain of anxiety, researchers started developing such methods [34–36]. The resulting training paradigms are typically based on assessment versions of reaction-time tasks used to measure the targeted cognitive bias, with a built-in stimulus-response contingency to manipulate the bias [18, 37].

For example, to manipulate selective attentional processes toward salient cues, researchers adjusted the visual-probe task [34]. In this task, participants have to respond to a probe presented at the location of one of two stimuli displayed next to each other on the computer screen (e.g., an addiction-related picture and a neutral picture). In the assessment version of the task, the probe is presented equally often after both stimuli. The idea is that participants show a faster response when the probe appears at the location on which their attention was already focused [38]. In the training version of the task, the stimulus-probe contingency is manipulated so as to consistently present the probe at the location of the neutral stimulus, thus training participants to consistently shift attention away from addiction-related cues and to attend to neutral cues instead. Similar contingencies are added to other tasks used to train different biases (e.g., approach bias and memory associations) and to stimulate learning of a new stimulus-response association counteracting the previously learned, dysfunctional implicit associations. The underlying idea is that repeated training can reduce or even invert biases and lead to behavioral change [18].

10.2.2.1 Attentional Bias Modification

Motivationally salient cues have the ability to grasp our attention over neutral cues and interfere with the processing of our surrounding environment by "hijacking" our cognitive resources. This attentional preference has been called attentional bias [18]. While mostly studied in the domain of anxiety, where threatening stimuli seem to grab the attention of anxious participants more than neutral or positive cues [39], the role of attentional bias has also been more recently explored in addictive behaviors by using training varieties of two reaction-time tasks: the emotional Stroop task [40] and the visual-probe or dot-probe task [41]. Both tasks measure the attentional interference induced by salient (i.e., addiction-related) cues [42]. Using these two tasks, attentional bias toward addiction-related cues has been found in tobacco [43, 44], alcohol and drugs [45, 46], cannabis [47], heroin [48], cocaine [49], and in the eating domain [50]. Moreover, attentional bias has been found to be related to addiction severity ([51–53]; but for a critical review, see [54]).

A few studies have investigated the role of selective attentional processes in GD as well (for a review, see [30]). Consistent with other addiction disorders, problematic and pathological gamblers show generally faster reaction times toward gambling-related cues, compared to other stimulus categories [55–60]. This attentional preference for gambling-related cues was also found in other behavioral measures of attention [29, 57, 61]. Further, neuroimaging studies on cue reactivity for gambling stimuli found increased activations in fronto-striatal reward circuitry and brain areas related to attentional processing in pathological and problematic gamblers compared to healthy controls [62, 63]. Importantly, some research suggests gamblers' attentional bias is specific to their preferred gambling activity [64, 65].

Building upon this knowledge, researchers tried to manipulate and retrain selective attentional processes using adjusted versions of the same tasks used to measure this bias, i.e., attention bias modification (ABM) paradigms. A first group of experimental studies on ABM for alcohol successfully manipulated the attentional bias toward alcohol or neutral cues, with participants trained to avoid alcohol cues reporting less craving for alcohol compared to participants trained to attend to alcohol cues [66, 67]. However, manipulation of alcohol attentional bias did not affect alcohol consumption after the training. In a further study with heavy drinkers trained to avoid alcohol cues, ABM was successful in decreasing alcohol attentional bias [68]. However, this effect did not generalize, as participants did not show reduced attentional bias for untrained alcohol cues. No effects on craving were found either. Following these early preliminary lab studies, in a first clinical study with alcohol-dependent patients, 5 ABM sessions were offered as an add-on intervention atop treatment as usual (3–6 months of CBT [69]). Patients were randomized to either ABM training or sham training. Results indicated that ABM was successful in reducing alcohol attentional bias in the experimental condition, and this effect did generalize to novel alcohol stimuli. As in the previous studies, a reduced attentional bias did not result in less craving. However, participants who received the ABM training were discharged faster and took significantly longer to relapse. Other studies using different training paradigms (i.e., the Alcohol Attention-Control Training Program based on the emotional Stroop task) over multiple sessions found similar results: reduced attentional bias after ABM training, resulting in reduced alcohol consumption and increased motivation to change drinking habits [70], but results are hard to interpret and not conclusive due to the lack of a control group. In a more recent study, this training was combined with a motivational intervention in a full factorial design, with ABM yielding primarily short-term reductions in drinking, while motivational enhancement yielded more long-term changes [71].

The investigation of ABM interventions with smokers has produced rather mixed results, with ABM not always successfully reducing attentional bias toward smoking cues [72, 73]. Smoking-related attentional bias can be manipulated, albeit not always resulting in sustained effects or changes in craving and smoking rate [74, 75]. In contrast, one study in a more natural environment did find effects of ABM on smoking attentional bias and craving in participants not seeking help [76]. However, the reduction in attentional bias and craving did not result in decreased smoking behavior, which is not surprising given the fact that the participants did not want to quit smoking. A longitudinal study including help-seeking smokers varied the number of ABM sessions (0–3) across participants [77]. Results indicated ABM successfully reduced attentional bias, and the sustainability of this effect was dependent on the number of sessions (up to 6 months for participants receiving three ABM sessions). However, reduced attentional bias once again did not result in reduced craving or abstinence. A recent study obtained more promising results: smokers who wanted to quit were invited to participate in an online ABM program, based on the visual-probe task [78]. Participants were selected based on motivation to quit: only those who confirmed an actual quit attempt were included. While the clinical trial did not result in significant effects in the whole group, it did significantly increase 6-month abstinence in the subgroup of heavier smokers.

ABM studies have also been conducted in the field of eating disorders, with similar findings: reversed attentional bias for unhealthy foods with generalization to novel food cues [79]. Moreover, manipulating attentional bias for food-related cues affected craving for and consumption of unhealthy foods [80, 81]. ABM has also been used to promote healthy food choice by increasing attentional bias for healthy food cues, with a related increase in consumption of healthy food [82].

To our knowledge, no study has been published on the effects of ABM in gambling disorder yet. However, a first pilot randomized clinical trial is currently ongoing [83], where an online ABM program including 6 sessions of training is being tested with a sample of problematic and disordered gamblers. The researchers hope to answer the question as to whether ABM is potentially effective in reducing gambling-related attentional bias and gambling problems.

All in all, ABM seems to be effective in altering attentional bias for motivationally salient cues in addictive behaviors. Results on the effectiveness of ABM in reducing craving or actual consumption, however, are mixed. It should be taken into account that most of the research done on ABM in addictive behaviors can be considered experimental, often using just one session of training, whereas in the first, albeit very few, clinical studies with motivated patients receiving multiple ABM sessions on top of treatment as usual, ABM does seem to have clinically significant effects. In the light of the psychopathological and endophenotypical similarities between GD and other addictive behaviors and the evidence on cue-induced selective attentional processes in problem gamblers, ABM holds promise as an innovative (add-on) treatment approach for GD targeting conditioned attentional processes.

10.2.2.2   Approach Bias Modification

As mentioned in Sect. 10.1, through conditioning, addiction-related cues and behaviors acquire incentive salience properties for triggering impulsive, automatic, and involuntary motivational states [27, 28]. As a result, these cues not only grab our attention, but they can also induce a state of behavioral preparedness and approach tendencies toward those cues signaling the upcoming reward, i.e., approach bias. Approach bias has received increasing interest over the last few years, since it appears to play a crucial role in the onset and maintenance of addictive behaviors [18]. Addiction-related cues do gain increasing motivational incentive salience over time, in turn resulting in an increased tendency to reach for or move toward these cues.

Reaction-time assessment tasks of approach bias generally require participants to either approach or avoid certain cues, based on specific stimulus characteristics. The cues themselves are often a mix of neutral (e.g., photos of flowers, animals, landscapes, daily objects or activities, etc.) and addiction-related cues (e.g., photos of slot machines or alcoholic beverages). Depending on the type of task, stimulus features on which the approach or avoid decision has to be made can be either related or unrelated to the contents of the stimulus (i.e., relevant- or irrelevant-feature tasks, see [84–86]). Frequently used tasks to measure approach bias are the relevant-feature manikin and stimulus-response compatibility task [87, 88] and the irrelevant-feature Approach Avoidance Task (AAT [89]). Using these tasks, addiction-related approach bias has been documented in different addictive behaviors, including smoking [90–92], cannabis use [47, 93], drinking [42, 89, 94], and even toward unhealthy foods in overeaters and overweight individuals [95–99]. Moreover, the strength of the approach bias seems to be related to addiction severity and addictive behavior escalation across substances [91–93, 98]. A study in the alcohol domain has also associated the strength of an approach bias to a genetic variation: male carriers of the G allele in the OPRM1 gene showed a stronger approach bias for alcohol and other appetitive cues, compared to noncarriers [89].

A first set of studies has been recently conducted to examine the role of gambling-related approach bias in Canadian and Dutch problem and non-problem gamblers, using an adapted version of the AAT with gambling stimuli tailored to participants' gambling preferences [100, 101]. Results demonstrated the presence of approach bias toward gambling cues among Dutch gamblers with moderate-to-high severity of gambling problems, compared to non-problem gamblers [101], but not for Canadian problem gamblers [100]. Moreover, gambling approach bias predicted frequency and duration of prospective gambling episodes, over and above baseline neutral approach bias and gambling frequency and duration, respectively [101]. Even though not yet replicated, these results are consistent with findings in other addictive behaviors and support the hypothesis that automatic approach tendencies also play a role in problematic gambling behavior.

Similar to ABM, assessment tasks used to measure approach bias have been adapted to retraining paradigms, falling under the category of approach bias modification (ApBM). The first experimental study delivered one session of ApBM with a training version of the AAT, to train participants to either approach or avoid alcohol [94]. At posttest, participants who were trained to approach alcohol cues proved to be faster to approach (i.e., pull the joystick) alcohol cues, while those who were trained to avoid (i.e., push the joystick) alcohol cues showed an increased avoidance bias toward alcohol. These results also generalized to novel cues and to another implicit task using words instead of pictures (i.e., the approach-avoid Implicit Association Test [102, 103], based on [104]). Moreover, heavier drinkers who were successfully trained to avoid alcohol cues drank less alcohol during a subsequent taste test [94].

Consecutive clinical studies on AppBM in alcohol showed similar results (for a recent review and meta-analysis, see [105, 106]). Two large-scale randomized clinical trials have been published [24, 25]. In both studies, ApBM was implemented as an add-on to treatment as usual (primarily CBT therapy). The first of these studies ($n = 214$) found that 4 sessions of ApBM had a long-term positive effect on relapse rate in alcohol-dependent participants 1 year after treatment completion [24], with 13% less relapse in trained patients compared to controls, who were either assigned to a no-training control group or to a sham-training (continued assessment) control group. A second replication study ($n = 509$) with 12 sessions of training found similar results, with 9% lower relapse rate after 1 year in the experimental group. The large sample size allowed for determination that the clinical effect was mediated by the change in alcohol approach bias. Moreover, a moderation effect was also found: participants with a strong alcohol approach bias prior to treatment and of older age benefited most from the ApBM training [25].

A reduced relapse rate in the experimental group was also found when 4 sessions of ApBM or sham training were offered to inpatients during the early week of detoxi-fication phase before treatment as usual [107]. It is interesting to note that an optimal dosage of AppBM is not yet known. In a re-analysis of Eberl et al.'s data [25], the same authors investigated the dose-response relationship of ApBM intervention and found 6 ApBM sessions to be the mean optimum dosage but also indicated that a proportion of participants showed further improvement after 9 and 12 sessions [108].

The implementation of ApBM for smoking behavior provided promising initial results, with participants receiving one session of online ApBM showing reduced levels of smoking after 4 weeks [109] and after 3 months [110]. However, these results should be considered preliminary. Other results of ApBM in smoking are somewhat mixed and appear to be dependent on the setting and the motivation of participants (e.g., [111]) and the amount of behavior change in studies is still very limited [106]. A few studies have started exploring the efficacy of ApBM in other addictive behaviors, such as unhealthy food intake [112–114]. However, when the approach bias toward unhealthy foods was not successfully modified, ApBM did not have any behavioral effect [115], consistent with the mediation effect demon-strated in the alcohol domain. A preliminary study in a different form of behavioral addiction, namely, online gaming, reported that a single session of ApBM resulted in a reduced approach bias to gaming cues, subjective urges, intention to play, and game-seeking behavior [116].

To our knowledge, there is as yet no published study on ApBM in GD. First attempts are however under way encouraged by the discovery of an approach bias in problem gamblers [101]. An online ApBM program is currently being tested with Belgian and Dutch problem and disordered gamblers (the randomized clinical trial has a parallel-group design testing both ABM and ApBM interventions [83]). Personalized motivational feedback has been added to the training program to increase training adherence and prevent dropout. The same research group also launched a second web-based study combining online ApBM with internet-based CBT program with chat-based guidance from a trained therapist [117]. Participants receive nine CBT sessions through online chat with the therapist and, concurrently, nine sessions of AppBM. The same Canadian-Dutch group that found an approach bias in problem gamblers [101] also launched a subsequent study investigating whether problem gambling symptoms can be reduced trough an online program combining 4 sessions of ApBM with dynamic personalized motivational feedback, the latter added to increase adherence (Stewart, S.H., personal communication, March 2017).

The evidence suggesting a role of approach bias in addictive behaviors is accu-mulating and already quite extensive, with first results pointing to similar automatic associative processes in disordered gambling. The use of ApBM paradigms to decrease or reverse approach bias toward addiction-related appetitive cues has pro-vided promising results and is also currently tested in the gambling population. ApBM has the potential to become an innovative add-on treatment program, when used in addition to regular treatment or as low threshold and not too intensive train-ing program for motivated participants. Future research is warranted to further investigate the clinical effectiveness of AppBM, hopefully leading to a better under-standing of its working mechanisms and operational optimization.

10.2.2.3 Evaluative Conditioning

The last CBM paradigm is evaluative conditioning (EC), which is based on the assumption that behavior is influenced by implicit attitudes or associations [118]. These implicit attitudes are formed through experience and are activated whenever coming in contact with (addiction-related) environmental cues that have been associated with a strong emotional valence and anticipatory expectation of reward.

Indeed, there is some evidence for implicit evaluative associations to predict unique variance in additive behaviors [119]. For example, implicit positive attitudes have been found to predict escalation of alcohol consumption [120], to correlate with nicotine dependence and predict relapse in smoking [121], and to predict food choice [122]. In gambling, implicit positive attitudes seem to be associated with greater gambling involvement and more gambling-related problems and uniquely predict gambling behavior above and beyond explicit outcome expectancies [123–126] and to be a hallmark of problem gamblers [127].

EC has been designed to target these dysfunctional attitudes, based on the assumption that, similarly to how these attitudes are developed, repeatedly pairing addiction cues with emotional or valenced cues results in dominant evaluative associations. EC can work both ways by creating new positive or negative valence associations and has previously been used in, among others, the areas of advertising, racial prejudice, and anxiety and phobias [118, 128, 129].

More recently, researchers have begun assessing the effectiveness of EC in addictive behaviors. In alcohol, EC resulted in stronger implicit and explicit negative attitudes toward alcohol, less craving for alcohol, and less alcohol consumption directly after and 1 week following the intervention [130, 131]. Interestingly, one study found EC was only effective in changing implicit alcohol attitudes when general negative images were used and not when photos of frowning faces were used [130]. This implies implicit alcohol attitudes are perhaps more strongly influenced by experiencing affective states than by social feedback.

In the eating domain, EC increased implicit negative attitudes toward unhealthy foods [132–135] while leaving explicit attitudes and cognitions intact [132, 136]. In a number of studies, EC also resulted in reduced unhealthy food intake [132], possibly through a mediating role of implicit attitudes [134]. However, in other studies, EC did not produce any behavioral result [133, 135]. Interestingly, the effectiveness of EC in changing implicit attitudes also appears to be greatest in those with prior stronger implicit attitudes and those with low emotional control [132, 134, 135], partially similarly to the moderation effects observed in AppBM for alcohol [25]. It should be noted that a lot of research done on EC in the food domain demoted unhealthy food choices while simultaneously promoting healthy food choices. Hence, behavioral effects of EC (choosing to eat a healthy snack vs. an unhealthy snack in a subsequent taste test) should be interpreted with caution since it is unclear whether these effects are due to devaluation or promotional effects, or perhaps even both.

These first proof-of-principle studies in alcohol and food intake have pinpointed the positive effects of EC in reducing the strength of positive memory associations with addictive cues. The deployment of EC as a therapeutic approach is still in the experimental phase, and more studies are necessary to further prove its validity as an effective training program. To our knowledge, no studies have yet explored the effects of an EC program in GD.

10.2.3 General Cognitive Training

General cognitive control training aims at improving the ability to self-control. We can better visualize the role of self-control by using the metaphor of a rider riding a horse and trying to steer it in an intended direction. The horse represents our impulses and urges striving for immediate gratification and the rider our intentional plans of action and ideas of where to go. In spite of the clear goal of reaching the destination, the rider needs to be able to tame and guide the horse, preventing it from taking over whenever something interesting and appetitive appears along the path. General cognitive training helps in improving the rider's strength to tame the horse and guide it in the intended direction [137].

This class of training targets executive functions often used to exert self-control and guide behavior, such as working memory and response inhibition. However, sometimes a training may have different effects than one might expect; for example, selective inhibition training has often been classified as a variety of cognitive control training, but in fact, a specific response to a cue can also be trained (e.g., a no-go response to an addiction-related cue), which makes the addiction-related associations more negative (e.g., [138, 139]) but does not increase general inhibition capacity [138].

10.2.3.1 Working Memory Training

Working memory training (WMT) is used to improve working memory capacity (WMC), which refers to the ability of transiently holding, processing, and manipulating information. WMC is a core executive function and a crucial factor in cognitive processes such as monitoring, planning, problem-solving and decision-making, and performing complex cognitive tasks such as learning, reasoning, and comprehension [140]. As such, WMC appears to be heavily involved in top-down control and guidance of behavioral processes.

WMC deficits are seen in a number of unhealthy and addictive behaviors. In smokers, for example, WMC has been found to be impaired after a period of abstinence [141], and impaired WMC during abstinence was a predictor of relapse [142, 143]. In alcohol, WMC interacts with impulsivity and cognitive biases in predicting alcohol consumption, in line with the role of WMC in top-down processes (see review by Wiers et al. [144]). WMC deficits indeed predict alcohol use in those with strong cognitive biases or high impulsivity [145–147]. Moreover, a longitudinal study on early alcohol use in adolescence showed that WMC deficits preceded impulsivity, which in turn predicted alcohol use [148]. This same interaction has been reported in predicting drug use [149]. Results in cannabis use and unhealthy food intake show similar patterns [150, 151].

In problem gambling, the role of WMC seems to be more complex. In a number of studies, problem gamblers did not differ from healthy controls on measures of WMC [152–154] while one study did find WMC deficits in problem gamblers [155]. It is also unclear whether or not WMC can predict gambling or gambling relapse after treatment.

Considering the role of WMC in addictive behaviors, training programs aiming to increase WMC could be a promising and efficient addition to regular therapy

[140]. A meta-analysis indicated that improving WMC is in fact possible through WMT [156], and WMT seems especially effective in those with low WMC [157–159], although one critical meta-analysis expressed concerns regarding these results [160]. WMT paradigms generally consist of several visuospatial or sequence recall tasks in which participants are required to mentally store and recall increasingly complex information [32, 33, 161].

WMT interventions have been experimentally tested in individuals who heavily consume, or have problems with, a variety of substances. In alcohol, WMT was effective in improving WMC and reducing drinking at 1-month follow-up [33], with the strongest effects in participants with strong automatic impulses or associations. One study assessing the effects of WMT in stimulant addiction reported that WMT did not produce any effect on a number of cognitive measures, including a measure of WMC, but WMT did improve performance on a delay discounting task [32]. In a follow-up study, the authors proposed delay discounting to be closely related to WMC [162]. The effects of WMT have also been studied in unhealthy eating [163]. In obese adolescent inpatients, WMT resulted in enhanced WMC but did not improve weight loss at discharge. However, those who received WMT better maintained their weight loss 8 weeks after discharge. At 12 weeks after discharge, the advantage of the WMT subsided [163]. In a study with adult overweight individuals, WMT effectively reduced eating-related thoughts, overeating in response to negative emotions, and food intake among participants with strong dietary restraint goals, but no changes in BMI, craving or hunger in the laboratory were observed [164]. To the best of our knowledge, no studies exist assessing the effects of WMT interventions for disordered gambling.

Considering the role of WMC in decision-making processes and in regulating behavior and the preliminary results of WMT in other addictive behaviors, WMT would seem a promising addition to existing therapy for gambling problems. However, results so far are mixed, and some authors are concerned with the generalized effectiveness of WMT [160]. Future research is therefore needed to further investigate the role of different WMC components in addictive behaviors and particularly in disordered gambling, due to the absence of exogenous neurotoxin intake, which possibly leads to different patterns of neuropathology in disordered gambling vs. substance addiction. Broadening the understanding of the role of WMC in behavioral addictions would then also result in more refined training programs efficiently manipulating it.

10.2.3.2 Selective Inhibition Training

Research shows that, similarly to SUDs, inhibitory control plays a crucial role in the formation and continuation of GD [165, 166]. Indeed, problem gamblers tend to score lower on measures of general inhibitory control [63, 152, 167–172]. The notion that deficits in inhibitory control play an important role in addictive behaviors led to the idea that training and improving general inhibition could reduce addictive behavior. However, results of general inhibition training on addictive behavior are mixed and effects limited (e.g., [173–175]; for a review, see [176]).

Interestingly, some theories have taken a different approach in explaining the relation between inhibitory control and addictive behavior. These theories state that inhibitory control should be considered a fluctuating state dependent on internal and external momentary states and conditions, including the influence of environmental cues [177, 178]. In support of this idea, studies in addictive and eating behaviors have shown that states of impaired inhibitory control can be induced by addiction- and food-related cues [179–182]. This state, in turn, has been shown to prospec- tively predict addictive behavior [180].

Further support for the role of selective inhibition in addictice behaviors, as opposed to general inhibition, comes from studies trying to train inhibitory control in addiction using adapted tasks used to measure response inhibition or impulsivity, such as the go/no-go task [183] or the stop-signal task [184]. While quite similar in task structure and purpose (i.e., assessing response impulsivity), it has been argued these tasks measure two distinct processes: a more associative and bottom-up form of cognitive inhibition (go/no-go task) and a more controlled and top-down form of motor inhibition (stop-signal task; for a moredetailed explanation of differences between the processes underlying the two tasks, see [185]). Inhibition training in addictive behavior is, in general, more effective when using the go/no-go task [176, 186], as automatic inhibition leads to devaluation of no-go cues [187], whereas there is no evidence that controlled inhibition devalues stop-signals. These results and the differential effects of using addiction-specific cues as targets [178], led to a reconceptualization of inhibition training, separating (top-down) general inhibition training and (bottom-up) selective inhibition training (SIT) [188].

Most research into SIT has been conducted in the eating domain, wherein research- ers were interested in reducing the intake of unhealthy foods. The majority of the stud- ies are proof-of-principle lab studies comprising a single session of an adapted go/ no-go training paradigm. Results indicate that SIT is effective in increasing inhibition for food cues [189, 190] and, more importantly, is effective in reducing the intake of unhealthy foods post-training [189–193]. Interestingly, the effects of SIT were espe- cially strong for participants who were hungry or regularly ate unhealthy foods [193] and for participants who had a high BMI or were chronic dieters [190]. Effects on crav- ing are mixed, with some studies indicating reduced craving after SIT [189], while others do not [192]. One study using training with the adapted stop-signal training found the same pattern of decreased unhealthy food intake after SIT training, albeit only for participants who scored high on general impulsivity prior to training [194].

A small number of studies have looked at the effects of multiple SIT sessions on unhealthy eating behavior. Studies using the go/no-go training task found SIT resulted in greater weight loss and a reduction in intake and liking of unhealthy foods directly after treatment [175, 195]. The effect of SIT on weight loss was still present after 6 months [195] and was strongest in participants with a high BMI prior to treatment [175]. However, no behavioral effects were observed. One study using a stop-signal training task found SIT resulted in increased inhibitory control directly after treatment, but not at a 1-week follow-up [174]. Furthermore, effects of SIT on weight loss were mixed, and no behavioral effects were found.

Few studies have looked at the effects of SIT on (heavy) drinking. One study using a one-session go/no-go SIT found heavy drinkers developed negative attitudes toward alcohol and reduced their alcohol consumption in the week following training [139]. A second study in heavy drinkers found one session of stop-signal SIT reduced craving and alcohol consumption directly after training but not in the week following training [173].

In the field of behavioral addiction, there is a paucity of research on SIT. Only one study in sex addiction presented one session of go/no-go SIT training with sexually appealing cues. SIT resulted in cues being rated as less appealing and a reduced sex approach bias directly after training [196]. To our knowledge, no studies have been reported on the effectiveness of SIT in GD, nor are we aware of any such studies presently being conducted or proposed.

Two recent meta-analyses summarized the effectiveness of SIT, concluding it does produce a contingent effect on addictive behavior but that evidence of long-term effectiveness is still mixed [174, 188]. SIT effectiveness does not appear to depend on the number of training trials and training programs using the go/no-go paradigm as the training task showed more positive effects than studies using the stop-signal task. Furthermore, participants who are motivated to change their behavior seem to benefit the most from SIT.

To conclude, the revised conceptualization of SIT working mechanisms encourages the endorsement of SIT as a potential candidate for future research on innovative treatments for GD, since GD is characterized by fluctuations of selective cue-induced states of impaired inhibitory control, rather than general response inhibition problems [159]. SIT works by increasing selective inhibitory control and is especially effective in motivated participants with low selective inhibitory control for addiction-specific cues [175, 190, 191], consistent with findings in CBM for alcohol approach bias [25].

10.3 Brain Stimulation

In the past decade, there has been a surge of interest in the use of neuromodulating interventions in the treatment of a broad range of both neurological and psychiatric disorders, such as depression, anxiety, and addiction [197–199]. The concept of neuromodulation refers to the temporal (noninvasive) modulation of brain neurophysiology within specific regions and circuitries, aimed at changing related emotional and behavioral patterns. Two main neuro-technologies have been commonly used to externally modulate cortical excitability: repetitive transcranial magnetic stimulation (rTMS) and transcranial direct current stimulation (tDCS).

rTMS generates repeated pulses of high-intensity magnetic field by passing a brief electric current through an inductive coil placed on the scalp. This magnetic field induces an electrical current in the brain tissue beneath the coil, resulting in alterations of neural excitability (i.e., neuron depolarization). In addition to its cortical action and as a function of the placement of the coil, rTMS may act remotely on deeper brain structures via brain circuits and interhemispheric connections [200, 201]. tDCS is another method capable of modulating cortical excitability. It consists of delivering a low-intensity electric field (1–2 mA) through the brain between two external electrodes placed on the scalp and inducing a subthreshold modulation of neuronal membrane potentials.

rTMS and tDCS can have both enhancing and inhibiting effects. Anodal tDCS over the dorsolateral prefrontal cortex (DLPFC) increases excitability, while cathodic tDCS reduces it. Likewise, high-frequency rTMS exerts an enhancing effect, while low-frequency rTMS has an inhibitory effect. Increasing (prefrontal) cortical excitability is hypothesized to enhance cognitive functioning. Specifically, noninvasive brain stimulation over the prefrontal cortex region is increasingly shown to (transiently) modify impulsivity and its different components, such as decision-making and delay discounting [202, 203]. Of importance, impulsivity is strongly linked with the pathogenesis (initiation and continuation) of GD [204, 205] and as such might represent an important target for therapeutic interventions. Within this context, neurostimulating interventions such as rTMS and tDCS applied to the DLPFC may indirectly modulate dopaminergic pathways and consequently have an impact on the symptoms of addiction, i.e., improving cognitive control and reducing craving [197].

Within clinical samples, tDSC and rTMS have shown clinically relevant effects specifically on reducing craving for alcohol, cocaine, and nicotine [197, 206]. However, their temporal effect indicates the need of repetitive treatment. In contrast to SUDs, hardly any studies have currently been done on GD, although from a viewpoint of etiology/pathogenesis, the similarity with SUDs might suggest that these interventions could be of use in patients suffering from GD and/or other behavioral addictions. With regard to rTMS, a recent small study showed that high-frequency rTMS of the medial prefrontal cortex (PFC) and continuous theta burst stimulation (cTBS) of the right dorsolateral PFC, can reliably reduce motivational and physiological reinforcement effects of slot machine gambling in men diagnosed with GD [207]. These positive findings contrast an earlier, even smaller study showing no effect of deep TMS on gambling behavior [208].

Taken together, based upon the hypothesized neurophysiological working mechanisms associated with noninvasive neuromodulation techniques and the findings from clinical studies in SUDs, neuromodulation interventions can be expected to be effective within the treatment of GD. As such, they represent a novel line of interventions. However, at this point in time, studies are few and findings preliminary. In addition to the clinical effectiveness, many questions remain to be explored. These include, among others, exploring the exact components of gambling behavior (and cognitions) that are affected, the location of the coils, depth and intensity of the stimulation, and the ideal repetition time. Indeed, although neurostimulation has been suggested to initiate a process of neuroplasticity [209], and as such a more sustainable change, questions remain about how long a stimulation period is necessary and indeed whether the initial effects will hold up. Finally, there is a need for future studies exploring whether neuromodulation as an add-on to cognitive treatment can enhance the treatment effect. First studies, albeit in heavy alcohol drinking populations, point in that direction [210, 211]. Whether this holds for the treatment of GD remains to be explored.

10.4   Digital Interventions

Overcoming barriers to treatment is one of the primary challenges for healthcare providers when designing, evaluating, and delivering evidence-based care in an accessible and cost-efficient fashion. Broadening the outreach and offering low-threshold programs, tailored to the demands for privacy and self-reliance, and ensuring sensitivity to the socioeconomic conditions of problem gamblers [10, 11] could potentially decrease treatment-seeking stigma and stimulate behavior change on a larger scale. In order to achieve such goals, research in innovative interventions for GD has recently began exploring new mediums of administering treatment. One such a medium sparking researchers' interest is also increasingly being used by gamblers to engage in their activities: the Internet and, more generally, digital technology [212–214].

In the past decade, digital technologies have increasingly become pervasive in all aspects of our daily lives. Mobile and wireless technologies, including laptops, smartphones, tablets, and embedded cameras, promote real-time connectivity in every moment of our lives and provide instant access to a monstrous amount of information, news, documents, and services available nonstop. For health and healthcare, the Internet infrastructure provides a compelling profusion of possibilities to develop and integrate digital health products, services, apps, and platforms, into care protocols complying with the advances in technology, new findings about the determinants of health and illness, and changing modalities of healthcare and recipients' needs.

10.4.1 What Is E-health?

The World Health Organization defines *E-health* as the use of information and communication technologies for health purposes, in which health resources and healthcare are being communicated and transferred by electronic means, facilitating healthcare management and promotion, the confidential communication between caregivers and clients, and a wide outreach of health services to a large scale. Digital health interventions also fall under the field of E-health and refer to "interventions that employ digital technology to promote and maintain health, through primary or secondary prevention and management of health problems" ([215], p. 814). They include web-based programs accessible via smartphone, laptop, and tablet devices but can also employ automated healthcare and communication systems, mobile "apps" (m-health), virtual reality and serious games, and mobile, wearable, and environmental sensors that can provide intelligent monitoring and feedback as and when needed (e.g., ecological momentary assessment and interventions [216]).

It is important to note here that "digital interventions" generally refers to the implementation of therapeutic principles in a digital environment rather than an entirely novel type of interventions [217–219]. In doing so, digital interventions expand the reach of traditional interventions, building upon existing therapeutic principles and harnessing the potential of increasingly sophisticated new technologies, whether it is through serious games, web-based craving diaries, or cognitive training applications. Digital health interventions are typically automated, interactive, and personalized, employing user input or sensor data to tailor feedback or treatment pathways without the need for direct health professional input, although they may still include elements of tele-healthcare (i.e., remote interaction with or monitoring by health professionals). Digital interventions can then facilitate healthy behaviors and lifestyles by supporting the individual in the "real world," outside the highly protected clinical setting, to promote change in behaviors associated with specific contexts in the individual's daily life. Compared to standard face-to-face treatment, digital interventions give users the opportunity to empower self-reliance and self-management skills in a setting that is immediately and intrinsically linked to their health problem and guarantee convenience, 24/7 accessibility, and availability. These features are particularly relevant for hard-to-reach populations and users who seek help but are not inclined to use traditional services, such as at-risk or problem gamblers. Furthermore, as problem recognition and desire for anonymity also appear to be an important barrier to prevention and treatment access, Internet-based screening and support tools for problem gamblers are one way of increasing accessibility due to the confidentiality and nonjudgmental quality of digital interventions [220].

A number of recent systematic reviews have demonstrated the beneficial effects of digital interventions stand-alone or in combination with standard treatment, including Internet-based programs [221–224], mobile applications [225–227], serious games [228–230], and virtual reality environments [231, 232], to promote healthy behaviors and lifestyle (e.g., smoking cessation, healthy eating, physical activity, or alcohol consumption); improve treatment adherence, self-management, and outcomes in people with long-term health conditions (e.g., depression, anxiety, diabetes, asthma, or chronic pain); and provide remote access to effective treatments (e.g., digitally delivered CBT or motivational interviewing for different mental and somatic disorders).

10.4.2 Web-Based and Smartphone Interventions

A general Google search on "how to stop gambling online" gives about 2,930,000 results (November 2016), listing a myriad of websites providing help tools ranging from educational information such as books, brochures, checklists, and functional guidelines, self-assessment instruments, forums for gamblers, and modular self-directed programs to online counseling and chats with therapists. However, until recently only a few studies systematically examined the potential effects of digital interventions for GD, thus providing scientific evidence for their value as an effective and solid treatment option. Most of them created self-directed, web-based interventions based on motivational interviewing and CBT protocols described in existing self-help books [233, 234].

Carlbring and Smit [235] examined the efficacy of a therapist-assisted, 8-week Internet-based CBT program with minimal therapist contact via e-mail and weekly telephone calls of less than 15 min, relative to a wait-list control condition in a sample of 66 pathological gamblers. Participants randomized to the online intervention reported significant improvements in gambling problems, anxiety, depression, and quality of life, compared to the wait-list group at the posttreatment assessment. Treatment effects were sustained in follow-ups at 6, 18, and 36 months, but no medium- and long-term between-group comparison at follow-up was possible given that participants in the waiting list received treatment before the follow-up data collection [236].

Similarly, Castren et al. [237] delivered an online 8-week CBT program for gamblers in Finland, comprising 8 modules containing psychoeducational, motivational, and cognitive-behavioral exercises, relapse prevention information and exercises, homework assignments, and a maximum of 30 min of weekly telephone support provided by 4 trained therapists. The participants could also join online discussion groups. Significant decreases in gambling expenditure, gambling-related problems and erroneous thoughts, and impaired control over gambling from baseline to post-treatment were observed. Gambling urges also decreased after the intervention and sustained after 6 months.

Fully online supporting materials have also been designed to increase accessibility to healthcare, such as the brief personalized feedback screener for problem gamblers Check Your Gambling (www.checkyourgambling.net [238]). The feedback included a summary of gambling severity, gambling-related cognitive distortions, and a list of techniques to lower the risk associated with gambling, personalized to the participant's responses to an extensive screening survey. The screening tool was further tested compared to a wait-list control with Ontario-based gamblers with moderate to severe gambling problems, with or without the addition of normative feedback [220]. The study reported mixed results: none of the two interventions affected gambling expenditure, with all conditions reporting reduced amount of money spent from baseline to the 12-month follow-up, but the personalized feedback intervention without norms reported a lower number of days gambled, compared to the normative personalized feedback and the wait-list control. The authors concluded that despite the modest positive results, a personalized feedback intervention may have a limited, short-term impact on the severity of problem gambling. Further, it shows potential for a wider outreach of the gambling population and for motivating gamblers to seek further help online or in person [220]. Noteworthy, in the first 15 months the website was active, 1321 tests were recorded, and 78% of respondents were screened as severe problem gamblers, indicating that the online screener reached the population it had been designed for.

More recently, Luquiens et al. [239] conducted a large-scale randomized clinical trial with 1122 non-help-seeking online problem gamblers, in particular poker players, testing three web-based psychotherapy modalities compared to a wait-list control condition: (1) personalized normalized feedback on gambling status by e-mail, (2) a downloadable self-help book adapted from the six-step CBT program by Ladouceur and Lachance [234] with no guidance, and (3) the same CBT program e-mailed weekly by a trained psychologist with personalized guidance. The program lasted 6 weeks, and the main outcome measure was a change in problem gambling severity. At the end of treatment, no significant differences were found between any of the groups. Importantly, high dropout rates were observed, particularly in the group receiving the CBT intervention with guidance. The authors concluded that web-based treatment in nontreatment-seeking populations may have poor acceptability if it requires a large investment of time and participants have no motivation to change their behavior.

Another recent randomized clinical trial tested an online intervention for disordered gambling with a sample of high school students in Italy [240]. Twelve classes were randomized to either an online personalized feedback control group or an intervention group that participated in a 3-week online training in addition to the same feedback. The extended web intervention included question-and-answer games and quizzes, which educated students about gambling activities and concepts such as luck and probability, as well as gambling-related characteristics, such as prevalence of problem gambling and cognitive distortions. At the 2-month follow-up, the intervention group reported significantly fewer gambling problems compared to the control group. However, only participants who were frequent gamblers at baseline showed a significant decrease in proxy measures of gambling severity such as gambling frequency, expenditure, and attitudes.

Currently, there are multiple ongoing randomized clinical trials testing the effectiveness of a variety of treatment programs for gambling problems delivered via the web [83, 117, 241, 242]. Hodgins et al. [242] are evaluating the effectiveness of a fully online version (*Self-change Tools*) of the self-directed CBT program developed by Hodgins [233], incorporating workbook materials, relapse prevention, and motivational interviewing elements, in comparison with the online screener Check Your Gambling developed by Cunningham et al. ([241]; both tools are available at www.problemgambling.ca). The same research group is also testing the same online self-directed CBT program versus an extended version additionally including an intervention for anxiety and depression, with a sample of problematic gamblers with and without co-occurring mental health problems, disclosing interest in online self-help materials [241].

Motivational interviewing interventions for gambling problems have also started being adapted to the web [243]. A text-based, online self-directed motivational enhancement intervention (iMET) has been implemented based on a previous study on brief motivational interventions for problem gamblers [244], with the goal of building commitment to change. Participants received a final report with a review of their gambling behavior and concerns, gambling severity, motivation and confidence to change, values, decisional matrix, and goals. A randomized clinical trial is currently testing the iMET versus the online screener Check Your Gambling. Although the study is still ongoing, preliminary results for the first 40 participants randomized to the two conditions show, similar to the RCT by Cunningham et al. [220], that both groups reported decreases in gambling involvement over the 3-month follow-up and increases in motivation to change, irrespective of received intervention. However, there is a first indication that iMET may positively affect gambling severity, as shown by a marginally greater reduction in problem gambling severity compared to the group completing the Check Your Gambling online screener [243].

Computerized CBM interventions, previously presented in this chapter, are also suitable to be administered online, thus showing potential of being a low-cost, low-threshold addition to conventional treatments. However, it should be noted that in general, CBM has shown to be less effective in online interventions than in a clinical setting, presumably because in an online intervention, it is harder to effectively change the cognitive bias (which requires focused attention [245]). This pattern can also be observed in CBM for addiction [246]. Currently, there is one ongoing study testing the effectiveness of a stand-alone online CBM program targeting selective attention and automatic approach tendencies toward gambling cues in a sample of Dutch and Belgian problematic and pathological gamblers [83]. The program consists of 6 sessions of training, combined with brief automated personalized feedback on gambling motives and reasons to quit or reduce gambling at baseline and at the start of each training session, similarly to Swan and Hodgins et al.'s studies [243, 244]. Another online study by the same research group is launching soon, combining an online CBT program specific for gambling problems with 9 chat sessions with a therapist and 9 sessions of ApBM in parallel [117].

Despite advancements in the implementation and deployment of online interventions for gambling problems, it should be noted that there is still a paucity of published literature about the use of smartphone applications to deliver gambling interventions. It is noteworthy to mention, though, that ongoing research and technological development are focusing on exploiting the benefits of mobile technology to provide gamblers with tools to monitor and support their goals of behavioral change. For example, the Problem Gambling Institute of Ontario developed and published a free online app to help cutting down or quitting gambling, *Mobile Monitor Your Gambling & Urges* (MYGU; http://www.problemgambling.ca/gambling-help/mygu-getmobile/). MYGU promotes self-awareness of gambling behaviors, i.e., it gathers information about gambling behaviors, such as money expenditure, and reports back to the gambler the date and time of craving episodes and their triggers, alternative activities they perform instead of gambling, wins and losses when they gambled, and feelings and consequences if they gambled or did not gamble. The app also complements counseling sessions and provides information to therapists. Another smartphone application has been recently developed and preliminarily evaluated by researchers at the University of Auckland [247]. *SPGETTI* (*Smartphone-Based Problem Gambling Evaluation and Technology Testing Initiative*) was designed to support people with a gambling problem who are seeing counselors and accessing services to receive "just in time" and "at the right place" support, specifically to prevent relapse and remain abstinent from harmful gambling on electronic gambling machines.

There is an emerging body of literature demonstrating the promising efficacy of online cognitive-behavioral and motivational interventions. However, despite the existence of various treatment paradigms, there are only a few methodologically sound, empirical studies comparing the differential, long-term efficacy of these therapeutic approaches. Further studies and development efforts, particularly in the field of m-Health, are currently exploring new venues of treatment programs and modalities, in terms of their effectiveness comparability, clinical feasibility, and utility.

10.4.3 Virtual Reality Interventions

Virtual reality (VR) technology allows the user to navigate and to interact in real time with a virtual three-dimensional environment. VR has mainly been used to deliver cue exposure therapy by using a head-mounted display (HMD or helmet), which is a pair of goggles allowing the presentation of images in stereoscopy, combined with audio stimuli and a motion tracker that follows the user's head — and sometimes also eye — movements. VR offers great control over different types of stimuli and the rhythm of their presentation and provides the opportunity to conduct exposure as well as relapse prevention in various locations (e.g., a bar or casino) that could provoke different reactions in the same person. The fact that VR is interactive and very similar to real-life situations also adds to the acceptability and ecological validity of therapy, thereby lowering the threshold for seeking treatment.

A pilot clinical trial comparing the use of standard imaginal exposure with immersions in a VR bar was conducted with 28 pathological gamblers participating in a 28-day residential CBT program [248]. The first and the last session of the CBT program were modified to include VR. Results revealed that the first VR immersion uncovered significantly more high-risk situations and more dysfunctional thoughts than the standard imaginal exposure exercise. In the second session, devoted to relapse prevention, immersion in the virtual bar was associated with stronger changes in urges to gamble compared with the imaginal exposure condition. Furthermore, changes in urges to gamble induced during the relapse prevention session significantly predicted patient improvements. No ethical issue or adverse events were reported following the use of VR (e.g., inducing too intense craving or cybersickness).

Another study explored the effects of a one-session VR cue exposure paradigm for disordered gamblers [249]. Ten participants moved throughout a virtual bar with 5 video lottery terminals for 5 times. Although the desire to gamble significantly increased when participants transitioned from the practice environment to the gambling environment, this study was unable to confirm the process of extinction because it consisted of only a single 20-min session. A more recent experimental study included 5 sessions of VR exposure and relaxation training with a small sample of 12 recreational gamblers [250]. All virtual environments with casino-related cues triggered subjective gambling urges, albeit with no associated psychophysiological arousal response. Urges to gamble decreased after repeated exposure to two main VR cues, playing a casino game and discussing gambling with a colleague, while psychophysiological arousal measures did not significantly change across sessions.

The investigation of VR for gambling problems is still in its infancy. However, despite the preliminary nature of the first experimental studies, alongside the lack of control conditions and long-term follow-up assessments, the use of VR seems to be a viable and promising medium to safely deliver exposure interventions for addictive behaviors without all the inconveniences of in vivo exposure techniques.

10.4.4 Serious Games for Behavioral Change

The term gamification is widely used to indicate the application of gaming elements in nongame contexts to influence behavior, improve motivation, and enhance engagement, such as adding progress bars to a website to show how much of your profile you have filled in, adding points, badges, leaderboards, peer pressure, quests or missions, social interactions, and more to things that normally would not have them. Serious games take this concept one step further: they contain gameplay elements commonly found in video games and, most importantly, are designed for a specific purpose besides mere entertainment.

Currently, there is only one published pilot study looking at the effects of using a serious game as a therapeutic intervention for gambling disorder [251]. The authors explored the feasibility and effectiveness of a serious game specifically designed to treat impulse control disorders like gambling disorder. The overall goal of the serious game, *PlayMancer*, was to train emotion regulation and impulsivity control by improving problem-solving and planning skills, as well as control over general impulsive behaviors and relaxation skills via three mini-games of increasing difficulty. The serious game was incorporated as a complementary therapy tool into a CBT program in a male sample of 16 treatment-seeking participants with severe gambling disorder. The intervention consisted of 16 weekly group CBT sessions and, concurrently, 10 additional 20-min weekly sessions of the serious game. After the intervention, significant changes were observed in severity of gambling problems, several measures of impulsivity, state anxiety, and general psychological distress. Furthermore, dropout and relapse rates during treatment were similar to those described in the CBT literature.

While this is the first semi-experimental study to describe the results of an intervention for gambling problems based on a serious game, the application of gamification and serious games for health and behavior change has become more and more widespread [229]. The exploitation of gamification techniques and the development of serious games as a low-threshold intervention, or as a complement to or enhancer of conventional treatments, could prove to be an interesting and innovative tool to promote users' motivation and engagement in behavior change, and a viable training tool, especially when designed to target concrete problems or specific skills, such as monitoring gambling expenditure or improving risky decision-making and impulse control.

10.5 Innovative Approaches on Existing Treatment

10.5.1 Tailoring

Personalized medicine has been gaining a stronger interest and endorsement in all areas of healthcare, including addiction [252]. Inter- and intraindividual heterogeneity in the gambling population and different clinical profiles of GD strongly confronts researchers and clinical practitioners with the necessity of shifting treatment approaches and methods from a "one-size-fits-all" to a more tailored variety. This implies a targeted focus on the patient's individual, cultural, and environmental characteristics and a better selection of treatment strategies to increase positive outcomes and reduce misdiagnoses and costs.

For example, personalized treatment programs for GD have been recently explored that use available research information on problem gambler subtypes to develop and test novel "matched treatments." These treatments utilize intervention techniques that target each subtype's unique treatment needs [253]. This work is informed by the successes of such matched treatments when applied in other areas of addiction treatment. For example, Conrod and colleagues [254, 255] have developed novel personality-matched interventions for SUD treatment and prevention, which involve unique interventions for individuals at risk for SUDs as a function of their personality features and associated risky motives for use. In this approach, the interventions provided to a sensation seeker (i.e., one who prefers novelty and intense stimulation) are quite different from those provided to a hopeless (i.e., depression-prone, negative thinking) individual, for example. Relative to a variety of controls, in a series of randomized controlled trials, these personality-matched treatments have been shown to reduce substance misuse among those with existing SUDs and to reduce substance use and delay uptake of substance use in youth when used in a school-based prevention context (e.g., [254, 255]).

This type of approach has recently been adapted for use in the problem gambling treatment context. Studies have repeatedly shown that there are valid subtypes of gamblers that differ in characteristics such as psychiatric comorbidity and their primary motivations for gambling (e.g., [6, 256]). In particular, at least two distinct subtypes have been identified: a subtype that gambles primarily for coping motives or to "escape" (i.e., gambling to reduce or avoid negative affective states) and another distinct subtype that gambles primarily for enhancement motives or for "action" (i.e., gambling to achieve pleasurable states or for stimulation) ([6, 257]; see review by Milosevic and Ledgerwood [7]). Reasoning that interventions for problem gamblers could be made more meaningful, efficient, and efficacious by developing interventions that are unique to each of these gambler subtypes, Stewart and colleagues developed the Brief Escape and Action Treatments for problem gambling (i.e., the BEAT Gambling program [258]). Drawing upon a cognitive-behavioral framework, the objective of BEAT Gambling was to expand on traditional CBT for problem gamblers [259] by including intervention components that specifically target psychological factors (e.g., maladaptive beliefs) related to the gambling exhibited by each gambler subtype (action vs. escape). This 6-session motivation-matched treatment was designed to target the distinct beliefs and behavioral patterns that impede control of gambling behavior that are characteristic of each subtype of problem gambler. Problem gamblers of each subtype are taught to identify and challenge their unique thinking errors and to engage in distinct behavioral strategies as means of overcoming their problem gambling. For example, escape gamblers are trained in more adaptive means of relieving distress, whereas action gamblers are trained in less risky means of achieving excitement and stimulation.

Stewart and colleagues recently published a case series that was designed as a preliminary assessment of the effectiveness of this novel, motivation-matched treatment for problem gambling [260]. On the basis of their primary underlying motivations for gambling (as assessed with the Gambling Motives Questionnaire [261]), 6 problem gamblers received either a 6-session escape-motivated ($n = 2$) or a 6-session action-motivated ($n = 4$) treatment from the manualized BEAT gambling intervention. Assessments were conducted at baseline, immediate posttreatment, and at 3- and 6-month follow-ups. Primary outcome measures included gambling involvement (i.e., gambling frequency, and time and money spent gambling), problem gambling severity, and gambling-related disability. The secondary outcome measures included gambling abstinence self-efficacy, craving to gamble, high-risk gambling situations, and gambling expectancies. Overall, these pilot participants showed significant improvements from pre- to posttreatment on most of these measures, with relatively less immediate posttreatment gains seen on measures that assessed excessive gambling in specific high-risk situations (i.e., positive situations for action gamblers, negative situations for escape gamblers) and gambling-related disability. However, treatment gains were observed for most participants on these latter measures by the follow-ups [260]. The next step was to conduct a randomized controlled trial to compare the efficacy of the motivation-matched treatment with treatment as usual. Preliminary results regarding short-term outcomes show that, relative to treatment as usual in the community, the BEAT gambling treatment showed statistically superior outcomes on several outcome variables: reduction in gambling frequency, improvement in readiness to change, reduction in gambling craving, and improvements in severity of gambling problems. The matched treatment also showed superior retention relative to treatment as usual suggesting that the BEAT gambling treatment may be more engaging to problem gambling clients (possibly due to these interventions being very relevant to their unique treatment needs), resulting in an increased willingness to remain in treatment (see [262]). The results from this case series and preliminary outcomes from the RCT certainly suggest promise for this novel treatment approach.

The large variety of gambling games and the differences in the legalization and normative regulation of gambling practices among countries bring to the table another level of heterogeneity at the macro level: culture (please also see Chap. 13). Distinctive types of gambling activities, games, design, and locations play a role in shaping gambling behavior and preferences: for example, gambling games and practices in the Netherlands are different than those in Canada, resulting in Dutch and Canadian gamblers becoming highly familiar with the gambling instances available and common in their environment. This element is of particular importance for training programs aimed at reducing maladaptive reward-related associative processes toward gambling, such as CBM interventions.

As mentioned earlier, the first set of studies examining gambling-related approach bias attempted to validate a new gambling AAT task by evaluating its correlates cross-culturally in the Netherlands and Canada [100, 101]. Results for Dutch gamblers revealed the hypothesized gambling approach bias only among problem gamblers [101], compared to non-problem gamblers. Unexpectedly, Canadian gamblers appeared to show an avoidance bias, rather than an approach bias, toward the gambling stimuli, and approach bias showed a significant negative (rather than positive) correlation with gambling severity [100].

A potential explanation for what may at first look like an important cross-cultural difference is that these discrepancies may be due to the pictures used for the Canadian version of the gambling AAT. The Canadian researchers were not granted access to local casinos and play halls to create relevant stimuli for their gambling AAT and thus opted to use the original Dutch gambling stimuli or to process using Photoshop any Dutch stimuli that were deemed to be not cross-culturally appropriate. The observed differences may be the result of an effect akin to "the uncanny valley effect," in which subtle imperfections in the visual familiarity of a specific object, in this case the gambling stimuli, result in an aversion toward that specific object or stimuli [263]. Perhaps the Dutch gambling stimuli were close but not close enough to what Canadian gamblers typically see when they gamble, and this close but not perfect appearance put Canadian gamblers in a situation similar to the "uncanny valley" originally evidenced in the domain of humanoid robotics design [264], generating an associated aversion toward the gambling stimuli. Presumably, these subtle discrepancies would be most evident to the problem gamblers with a greater history of gambling exposure, leading to a stronger "uncanny valley" and associated aversion bias to Dutch and photoshopped gambling stimuli among the Canadian problem gamblers [100]. To confirm such a culture-based effect, the study is currently being repeated with new, localized pictures for the Canadian gambling AAT that are more culturally appropriate to the Canadian gambling context.

Salmon et al. [100] is not the first study to observe aversion to addiction-relevant stimuli when adapting a computerized implicit association task across cultures. Specifically, Larsen et al. [264] examined approach bias differences between Dutch and American teenagers toward smoking stimuli. The study used smoking and control stimuli that were validated among American but not Dutch teenagers. Dutch teens exhibited an avoidance bias toward smoking and control stimuli while American teens did not. While this could represent a cross-cultural difference, it is possible that this difference may have resulted from an "uncanny valley" effect – an aversion toward the stimuli, which were familiar but not quite right to the Dutch adolescents.

Given emerging work on the utility of implicit association-type tasks in the gambling research area (e.g., [123, 125]), these early results highlight the importance of using culturally appropriate stimuli in implicit cognition studies. An appropriate selection of stimuli representing common gambling activities in the local participants' context would also allow for a more refined matching of relevant stimuli to the individual gambling preferences.

10.5.2 Mindfulness

In the last decade, a new group of treatment approaches has emerged, combining CBT techniques with Buddhist principles. This group of interventions is part of a body of newly developed methods which is commonly referred to as the "third wave" of cognitive-behavioral interventions [265]. While traditional CBT focuses on controlling and modifying cognitions, third-wave approaches focus on mechanisms of awareness and acceptance of and re-distancing from cognitions [266]. Moreover, these approaches offer a new perspective on different psychopathologies, such as addiction, and add new techniques based on meditation and Buddhist philosophy [267]. Within the group of third-wave approaches, mindfulness-based interventions (MBI) take a prominent place.

Mindfulness has been defined as "the process of observing body and mind intentionally, of letting […] experiences unfold from moment to moment and accepting them as they are" [268]. It is both a trait and a process, a form of meditation [269]. MBI encompass a spectrum of interventions, including mindfulness-based relapse prevention, mindfulness-based cognitive therapy, dialectical behavior therapy, and acceptance and commitment therapy [270]. Since a review of these individual interventions is beyond the scope of this chapter, we will refer to them collectively.

MBI have been employed in the treatment of, among others, mood and anxiety disorders and seem especially effective as an adjunct to regular treatment and in patients who respond poorly to previous treatments [271]. MBI have also been used in substance and behavioral addictions, showing some promising preliminary results such as reduced substance use and increased positive psychosocial outcomes [266, 272, 273]. Inspired by these results, interest has grown in the applicability of MBI in the treatment of problem gambling. This interest is further fueled by the high relapse rates and large numbers of treatment nonresponders in the disordered gambling population [269]. In further support of the potential of MBI in problem gambling, trait mindfulness has been found to be inversely related to problem gambling, gambling severity, gambling cue reactivity and urge, and psychological distress [274–277]. Interestingly, there is some evidence that this relation might be mediated by impulsivity [274], rumination, emotion dysregulation, and thought suppression [275].

A number of case studies have provided initial, preliminary insights into the effectiveness of MBI in the treatment of gambling problems [270, 278, 279]. These studies used MBI combined with CBT in patients who did not respond to previous usual treatment. Results indicate that MBI could increase trait mindfulness, reduce craving, and decrease anxious and depressive symptomatology, decrease problem gambling severity, help gamblers reach abstinence, and improve re-distancing from obtrusive thoughts [270, 278, 279]. These results were maintained up to 3 months after treatment [278], but only when patients continued practicing mindfulness after treatment ended [270]. However, due to the nonexperimental nature of case studies, these results should be interpreted with caution.

A few initial clinical studies have explored systematically the effects of MBI in disordered gambling [280–283]. These studies have generally included a small number of inpatients not responding to previous treatments and employed different types of MBI, most commonly dialectical behavioral therapy or mindfulness-based cognitive therapy. Despite not evaluating effects on gambling severity, one study found that MBI improved trait mindfulness in the short term [283]. Another study confirmed MBI to increase trait mindfulness in problem gamblers and found that 83% of participants were abstinent or had reduced gambling after treatment [281]. However, both studies did not include a control group and had moderately high dropout rates. When employing a group-controlled experimental design, MBI was shown to reduce severity of gambling, gambling urges, and psychiatric symptoms directly after treatment and with sustained effects after 3 months [282]. This study also found that those participants who continued to practice mindfulness after treatment had better clinical outcomes. The latter results are in line with findings from an earlier study, in which MBI in problem gamblers resulted in reduced psychopathological symptoms 14 weeks after treatment, compared to treatment as usual [280]. Some of the methodological limitations of these studies, mainly due to small sample size and the lack of proper control comparisons, still prevent us from drawing any firm conclusion, and results should thus be interpreted with caution.

Altogether, MBI have shown several beneficial advantages when used as an alternative or adjunct treatment of gambling problems, especially with patients who respond poorly to usual treatment. This claim is supported by the inverse relation between trait mindfulness and gambling severity as well as preliminary findings on the effectiveness of MBI in the treatment of gambling disorder. Interestingly, the inverse relationship between trait mindfulness and, for example, impulsivity, can help explain the underlying working mechanisms of MBI within the framework of dual-process theories [274]. What sets MBI apart from standard treatment programs such as CBT is the focus on changing the individuals' relation to their cognition instead of changing the cognition itself [284]. Considering the role of rumination, obtrusive irrational beliefs, and cognitive distortions in the development and maintenance of disordered gambling [279], MBI may offer a new way of dealing with these beliefs and cognitions. Finally, MBI can effectively be administered online, meeting the need for more accessible, low-threshold, and cost-efficient treatment programs [285].

10.6 Conclusion

In this chapter, we explored a number of innovative approaches for the treatment of GD. Although the resulting assemblage is arguably quite diverse, there is a common denominator: they expand upon existing interventions by trying to fill in current voids and by extending the reach of existing treatments. They achieve this by exploring new media and techniques, providing new routes for caregivers to reach patients and vice versa, building upon new psychological and neurobiological insights, thereby increasing intervention effectiveness and suitability, and by translating scientific knowledge into practical solutions at the individual level. More importantly, they force us to reconsider the very way we understand and treat GD. In light of this, it may come as no surprise that none of the interventions discussed in this chapter should be considered alone as the answer to GD. They should rather be perceived as different but complementary modules sharing a common ambition. For clinical practice, this means that the true innovation in the treatment of GD would be an integrative approach, building upon existing knowledge, harnessing the power of new techniques and technologies, and tailoring interventions to meet individual needs.

Acknowledgements Preparation of this chapter was partly supported by grants from the National Belgian Lottery (grant: A15/0726) and the US National Center for Responsible Gaming. Additional support has been provided by the Nova Scotia Department of Health and Wellness and the Nova Scotia Health Research Foundation (grant: PSO-SSG-2015-10,036). The contents of this manuscript are solely the responsibility of the authors and do not necessarily represent the official views of any of the funding agencies.

References

1. Grant JE, Odlaug BL, Chamberlain SR. Neural and psychological underpinnings of gambling disorder: a review. Prog Neuro-Psychopharmacol Biol Psychiatry. 2016;65:188–93.
2. Hodgins DC, Stea JN, Grant JE. Gambling disorders. Lancet. 2011;378(9806):1874–84.
3. Romanczuk-Seiferth N, Van Den Brink W, Goudriaan AE. From symptoms to neurobiology: pathological gambling in the light of the new classification in DSM-5. Neuropsychobiology. 2014;70(2):95–102.
4. Thomsen KR, Fjorback LO, Møller A, Lou HC. Applying incentive sensitization models to behavioral addiction. Neurosci Biobehav Rev. 2014;45:343–9.
5. American Psychiatric Association. Diagnostic and statistical manual of mental disorders. 5th ed. Arlington, VA: American Psychiatric Publishing; 2013.
6. Stewart SH, Zack M, Collins P, Klein RM, Fragopoulos F. Sub-typing pathological gamblers on the basis of affective motivations for gambling: relations to gambling problems, drinking problems, and affective motivations for drinking. Psychol Addict Behav. 2008;22:257–68.
7. Milosevic A, Ledgerwood DM. The subtyping of pathological gambling: a comprehensive 1101 review. Clin Psychol Rev. 2010;30:988–98.
8. Cunningham JA. Little use of treatment among problem gamblers. Psychiatr Serv. 2005;56(8):1024–5.
9. Suurvali H, Hodgins DC, Toneatto T, Cunningham JA. Treatment-seeking among Ontario problem gamblers: results of a population survey. Psychiatr Serv. 2008;59:1343–6.
10. Gainsbury S, Hing N, Suhonen N. Professional help-seeking for gambling problems: awareness, barriers and motivators for treatment. J Gambl Stud. 2014;30(2):503–19.
11. Suurvali H, Cordingley J, Hodgins DC, Cunningham J. Barriers to seeking help for gambling problems: a review of the empirical literature. J Gambl Stud. 2009;25(3):407–24.
12. Cowlishaw S, Merkouris S, Dowling N, Anderson C, Jackson A, Thomas S. Psychological therapies for pathological and problem gambling. Cochrane Database Syst Rev. 2012;11:CD008937.
13. Bechara A. Decision making, impulse control and loss of willpower to resist drugs: a neurocognitive perspective. Nat Neurosci. 2005;8(11):1458–63.
14. Wiers RW, Bartholow BD, van den Wildenberg E, Thush C, Engels RCME, Sher KJ, et al. Automatic and controlled processes and the development of addictive behaviors in adolescents: a review and a model. Pharmacol Biochem Behav. 2007;86(2):263–83.
15. Keren G, Schul Y. Two is not always better than one a critical evaluation of two-system theories. Perspect Psychol Sci. 2009;4(6):533–50.
16. Cunningham WA, Zelazo PD. Attitudes and evaluations: a social cognitive neuroscience perspective. Trends Cogn Sci. 2007;11(3):97–104.
17. Gladwin TE, Figner B, Crone EA, Wiers RW. Addiction, adolescence, and the integration of control and motivation. Dev Cogn Neurosci. 2011;1(4):364–76.
18. Wiers RW, Gladwin TE, Hofmann W, Salemink E, Ridderinkhof KR. Cognitive bias modification and cognitive control training in addiction and related psychopathology: mechanisms, clinical perspectives, and ways forward. Clin Psychol Sci. 2013a;1:192–212.
19. Gladwin TE, Wiers CE, Wiers RW. Interventions aimed at automatic processes in addiction: considering necessary conditions for efficacy. Curr Opin Behav Sci. 2017;13:19–24.
20. Kopetz CE, Lejuez CW, Wiers RW, Kruglanski a W. Motivation and self-regulation in addiction: a call for convergence. Perspect Psychol Sci. 2013;8(1):3–24.
21. Lewis M. The biology of desire: why addiction is not a disease. NY: Public Affairs; 2015.
22. Miller W, Rollnick G. Motivational interviewing: helping people change. NY: Guilford; 2013.
23. Stacy AW, Wiers RW. Implicit cognition and addiction: a tool for explaining paradoxical behavior. Annu Rev Clin Psychol. 2010;6:551–75.
24. Wiers RW, Eberl C, Rinck M, Becker ES, Lindenmeyer J. Retraining automatic action tendencies changes alcoholic patients' approach bias for alcohol and improves treatment outcome. Psychol Sci. 2011;22(4):490–7.

25. Eberl C, Wiers RW, Pawelczack S, Rinck M, Becker ES, Lindenmeyer J. Approach bias modification in alcohol dependence: do clinical effects replicate and for whom does it work best? Dev Cogn Neurosci. 2013;4:38–51.
26. Franken IHA. Drug craving and addiction: integrating psychological and neuropsychopharmacological approaches. Prog Neuro-Psychopharmacol Biol Psychiatry. 2003;27(4):563–79.
27. Robinson TE, Berridge KC. The neural basis of drug craving: an incentive-sensitization theory of addiction. Brain Res Rev. 1993;18(3):247–91.
28. Robinson TE, Berridge KC. The incentive sensitization theory of addiction: some current issues. Philos Trans R Soc Lond Ser B Biol Sci. 2008;363(1507):3137–46.
29. Hudson A, Olatunji BO, Gough K, Yi S, Stewart SH. Eye on the prize: high-risk gamblers show sustained selective attention to gambling cues. J Gambl Iss. 2016:100–19.
30. Hønsi A, Mentzoni RA, Molde H, Pallesen S. Attentional bias in problem gambling: a systematic review. J Gambl Stud. 2013;29(3):359–75.
31. Bickel WK, Landes RD, Kurth-Nelson Z, Redish AD. A quantitative signature of self- control repair: rate-dependent effects of successful addiction treatment. Clin Psychol Sci. 2014;2(6):685–95.
32. Bickel WK, Yi R, Landes RD, Hill PF, Baxter C. Remember the future: working memory training decreases delay discounting among stimulant addicts. Biol Psychiatry. 2011;69(3):260–5.
33. Houben K, Wiers RW, Jansen A. Getting a grip on drinking behavior: training working memory to reduce alcohol abuse. Psychol Sci. 2011;22(7):968–75.
34. MacLeod C, Rutherford E, Campbell L, Ebsworthy G, Holker L. Selective attention and emotional vulnerability: assessing the causal basis of their association through the experimental manipulation of attentional bias. J Abnorm Psychol. 2002;111(1):107–23.
35. MacLeod C, Mathews A. Cognitive bias modification approaches to anxiety. Annu Rev Clin Psychol. 2012;8:189–217.
36. Taylor CT, Amir N. Modifying automatic approach action tendencies in individuals with elevated social anxiety symptoms. Behav Res Ther. 2012;50(9):529–36.
37. Kakoschke N, Kemps E, Tiggemann M. Approach bias modification training and consumption: a review of the literature. Addict Behav. 2016;64:21–8.
38. Posner MI, Snyder CRR, Davidson BJ. Attention and the detection of signals. J Exp Psychol Gen. 1980;109(2):160–74.
39. Mathews A, MacLeod C. Cognitive vulnerability to emotional disorders. Annu Rev Clin Psychol. 2005;1(1):167–95.
40. Cox WM, Fadardi JS, Pothos EM. The addiction-stroop test: theoretical considerations and procedural recommendations. Psychol Bull. 2006;132(3):443–76.
41. MacLeod C, Mathews A, Tata P. Attentional bias in emotional disorders. J Abnorm Psychol. 1986;95(1):15–20.
42. Field M, Cox WM. Attentional bias in addictive behaviors: a review of its development, causes, and consequences. Drug Alcohol Depend. 2008;97:1–20.
43. Munafò M, Mogg K, Roberts S, Bradley BP, Murphy M. Selective processing of smoking-related cues in current smokers, ex-smokers and never-smokers on the modified Stroop task. J Psychopharmacol. 2003;17(3):310–6.
44. Bradley BP, Field M, Mogg K, De Houwer J. Attentional and evaluative biases for smoking cues in nicotine dependence: component processes of biases in visual orienting. Behav Pharmacol. 2004;15(1):29–36.
45. Johnsen BH, Laberg JC, Cox WM, Vaksdal A, Hugdahl K. Alcoholic subjects' attentional bias in the processing of alcohol-related words. Psychol Addict Behav. 1994;8(2):111–5.
46. Cox WM, Blount JP, Rozak AM. Alcohol abusers' and nonabusers' distraction by alcohol and concern-related stimuli. Am J Drug Alcohol Abuse. 2000;26(3):489–95.
47. Field M, Eastwood B, Bradley BP, Mogg K. Selective processing of cannabis cues in regular cannabis users. Drug Alcohol Depend. 2006;85(1):75–82.
48. Franken IHA, Kroon LY, Wiers RW, Jansen A. Selective cognitive processing of drug 1203 cues in heroin dependence. J Psychopharmacol. 2000;14(4):395–400.
49. Hester R, Dixon V, Garavan H. A consistent attentional bias for drug-related material in active cocaine users across word and picture versions of the emotional Stroop task. Drug Alcohol Depend. 2006;81(3):251–7.

50. Shafran R, Lee M, Cooper Z, Palmer RL, Fairburn CG. Attentional bias in eating disorders. Int J Eat Disord. 2007;40(4):369–80.
51. Townshend JM, Duka T. Attentional bias associated with alcohol cues: differences between heavy and occasional social drinkers. Psychopharmacology. 2001;157(1):67–74.
52. Bruce G, Jones BT. A pictorial Stroop paradigm reveals an alcohol attentional bias in heavier compared to lighter social drinkers. J Psychopharmacol. 2004;18(4):527–33.
53. Field M, Mogg K, Bradley BP. Cognitive bias and drug craving in recreational cannabis users. Drug Alcohol Depend. 2004;74(1):105–11.
54. Christiansen P, Schoenmakers TM, Field M. Less than meets the eye: reappraising the clinical relevance of attentional bias in addiction. Addict Behav. 2015;44:43–50.
55. Boyer M, Dickerson M. Attentional bias and addictive behaviour: automaticity in a gambling-specific modified Stroop task. Addiction. 2003;98(1):61–70.
56. Molde H, Pallesen S, Sætrevik B, Hammerborg DK, Laberg JC, Johnsen B-H. Attentional biases among pathological gamblers. Int Gambl Stud. 2010;10(1):45–59.
57. Brevers D, Cleeremans A, Bechara A, Laloyaux C, Kornreich C, Verbanck P, Noël X. Time course of attentional bias for gambling information in problem gambling. Psychol Addict Behav. 2011;25(4):675.
58. Ciccarelli M, Nigro G, Griffiths MD, Cosenza M, D'Olimpio F. Attentional bias in non-problem gamblers, problem gamblers, and abstinent pathological gamblers: an experimental study. J Affect Disord. 2016;206:9–16.
59. Ciccarelli M, Nigro G, Griffiths MD, Cosenza M, D'Olimpio F. Attentional biases in problem and non-problem gamblers. J Affect Disord. 2016;198:135–41.
60. Vizcaino EJV, Fernandez-Navarro P, Blanco C, Ponce G, Navio M, Moratti S, Rubio G. Maintenance of attention and pathological gambling. Psychol Addict Behav. 2013;27(3):861–7.
61. Brevers D, Cleeremans A, Tibboel H, Bechara A, Kornreich C, Verbanck P, Noël X. Reduced attentional blink for gambling-related stimuli in problem gamblers. J Behav Ther Exp Psychiatry. 2011;42(3):265–9.
62. Wölfling K, Mörsen CP, Duven E, Albrecht U, Grüsser SM, Flor H. To gamble or not to gamble: at risk for craving and relapse-learned motivated attention in pathological gambling. Biol Psychol. 2011;87(2):275–81.
63. van Holst RJ, van Holstein M, van den Brink W, Veltman DJ, Goudriaan AE. Response inhibition during cue reactivity in problem gamblers: an FMRI study. PLoS One. 2012;7(3):e30909.
64. McCusker CG. Cognitive biases and addiction: an evolution in theory and method. Addiction. 2001;96(1):47–56.
65. McGrath DS, Meitner A, Sears CR. The specificity of attentional biases by type of gambling: an eye-tracking study. PLoS One. 2018;13(1):e0190614.
66. Field M, Duka T, Eastwood B, Child R, Santarcangelo M, Gayton M. Experimental manipulation of attentional biases in heavy drinkers: do the effects generalise? Psychopharmacology. 2007;192(4):593–608.
67. Field M, Eastwood B. Experimental manipulation of attentional bias increases the motivation to drink alcohol. Psychopharmacology. 2005;183(3):350–7.
68. Schoenmakers TM, Wiers RW, Jones BT, Bruce G, Jansen ATM. Attentional re- 1254 training decreases attentional bias in heavy drinkers without generalization. Addiction. 2007;102(3):399–405.
69. Schoenmakers TM, de Bruin M, Lux IFM, Goertz AG, Van Kerkhof DHAT, Wiers RW. Clinical effectiveness of attentional bias modification training in abstinent alcoholic patients. Drug Alcohol Depend. 2010;109(1):30–6.
70. Fadardi JS, Cox WM. Reversing the sequence: reducing alcohol consumption by over- coming alcohol attentional bias. Drug Alcohol Depend. 2009;101(3):137–45.
71. Cox WM, Fadardi JS, Hosier SG, Pothos EM. Differential effects and temporal course of attentional and motivational training on excessive drinking. Exp Clin Psychopharmacol. 2015;23(6):445.
72. McHugh RK, Murray HW, Hearon BA, Calkins AW, Otto MW. Attentional bias and craving in smokers: the impact of a single attentional training session. Nicotine Tob Res. 2010;12(12):1261–4.

73. Begh R, Munafò MR, Shiffman S, Ferguson SG, Nichols L, Mohammed MA, Holder RL, Sutton S, Aveyard P. Lack of attentional retraining effects in cigarette smokers attempting cessation: a proof of concept double-blind randomised controlled trial. Drug Alcohol Depend. 2015;149:158–65.

74. Attwood AS, O'Sullivan H, Leonards U, Mackintosh B, Munafò MR. Attentional bias training and cue reactivity in cigarette smokers. Addiction. 2008;103(11):1875–82.

75. Field M, Duka T, Tyler E, Schoenmakers T. Attentional bias modification in tobacco smokers. Nicotine Tob Res. 2009;11(7):812–22.

76. Kerst WF, Waters AJ. Attentional retraining administered in the field reduces smokers' attentional bias and craving. Health Psychol. 2014;33(10):1232–40.

77. Lopes FM, Pires AV, Bizarro L. Attentional bias modification in smokers trying to quit: a longitudinal study about the effects of number of sessions. J Subst Abus Treat. 2014;47(1):50–7.

78. Elfeddali I, de Vries H, Bolman C, Pronk T, Wiers RW. A randomized controlled trial of web-based attentional bias modification to help smokers quit. Health Psychol. 2016;35(8):870–80.

79. Kemps E, Tiggemann M, Hollitt S. Biased attentional processing of food cues and modification in obese individuals. Health Psychol. 2014a;33(11):1391–401.

80. Kemps E, Tiggemann M, Orr J, Grear J. Attentional retraining can reduce chocolate consumption. J Exp Psychol Appl. 2014;20(1):94–102.

81. Kemps E, Tiggemann M, Elford J. Sustained effects of attentional re-training on chocolate consumption. J Behav Ther Exp Psychiatry. 2015;49:94–100.

82. Kakoschke N, Kemps E, Tiggemann M. Attentional bias modification encourages healthy eating. Eat Behav. 2014;15(1):120–4.

83. Boffo M, Willemen R, Pronk T, Wiers RW, Dom G. Effectiveness of two web-based cognitive bias modification interventions targeting approach and attentional bias in gambling problems: study protocol for a pilot randomised controlled trial. Trials. 2017;18(1):452.

84. Field M, Caren R, Fernie G, De Houwer J. Alcohol approach tendencies in heavy drinkers: comparison of effects in a relevant stimulus–response compatibility task and an approach/avoidance Simon task. Psychol Addict Behav. 2011;25(4):697–701.

85. Wiers RW, Gladwin TE, Rinck M. Should we train alcohol-dependent patients to avoid alcohol? Front Psych. 2013;4:33.

86. Kersbergen I, Woud ML, Field M. The validity of different measures of automatic alcohol action tendencies. Psychol Addict Behav. 2015;29(1):225.

87. Krieglmeyer R, Deutsch R. Comparing measures of approach–avoidance behaviour: the manikin task vs. two versions of the joystick task. Cognit Emot. 2010;24(5):810–28.

88. Field M, Mogg K, Bradley BP. Craving and cognitive biases for alcohol cues in social drinkers. Alcohol Alcohol. 2005;40(6):504–10.

89. Wiers RW, Rinck M, Dictus M, Van Den Wildenberg E. Relatively strong automatic appetitive action-tendencies in male carriers of the OPRM1 G-allele. Genes Brain Behav. 2009;8(1):101–6.

90. Bradley BP, Field M, Healy H, Mogg K. Do the affective properties of smoking-related cues influence attentional and approach biases in cigarette smokers? J Psychopharmacol. 2008;22(7):737–45.

91. Wiers CE, Kühn S, Javadi AH, Korucuoglu O, Wiers RW, Walter H, et al. Automatic approach bias towards smoking cues is present in smokers but not in ex-smokers. Psychopharmacology. 2013c;229(1):187–97.

92. Watson P, de Wit S, Wiers RW. Motivational mechanisms underlying the approach bias to cigarettes. J Exp Psychopathol. 2013;4(3):250–62.

93. Cousijn J, Goudriaan AE, Wiers RW. Reaching out towards cannabis: approach-bias in heavy cannabis users predicts changes in cannabis use. Addiction. 2011;106(9):1667–74.

94. Wiers RW, Rinck M, Kordts R, Houben K, Strack F. Retraining automatic action-tendencies to approach alcohol in hazardous drinkers. Addiction. 2010;105(2):279–87.

95. Veenstra EM, de Jong PJ. Restrained eaters show enhanced automatic approach tendencies towards food. Appetite. 2010;55(1):30–6.

96. Havermans RC, Giesen JCAH, Houben K, Jansen A. Weight, gender, and snack appeal. Eat Behav. 2011;12(2):126–30.

97. Kemps E, Tiggemann M. Approach bias for food cues in obese individuals. Psychol Health. 2015;30(3):370–80.
98. Kakoschke N, Kemps E, Tiggemann M. Combined effects of cognitive bias for food cues and poor inhibitory control on unhealthy food intake. Appetite. 2015;87:358–64.
99. Kakoschke N, Kemps E, Tiggemann M. Differential effects of approach bias and eating style on unhealthy food consumption in overweight and normal weight women. Psychol Health. 2017;32(11):1371–85.
100. Salmon JP, Boffo M, Smits R, Salemink E, de Jong D, Cowie M, Collins P, Stewart SH, Wiers RW. Measuring implicit biases towards gambling stimuli in problem gamblers from Canada and the Netherlands: lessons learned from cross-cultural internet research. Poster presented at the annual meeting of the National Centre for Responsible Gambling, Las Vegas, NV. 2016.
101. Boffo M, Smits R, Salmon JP, Cowie M, de Jong DTHA, Salemink E, Collins P, Stewart SH, Wiers RW. Luck, come here! Automatic approach tendencies toward gambling cues in moderate-to-high gamblers. Addiction. 2018;113(2):289–98.
102. Ostafin BD, Palfai TP. Compelled to consume: the implicit association test and automatic alcohol motivation. Psychol Addict Behav. 2006;20(3):322. 1327.
103. Palfai TP, Ostafin BD. Alcohol-related motivational tendencies in hazardous drinkers: assessing implicit response tendencies using the modified-IAT. Behav Res Ther. 2003;41(10):1149–62.
104. Greenwald AG, McGhee DE, Schwartz JL. Measuring individual differences in implicit cognition: the implicit association test. J Pers Soc Psychol. 1998;74(6):1464–80.
105. Wiers RW, Boffo M, Field M. What's in a trial? On the importance of distinguishing between experimental lab studies and randomized controlled trials: the case of cognitive bias modification and alcohol use disorders. J Stud Alcohol Drugs. 2018;79(3):333–43.
106. Boffo M, Zerhouni O, Gronau QF, van Beek RJJ, Nikolaou K, Marsman M, Wiers RW. Cognitive Bias Modification for behavior change in alcohol and smoking addiction: a Bayesian meta-analysis of individual participant data. Neuropsychol Rev. In press.
107. Manning V, Staiger P, Hall K, Garfield J, Flaks G, Leung D, et al. Cognitive bias modification training during inpatient alcohol detoxification reduces early relapse: a randomized controlled trial. Alcohol Clin Exp Res. 2016;40(9):2011–9.
108. Eberl C, Wiers RW, Pawelczack S, Rinck M, Becker ES, Lindenmeyer J. Implementation of approach bias re-training in alcoholism-how many sessions are needed? Alcohol Clin Exp Res. 2014;38(2):587–94.
109. Wittekind CE, Feist A, Schneider BC, Moritz S, Fritzsche A. The approach-avoidance task as an online intervention in cigarette smoking: a pilot study. J Behav Ther Exp Psychiatry. 2015;46:115–20.
110. Machulska A, Zlomuzica A, Rinck M, Assion HJ, Margraf J. Approach bias modification in inpatient psychiatric smokers. J Psychiatr Res. 2016;76:44–51.
111. Larsen H, Kong G, Becker D, Cavallo DA, Cousijn J, Salemink E, et al. Cognitive bias modification combined with cognitive behavioral therapy: a smoking cessation intervention for adolescents. Drug Alcohol Depend. 2015;146.
112. Brockmeyer T, Hahn C, Reetz C, Schmidt U, Friederich HC. Approach bias modification in food craving – a proof-of-concept study. Eur Eat Disord Rev. 2015;23(5):352–60.
113. Dickson H, Kavanagh DJ, MacLeod C. The pulling power of chocolate: effects of approach–avoidance training on approach bias and consumption. Appetite. 2016;99:46–51.
114. Kakoschke N, Kemps E, Tiggemann M. The effect of combined avoidance and control training on implicit food evaluation and choice. J Behav Ther Exp Psychiatry. 2017;55:99–105.
115. Becker D, Jostmann NB, Wiers RW, Holland RW. Approach avoidance training in the eating domain: testing the effectiveness across three single session studies. Appetite. 2015;85:58–65.
116. Rabinovitz S, Nagar M. Possible end to an endless quest? Cognitive bias modification for excessive multiplayer online gamers. Cyberpsychol Behav Soc Netw. 2015;18(10):581–7.
117. Snippe L, Boffo M, Willemen R, Dom G, Wiers RW. The added effectiveness of online approach bias modification atop internet-based CBT with chat-based guidance for problem gamblers. Manuscript in preparation.
118. Hofmann W, De Houwer J, Perugini M, Baeyens F, Crombez G. Evaluative conditioning in humans: a meta-analysis. Psychol Bull. 2010;136(3):390–421.

119. Rooke SE, Hine DW, Thorsteinsson EB. Implicit cognition and substance use: a meta-analysis. Addict Behav. 2008;33(10):1314–28.
120. Houben K, Wiers RW. Implicitly positive about alcohol? Implicit positive associations predict drinking behavior. Addict Behav. 2008;33(8):979–86.
121. Spruyt A, Lemaigre V, Salhi B, Van Gucht D, Tibboel H, Van Bockstaele B, et al. Implicit attitudes towards smoking predict long-term relapse in abstinent smokers. Psychopharmacology. 2015;232(14):2551–61.
122. Ellis EM, Kiviniemi MT, Cook-Cottone C. Implicit affective associations predict snack choice for those with low, but not high levels of eating disorder symptomatology. Appetite. 2014;77:122–30.
123. Stewart MJ, Yi S, Stewart SH. Effects of gambling-related cues on the activation of implicit and explicit gambling outcome expectancies in regular gamblers. J Gambl Stud. 2014;30:653–68.
124. Stewart MJ, Stewart SH, Yi S, Ellery M. Predicting gambling behaviour and problems from implicit and explicit positive gambling outcome expectancies in regular gamblers. Int Gambl Stud. 2015;15(1):124–40.
125. Stiles M, Hudson A, Ramasubbu C, Ames S, Yi S, Gough K, Stewart SH. The role of memory associations in excessive and problem gambling. J Gambl Iss. 2016;34:120–39.
126. Yi S, Kanetkar V. Implicit measures of attitudes toward gambling: an exploratory study. J Gambl Iss. 2010;24(24):140–63.
127. Brevers D, Cleeremans A, Hermant C, Tibboel H, Kornreich C, Verbanck P, Noël X. Implicit gambling attitudes in problem gamblers: positive but not negative implicit associations. J Behav Ther Exp Psychiatry. 2013;44(1):94–7.
128. de Houwer J, Thomas S, Baeyens F. Association learning of likes and dislikes: a review of 25 years of research on human evaluative conditioning. Psychol Bull. 2001;127(6):853–69.
129. Raes AK, De Raedt R. The effect of counterconditioning on evaluative responses and harm expectancy in a fear conditioning paradigm. Behav Ther. 2012;43(4):757–67.
130. Houben K, Havermans RC, Wiers RW. Learning to dislike alcohol: conditioning negative implicit attitudes toward alcohol and its effect on drinking behavior. Psychopharmacology. 2010;211(1):79–86.
131. Houben K, Schoenmakers TM, Wiers RW. I didn't feel like drinking but I don't know why: the effects of evaluative conditioning on alcohol-related attitudes, craving and behavior. Addict Behav. 2010;35(12):1161–3.
132. Hollands GJ, Prestwich A, Marteau TM. Using aversive images to enhance healthy food choices and implicit attitudes: an experimental test of evaluative conditioning. Health Psychol. 2011;30(2):195–203.
133. Lebens H, Roefs A, Martijn C, Houben K, Nederkoorn C, Jansen A. Making implicit measures of associations with snack foods more negative through evaluative conditioning. Eat Behav. 2011;12(4):249–53.
134. Hensels IS, Baines S. Changing "gut feelings" about food: an evaluative conditioning effect on implicit food evaluations and food choice. Learn Motiv. 2016;55:31–44.
135. Shaw JA, Forman EM, Espel HM, Butryn ML, Herbert JD, Lowe MR, Nederkoorn C. Can evaluative conditioning decrease soft drink consumption? Appetite. 2016;105:60–70.
136. Walsh EM, Kiviniemi MT. Changing how I feel about the food: experimentally manipulated affective associations with fruits change fruit choice behaviors. J Behav Med. 2014;37(2):322–31.
137. Friese M, Hofmann W, Wiers RW. On taming horses and strengthening riders: recent developments in research on interventions to improve self-control in health behaviors. Self Identity. 2011;10(3):336–51.
138. Houben K, Havermans RC, Nederkoorn C, Jansen A. Beer a no-go: learning to stop responding to alcohol cues reduces alcohol intake via reduced affective associations rather than increased response inhibition. Addiction. 2012;107(7):1280–7.
139. Houben K, Nederkoorn C, Wiers RW, Jansen A. Resisting temptation: decreasing alcohol related affect and drinking behavior by training response inhibition. Drug Alcohol Depend. 2011;116(1–3):132–6.

140. Otto MW, Eastman A, Lo S, Hearon BA, Bickel WK, Zvolensky M, et al. Anxiety sensitivity and working memory capacity: risk factors and targets for health behavior promotion. Clin Psychol Rev. 2016;49:67–78.
141. Mendrek A, Monterosso J, Simon SL, Jarvik M, Brody A, Olmstead R, et al. Working memory in cigarette smokers: comparison to non-smokers and effects of abstinence. Addict Behav. 2006;31(5):833–44.
142. Loughead J, Wileyto EP, Ruparel K, Falcone M, Hopson R, Gur R, Lerman C. Working memory-related neural activity predicts future smoking relapse. Neuropsychopharmacology. 2015;40(6):1311–20.
143. Patterson F, Jepson C, Loughead J, Perkins K, Strasser AA, Siegel S, et al. Working memory deficits predict short-term smoking resumption following brief abstinence. Drug Alcohol Depend. 2010;106(1):61–4.
144. Wiers RW, Boelema SR, Nikolaou K, Gladwin TE. On the development of implicit and control processes in relation to substance use in adolescence. Curr Addict Rep. 2015;2:141–55.
145. Ellingson JM, Fleming KA, Vergés A, Bartholow BD, Sher KJ. Working memory as a moderator of impulsivity and alcohol involvement: testing the cognitive-motivational theory of alcohol use with prospective and working memory updating data. Addict Behav. 2014;39(11):1622–31.
146. Sharbanee JM, Stritzke WGK, Wiers RW, Young P, Rinck M, MacLeod C. The interaction of approach-alcohol action tendencies, working memory capacity, and current task goals predicts the inability to regulate drinking behavior. Psychol Addict Behav. 2013;27(3):649–61.
147. Thush C, Wiers RW, Ames SL, Grenard JL, Sussman S, Stacy AW. Interactions between implicit and explicit cognition and working memory capacity in the prediction of alcohol use in at-risk adolescents. Drug Alcohol Depend. 2008;94(1–3):116–24.
148. Khurana A, Romer D, Betancourt LM, Brodsky NL, Giannetta JM, Hurt H. Working memory ability predicts trajectories of early alcohol use in adolescents: the mediational role of impulsivity. Addiction. 2013;108(3):506–15.
149. Grenard JL, Ames SL, Wiers RW, Thush C, Sussman S, Stacy AW. Working memory capacity moderates the predictive effects of drug-related associations on substance use. Psychol Addict Behav. 2008;22(3):426–32.
150. Becker MP, Collins PF, Luciana M. Neurocognition in college-aged daily marijuana users. J Clin Exp Neuropsychol. 2014.
151. Coppin G, Nolan-Poupart S, Jones-Gotman M, Small DM. Working memory and reward association learning impairments in obesity. Neuropsychologia. 2014;65:146–55.
152. Goudriaan AE, Oosterlaan J, De Beurs E, Van Den Brink W. Neurocognitive functions in pathological gambling: a comparison with alcohol dependence, Tourette syndrome and normal controls. Addiction. 2006;101(4):534–47.
153. Albein-Urios N, Martinez-González JM, Lozano Ó, Clark L, Verdejo-García A. Comparison of impulsivity and working memory in cocaine addiction and pathological gambling: implications for cocaine-induced neurotoxicity. Drug Alcohol Depend. 2012;126:1–2):1–6.
154. Yan WS, Li YH, Xiao L, Zhu N, Bechara A, Sui N. Working memory and affective decision-making in addiction: a neurocognitive comparison between heroin addicts, pathological gamblers and healthy controls. Drug Alcohol Depend. 2014;134(1):194–200.
155. Leiserson V, Pihl RO. Reward-sensitivity, inhibition of reward-seeking, and dorsolateral prefrontal working memory function in problem gamblers not in treatment. J Gambl Stud. 2007;23(4):435–55.
156. Karbach J, Verhaeghen P. Making working memory work: a meta-analysis of executive-control and working memory training in older adults. Psychol Sci. 2014;25(11):2027–37.
157. Klingberg T, Fernell E, Olesen PJ, Johnson M, Gustafsson P, Dahlström K, et al. Computerized training of working memory in children with ADHD—a randomized, controlled trial. J Am Acad Child Adolesc Psychiatry. 2005;44(2):177–86.
158. Buitenweg JIV, Murre JMJ, Ridderinkhof KR. Brain training in progress: a review of trainability in healthy seniors. Front Hum Neurosci. 2012;6(183).
159. Jaeggi SM, Buschkuehl M, Jonides J, Shah P, Morrison AB, Chein JM. Short-and long-term benefits of cognitive training. Proc Natl Acad Sci U S A. 2011;108(25):46–60.

160. Shipstead Z, Redick TS, Engle RW. Is working memory training effective? Psychol Bull. 2012;138(4):628–54.
161. Vugs B, Knoors H, Cuperus J, Hendriks M, Verhoeven L. Executive function training in children with SLI: a pilot study. Child Lang Teach Ther. 2016.
162. Wesley MJ, Bickel WK. Remember the future II: meta-analyses and functional overlap of working memory and delay discounting. Biol Psychiatry. 2014;75(6):435–48.
163. Verbeken S, Braet C, Goossens L, van der Oord S. Executive function training with game elements for obese children: a novel treatment to enhance self-regulatory abilities for weight-control. Behav Res Ther. 2013;51(6):290–9.
164. Houben K, Dassen FC, Jansen A. Taking control: working memory training in overweight individuals increases self-regulation of food intake. Appetite. 2016;105:567–74.
165. Jones A, Christiansen P, Nederkoorn C, Houben K, Field M. Fluctuating disinhibition: implications for the understanding and treatment of alcohol and other substance use disorders. Front Psych. 2013;4(140).
166. Nower L, Blaszczynski A. Impulsivity and pathological gambling: a descriptive model. Int Gambl Stud. 2006;6(1):61–75.
167. Goudriaan AE, Oosterlaan J, De Beurs E, Van Den Brink W. Decision making in pathological gambling: a comparison between pathological gamblers, alcohol dependents, persons with Tourette syndrome, and normal controls. Cogn Brain Res. 2005;23:137–51.
168. Fuentes D, Tavares H, Artes R, Gorenstein C. Self-reported and neuropsychological measures of impulsivity in pathological gambling. J Int Neuropsychol Soc. 2006;12(6):907–12.
169. Brevers D, Cleeremans A, Verbruggen F, Bechara A, Kornreich C, Verbanck P, Noël X. Impulsive action but not impulsive choice determines problem gambling severity. PLoS One. 2012;7(11).
170. Devos G, Clark L, Maurage P, Kazimierczuk M, Billieux J. Reduced inhibitory control predicts persistence in laboratory slot machine gambling. Int Gambl Stud. 2015;15(3):408–21.
171. Grant JE, Chamberlain SR, Schreiber LRN, Odlaug BL, Kim SW. Selective decision-making deficits in at-risk gamblers. Psychiatry Res. 2011;189(1):115–20.
172. Verdejo-García A, Lawrence AJ, Clark L. Impulsivity as a vulnerability marker for substance-1529 use disorders: review of findings from high-risk research, problem gamblers and genetic 1530 association studies. Neurosci Biobehav Rev. 2008;32(4):777–810.
173. Jones A, Field M. The effects of cue-specific inhibition training on alcohol consumption in heavy social drinkers. Exp Clin Psychopharmacol. 2013;21(1):8–16.
174. Allom V, Mullan B. Two inhibitory control training interventions designed to improve eating behaviour and determine mechanisms of change. Appetite. 2015;89:282–90.
175. Veling H, van Koningsbruggen GM, Aarts H, Stroebe W. Targeting impulsive processes of eating behavior via the internet. Effects on body weight. Appetite. 2014;78:102–9.
176. Allom V, Mullan B, Hagger M. Does inhibitory control training improve health behaviour? A meta-analysis. Health Psychol Rev. 2015;7199(6):1–38.
177. de Wit H. Impulsivity as a determinant and consequence of drug use: a review of underlying processes. Addict Biol. 2009;14:22–31.
178. Jones A, Christiansen P, Nederkoorn C, Houben K, Field M. Fluctuating Disinhibition: implications for the understanding and treatment of alcohol and other substance use disorders. Front Psych. 2013;4(140).
179. Gauggel S, Heusinger A, Forkmann T, Boecker M, Lindenmeyer J, Miles Cox W, Staedtgen M. Effects of alcohol cue exposure on response inhibition in detoxified alcohol-dependent patients. Alcohol Clin Exp Res. 2010;34(9):1584–9.
180. Jones A, Guerrieri R, Fernie G, Cole J, Goudie A, Field M. The effects of priming restrained versus disinhibited behaviour on alcohol-seeking in social drinkers. Drug Alcohol Depend. 2011b;113:55–61.
181. Houben K, Nederkoorn C, Jansen A. Eating on impulse: the relation between overweight and food-specific inhibitory control. Obesity. 2014;22(5):E6–8.
182. Jones A, Field M. Alcohol-related and negatively-valenced cues increase motor and oculomotor disinhibition in social drinkers. Exp Clin Psychopharmacol. 2015;23:122–9.
183. Fillmore MT, Rush CR, Marczinski CA. Effects of d-amphetamine on behavioral control in stimulant abusers: the role of prepotent response tendencies. Drug Alcohol Depend. 2003;71(2):143–52.

184. Logan G, Cowan W. On the ability to inhibit thought and action: a theory of an act of control. Psychol Rev. 1984;91:295–327.
185. Verbruggen F, Logan GD. Automatic and controlled response inhibition: associative learning in the go/no-go and stop-signal paradigms. J Exp Psychol Gen. 2008;137(4):649–72.
186. Jones A, McGrath E, Houben K, Nederkoorn C, Robinson E, Field M. A comparison of three types of web-based inhibition training for the reduction of alcohol consumption in problem drinkers: study protocol. BMC Public Health. 2014;14(1):796.
187. Veling H, Holland RW, van Knippenberg A. When approach motivation and behavioral inhibition collide: behavior regulation through stimulus devaluation. J Exp Soc Psychol. 2008;44(4):1013–9.
188. Jones A, Di Lemma LCG, Robinson E, Christiansen P, Nolan S, Tudur-Smith C, Field M. Inhibitory control training for appetitive behaviour change: a meta-analytic investigation of mechanisms of action and moderators of effectiveness. Appetite. 2016;7:16–28.
189. Houben K, Jansen A. Chocolate equals stop: chocolate-specific inhibition training reduces chocolate intake and go associations with chocolate. Appetite. 2015;87:318–23.
190. Veling H, Aarts H, Papies EK. Using stop signals to inhibit chronic dieters' responses toward palatable foods. Behav Res Ther. 2011;49(11):771–80.
191. Houben K, Jansen A. Training inhibitory control. A recipe for resisting sweet temptations. Appetite. 2011;56(2):345–9.
192. van Koningsbruggen GM, Veling H, Stroebe W, Aarts H. Comparing two psychological interventions in reducing impulsive processes of eating behaviour: effects on self-selected portion size. Br J Health Psychol. 2014;19(4):767–82.
193. Veling H, Aarts H, Stroebe W. Using stop signals to reduce impulsive choices for palatable unhealthy foods. Br J Health Psychol. 2013;18(2):354–68.
194. Houben K. Overcoming the urge to splurge: influencing eating behavior by manipulating inhibitory control. J Behav Ther Exp Psychiatry. 2011;42(3):384–8.
195. Lawrence NS, O'Sullivan J, Parslow D, Javaid M, Adams RC, Chambers CD, et al. Training response inhibition to food is associated with weight loss and reduced energy intake. Appetite. 2015;95:17–28.
196. Ferrey AE, Frischen A, Fenske MJ. Hot or not: response inhibition reduces the hedonic value and motivational incentive of sexual stimuli. Front Psych. 2012;3:575.
197. Jansen JM, Daams JG, Koeter MW, Veltman DJ, van den Brink W, Goudriaan AE. Effects of non-invasive neurostimulation on craving: a meta-analysis. Neurosci Biobehav Rev. 2013;37(10):2472–80.
198. Lefaucheur JP, André-Obadia N, Antal A, Ayache SS, Baeken C, Benninger DH, Cantello RM, Cincotta M, de Carvalho M, De Ridder D, Devanne H, Di Lazzaro V, Filipović SR, Hummel FC, Jääskeläinen SK, Kimiskidis VK, Koch G, Langguth B, Nyffeler T, Oliviero A, Padberg F, Poulet E, Rossi S, Rossini PM, Rothwell JC, Schönfeldt-Lecuona C, Siebner HR, Slotema CW, Stagg CJ, Valls-Sole J, Ziemann U, Paulus W, Garcia-Larrea L. Evidence-based guidelines on the therapeutic use of repetitive transcranial magnetic stimulation (rTMS). Clin Neurophysiol. 2014;125(11):2150–206.
199. Tortella G, Casati R, Aparicio LV, Mantovani A, Senço N, D'Urso G, Brunelin J, Guarienti F, Selingardi PM, Muszkat D, Junior BS, Valiengo L, Moffa AH, Simis M, Borrione L, Brunoni AR. Transcranial direct current stimulation in psychiatric disorders. World J Psychiatry. 2015;5(1):88–102.
200. De Ridder D, Vanneste S, Kovacs S, Sunaert S, Dom G. Transient alcohol craving suppression by rTMS of dorsal anterior cingulate: an fMRI and LORETA EEG study. Neurosci Lett. 2011;496(1):5–10.
201. Sauvaget A, Trojak B, Bulteau S, Jiménez-Murcia S, Fernández-Aranda F, Wolz I, Menchón JM, Achab S, Vanelle JM, Grall-Bronnec M. Transcranial direct current stimulation (tDCS) in behavioral and food addiction: a systematic review of efficacy, technical, and methodological issues. Front Neurosci. 2015;9.
202. He Q, Chen M, Chen C, Xue G, Feng T, Bechara A. Anodal stimulation of the left DLPFC increases IGT scores and decreases delay discounting rate in healthy males. Front Psych. 2016;7:1421.
203. Brevet-Aeby C, Brunelin J, Iceta S, Padovan C, Poulet E. Prefrontal cortex and impulsivity: interest of noninvasive brain stimulation. Neurosci Biobehav Rev. 2016;71:112–34.. He Q, Chen

M, Chen C, Xue G, Feng T, Bechara A. Anodal stimulation of the left DLPFC increases IGT scores and decreases delay discounting rate in healthy males. Front Psychol. 2016;7:1421

204. Goudriaan AE, Oosterlaan J, de Beurs E, Van den Brink W. Pathological gambling: a comprehensive review of biobehavioral findings. Neurosci Biobehav Rev. 2004;28(2):123–41.

205. van Holst RJ, van den Brink W, Veltman DJ, Goudriaan AE. Why gamblers fail to win: a review of cognitive and neuroimaging findings in pathological gambling. Neurosci Biobehav Rev. 2010;34(1):87–107.

206. Hone-Blanchet A, Ciraulo DA, Pascual-Leone A, Fecteau S. Noninvasive brain stimulation to suppress craving in substance use disorders: review of human evidence and methodological considerations for future work. Neurosci Biobehav Rev. 2015;59:184–200.

207. Zack M, Cho SS, Parlee J, Jacobs M, Li C, Boileau I, Strafella A. Effects of high frequency repeated transcranial magnetic stimulation and continuous theta burst stimulation on gambling reinforcement, delay discounting, and stroop interference in men with pathological gambling. Brain Stimul. 2016;9(6):867–75.

208. Rosenberg O, Klein LD, Dannon PN. Deep transcranial magnetic stimulation for the treatment of pathological gambling. Psychiatry Res. 2013;206(1):111–3.

209. Chervyakov AV, Chernyavsky AY, Sinitsyn DO, Piradov MA. Possible mechanisms underlying the therapeutic effects of transcranial magnetic stimulation. Front Hum Neurosci. 2015;9:303.

210. den Uyl TE, Gladwin TE, Rinck M, Lindenmeyer J, Wiers RW. A clinical trial with combined transcranial direct current stimulation and alcohol approach bias retraining. Addict Biol. 2017;22(6):1632–40.

211. den Uyl TE, Gladwin TE, Wiers RW. Electrophysiological and behavioral effects of combined transcranial direct current stimulation and alcohol approach bias retraining in hazardous drinkers. Alcohol Clin Exp Res. 2016;40(10):2124–33.

212. European Gaming and Betting Association. Market reality. 2017.

213. Gainsbury SM. Online gambling addiction: the relationship between internet gambling and disordered gambling. Curr Addict Rep. 2015;2(2):185.

214. Statista. Size of the online gaming market from 2003 to 2020 (in billion U.S. dollars). 2017.

215. Yardley L, Patrick K, Choudhury T, Michie S. Current issues and future directions for research into digital behavior change interventions. Am J Prev Med. 2016;51(5):814–5.

216. Versluis A, Verkuil B, Spinhoven P, van der Ploeg MM, Brosschot JF. Changing mental health and positive psychological Well-being using ecological momentary interventions: a systematic review and meta-analysis. J Med Internet Res. 2016;18(6):e152.

217. Khadjesari Z, Murray E, Hewitt C, Hartley S, Godfrey C. Can stand-alone computerbased interventions reduce alcohol consumption? A systematic review. Addiction. 2011;106(2):267–82.

218. Kraft P, Yardley L. Current issues and new directions in psychology and health: what is the future of digital interventions for health behaviour change? Psychol Health. 2009;24(6):615–218.

219. Murray E. Web-based interventions for behavior change and self-management: potential, pitfalls, and progress. Med 20. 2012;1(2):e3.

220. Cunningham JA, Hodgins DC, Toneatto T, Murphy M. A randomized controlled trial of a personalized feedback intervention for problem gamblers. PLoS One. 2012;7(2):e31586.

221. Andersson G, Cuijpers P, Carlbring P, Riper H, Hedman E. Guided internet-based vs. face-to-face cognitive behavior therapy for psychiatric and somatic disorders: a systematic review and meta-analysis. World Psychiatry. 2014;13(3):288–95.

222. Portnoy DB, Scott-Sheldon LA, Johnson BT, Carey MP. Computer-delivered interventions for health promotion and behavioral risk reduction: a meta-analysis of 75 randomized controlled trials, 1988–2007. Prev Med. 2008;47(1):3–16.

223. Shingleton RM, Palfai TP. Technology-delivered adaptations of motivational interviewing for health-related behaviors: a systematic review of the current research. Patient Educ Couns. 2016;99(1):17–35.

224. Webb T, Joseph J, Yardley L, Michie S. Using the internet to promote health behavior change: 1666 a systematic review and meta-analysis of the impact of theoretical basis, use of behavior change techniques, and mode of delivery on efficacy. J Med Internet Res. 2010;12(1):e4.

225. Fiordelli M, Diviani N, Schulz PJ. Mapping mHealth research: a decade of evolution. J Med Internet Res. 2013;15(5):e95.

226. Free C, Phillips G, Galli L, Watson L, Felix L, Edwards P, Patel V, Haines A. The effectiveness of mobile-health technology-based health behaviour change or disease management interventions for health care consumers: a systematic review. PLoS Med. 2013;10(1):e1001362.

227. Zhao J, Freeman B, Li M. Can mobile phone apps influence people's health behavior change? An evidence review. J Med Internet Res. 2016;18(11):e287.

228. DeSmet A, Van Ryckeghem D, Compernolle S, Baranowski T, Thompson D, Crombez G, et al. A meta-analysis of serious digital games for healthy lifestyle promotion. Prev Med. 2014;69:95–107.

229. Johnson D, Deterding S, Kuhn K-A, Staneva A, Stoyanov S, Hides L. Gamification for health and wellbeing: a systematic review of the literature. Internet Interv. 2016;6:89–106.

230. Primack BA, Carroll MV, McNamara M, Klem ML, King B, Rich M, et al. Role of video games in improving health-related outcomes: a systematic review. Am J Prev Med. 2012;42(6):630–8.

231. Turner WA, Casey LM. Outcomes associated with virtual reality in psychological interventions: where are we now? Clin Psychol Rev. 2014;34(8):634–44.

232. Valmaggia LR, Latif L, Kempton MJ, Rus-Calafell M. Virtual reality in the psychological treatment for mental health problems: an systematic review of recent evidence. Psychiatry Res. 2016;236:189–95.

233. Hodgins DC. Becoming a winner: defeating problem gambling: a self-help manual for problem gamblers. Calgary, AB, Canada: Calgary Regional Health Authority; 2002.

234. Ladouceur R, Lachance S. Overcoming pathological gambling. Oxford: Oxford University Press; 2006.

235. Carlbring P, Smit F. Randomized trial of internet-delivered self-help with telephone support for pathological gamblers. J Consult Clin Psychol. 2008;76(6):1090–4.

236. Carlbring P, Degerman N, Jonsson J, Andersson G. Internet-based treatment of pathological gambling with a three-year follow-up. Cogn Behav Ther. 2012;41(4):321–34.

237. Castren S, Pankakoski M, Tamminen M, Lipsanen J, Ladouceur R, Lahti T. Internet-based CBT intervention for gamblers in Finland: experiences from the field. Scand J Psychol. 2013;54(3):230–5.

238. Cunningham JA, Hodgins DC, Toneatto T, Rai A, Cordingley J. Pilot study of a personalized feedback intervention for problem gamblers. Behav Ther. 2009;40:219–24.

239. Luquiens A, Lagadec M, Tanguy M, Reynaud M. Efficacy of online psychotherapies in poker gambling disorder: an online randomized clinical trial. Eur Psychiatry. 2015;30:1053.

240. Canale N, Vieno A, Griffiths MD, Marino C, Chieco F, Disperati F, Andriolo S, Santinello M. The efficacy of a web-based gambling intervention program for high school students: a preliminary randomized study. Comput Hum Behav. 2016;55:946–54.

241. Cunningham JA, Hodgins DC, Bennett K, Bennett A, Talevski M, Mackenzie CS, Hendershot CS. Online interventions for problem gamblers with and without co-occurring mental health symptoms: protocol for a randomized controlled trial. BMC Public Health. 2016;16(1):624.

242. Hodgins DC, Fick GH, Murray R, Cunningham JA. Internet-based interventions for disordered gamblers: study protocol for a randomized controlled trial of online self-directed cognitive-behavioural motivational therapy. BMC Public Health. 2013;13(1):1.

243. Swan JL. The evaluation of an Internet-based self-directed motivational enhancement intervention for problem and pathological gamblers. Doctoral dissertation, University of Calgary. 2014.

244. Hodgins DC, Currie SR, Currie G, Fick GH. Randomized trial of brief motivational treatments for pathological gamblers: more is not necessarily better. J Consult Clin Psychol. 2009;77(5):950–60.

245. MacLeod C, Clarke PJ. The attentional bias modification approach to anxiety intervention. Clin Psychol Sci. 2015;3(1):58–78.

246. Wiers RW, Houben K, Fadardi JS, van Beek P, Rhemtulla MT, Cox WM. Alcohol cognitive bias modification training for problem drinkers over the web. Addict Behav. 2015b;40:21–6.

247. Bullen C, Rossen F, Newcombe D, Whittaker R, Strydom J. Smartphone-based Problem Gambling Evaluation and Technology Testing Initiative ('SPGETTI') feasibility study: final report. National Institute for Health Innovation & Centre for Addiction Research. Prepared for the Ministry of Health. Auckland, New Zealand: Auckland UniServices Limited, The University of Auckland. 2015.

248. Loranger C, Bouchard S, Boulanger J, Robillard G. Validation of two virtual environments for the prevention and treatment of pathological gambling. J Cyber Ther Rehabil. 2011;4:233–5.

249. Giroux I, Faucher-Gravel A, St-Hilaire A, Boudreault C, Jacques C, Bouchard S. Gambling exposure in virtual reality and modification of urge to gamble. Cyberpsychol Behav Soc Netw. 2013;16(3):224–31.
250. Park CB, Park SM, Gwak AR, Sohn BK, Lee JY, Jung HY, Choi SW, Choi JS. The effect of repeated exposure to virtual gambling cues on the urge to gamble. Addict Behav. 2015;41:61–4.
251. Tárrega S, Castro-Carreras L, Fernández-Aranda F, Granero R, Giner-Bartolomé C, Aymamí N, et al. A serious videogame as an additional therapy tool for training emotional regulation and impulsivity control in severe gambling disorder. Front Psych. 2015;6:1721.
252. van der Stel J. Precision in addiction care: does it make a difference? Yale J Biol Med. 2015;88(4):415–22.
253. Suomi A, Dowling NA, Jackson AC. Problem gambling subtypes based on psychological distress, alcohol abuse and impulsivity. Addict Behav. 2014;39:1741–5.
254. Conrod PJ, Stewart SH, Pihl RO, Côté S, Fontaine V, Dongier M. Efficacy of brief coping skills interventions that match different personality profiles of female substance abusers. Psychol Addict Behav. 2000;14:231–42.
255. Conrod PJ, Stewart SH, Comeau MN, Maclean M. Efficacy of cognitive behavioral interventions targeting personality risk factors for youth alcohol misuse. J Clin Child Adolesc Psychol. 2006;35:550–63.
256. Blaszczynski A, Nower L. A pathways model of problem and pathological gambling. Addiction. 2002;97:487–99.
257. Juodis M, Stewart S. A method for classifying pathological gamblers according to "enhancement," "coping," and "low emotion regulation" subtypes. J Gambl Iss. 2016;34:201–20.
258. Stewart SH, Buckley M, Darredeau C, Sabourin B, Zahradnik M, Hodgins D, Barrett SP. Brief escape and action treatment for gambling (BEAT gambling): action and escape therapist manuals. Halifax, Canada: Dalhousie University, Department of Psychology and Neuroscience; 2011.
259. Gooding P, Tarrier N. A systematic review and meta-analysis of cognitive behavioral interventions to reduce problem gambling: hedging our bets? Behav Res Ther. 2009;47:592–607.
260. Stewart MJ, Davis MacNevin PL, Hodgins DC, Barrett SP, Swansburg J, Stewart SH. Motivation-matched approach to the treatment of problem gambling: a case series pilot study. J Gambl Iss. 2016;33:124–47.
261. Stewart SH, Zack M. Development and psychometric evaluation of a three-dimensional gambling motives questionnaire. Addiction. 2008;103(7):1110–7.
262. Stewart SH. Short-term outcome of a motive-matched treatment for coping and enhancement gamblers: a randomized controlled trial. Invited presentation at the annual meeting of the Alberta Gambling Research Institute, Banff, Alberta, Mar 2013.
263. Ferrey AE, Burleigh TJ, Fenske MJ. Stimulus-category competition, inhibition, and affective devaluation: a novel account of the uncanny valley. Front Psych. 2015;6:249.
264. Larsen H, Kong G, Becker D, Cousijn J, Boendermaker W, Cavallo D, Khrishnan-Sarin S, Wiers RW. Implicit motivational processes underlying smoking in American and Dutch adolescents. Front Psych. 2014;5(51).
265. Hayes SC. Acceptance and commitment therapy and the new behavior therapies: mindfulness, acceptance, and relationship. In: Hayes SC, Follette VM, Linehan MM, editors. Mindfulness and acceptance: expanding the cognitive-behavioral tradition. New York: Guilford Press; 2004. p. 1–29.
266. Shonin E, Van Gordon W, Griffiths MD. Mindfulness as a treatment for behavioral addiction. J Addict Res Ther. 2014;5:e122.
267. Marlatt GA. Buddhist philosophy and the treatment of addictive behavior. Cogn Behav Pract. 2002;9(1):44–50.
268. Kabat-Zinn J. Coming to our senses: healing ourselves and the world through mindfulness. UK: Hachette; 2005.
269. Griffiths M, Shonin ÁE, Van Gordon ÁW. Mindfulness as a treatment for gambling disorder: current directions and issues. J Gambl Commer Gam Res. 2016;1(1):47–52.
270. de Lisle SM, Dowling NA, Sabura Allen J. Mindfulness-based cognitive therapy for problem gambling. Clin Case Stud. 2011;10(3):210–28.

271. Chiesa A, Serretti A. Mindfulness based cognitive therapy for psychiatric disorders: a systematic review and meta-analysis. Psychiatry Res. 2011;187(3):441–53.
272. Bowen S, Witkiewitz K, Dillworth TM, Chawla N, Simpson TL, Ostafin BD, et al. Mindfulness meditation and substance use in an incarcerated population. Psychol Addict Behav. 2006;20(3):343–7.
273. Toneatto T. Mindfulness. In: Miller PM, editor. Encyclopedia of addiction. London: Elsevier; 2013.
274. Lakey CE, Campbell WK, Brown KW, Goodie AS. Dispositional mindfulness as a predictor of the severity of gambling outcomes. Personal Individ Differ. 2007;43(7):1698–710.
275. de Lisle SM, Dowling NA, Allen JS. Mechanisms of action in the relationship between mindfulness and problem gambling behaviour. Int J Ment Heal Addict. 2014;12(2):206–25.
276. Riley B. Experiential avoidance mediates the association between thought suppression and mindfulness with problem gambling. J Gambl Stud. 2014;30(1):163–71.
277. McKeith CFA, Rock AJ, Clark GI. Trait mindfulness, problem-gambling severity, altered state of awareness and urge to gamble in poker-machine gamblers. J Gambl Stud. 2016:1–16.
278. Shonin E, van Gordon W, Griffiths MD. Cognitive behavioral therapy (CBT) and meditation awareness training (MAT) for the treatment of co-occurring schizophrenia and pathological gambling: a case study. Int J Ment Heal Addict. 2014;12(2):181–96.
279. Toneatto T, Vettese L, Nguyen L. The role of mindfulness in the cognitive-behavioural treatment of problem gambling. J Gambl Iss. 2007;19(19):91–100.
280. Korman L, Collins J, McMain S, Skinner W, Toneatto T. Concurrent gambling, substance use and anger: Development of a brief integrated treatment. Final Report. Ontario Problem Gambling Research Centre. 2005.
281. Christensen DR, Dowling NA, Jackson AC, Brown M, Russo J, Francis KL, Umemoto A. A proof of concept for using brief dialectical behavior therapy as a treatment for problem gambling. Behav Chang. 2013;30(2):117–37.
282. Toneatto T, Pillai S, Courtice EL. Mindfulness-enhanced cognitive behavior therapy for problem gambling: a controlled pilot study. Int J Ment Heal Addict. 2014;12(2):197–205.
283. Chen P, Jindani F, Perry J, Turner NL. Mindfulness and problem gambling treatment. Asian J Gambl Issues Public Health. 2014;4(1):2.
284. de Lisle SM, Dowling NA, Allen JS. Mindfulness and problem gambling: a review of the literature. J Gambl Stud. 2012;28(4):719–39.
285. Spijkerman MPJ, Pots WTM, Bohlmeijer ET. Effectiveness of online mindfulness-based interventions in improving mental health: a review and meta-analysis of randomised controlled trials. Clin Psychol Rev. 2016;45:102–14.

Similarities and Differences between Gambling Disorder and other Addiction-like Behaviors

Mira Fauth-Bühler

11.1 Introduction

Common behaviors such as shopping, food intake, sexual activities, gambling and Internet use may become maladaptive due to the high frequency or intensity at which they are performed. These activities have in common that they are viewed as pleasurable by most individuals. However, when these behaviors are conducted in excess and the ability to control the behavior is limited, these otherwise "normal" behaviors can cause deleterious consequences on the psychological, social and even somatic level.

A central characteristic of behavioral addictions is the failure to resist an impulse, drive or temptation to perform an act that is harmful to the person or to others [1]. Behavioral addictions are characterized by a recurrent pattern of behavior within a specific domain. The repetitive engagement in these behaviors ultimately interferes with functioning in other domains [2]. Unlike substance-related addictions, no chemical or substance intake is involved in behavioral addictions, although the behaviors conducted in excess may lead to withdrawal symptoms such as irritability and increased anxiety levels, resembling those of substance-related addictions (e.g., [3]).

The classification of gambling disorder as the first non-substance-related behavioral addiction in the Diagnostic and Statistical Manual of Mental Disorders, Fifth Edition (DSM-5 [1]), in the International Classification of Diseases (ICD-10 [4]) referred to by the term pathological gambling, has initiated a discussion on whether other behaviors conducted excessively can also be considered as "behavioral addictions." Phenomenological considerations reveal that substance-related and

M. Fauth-Bühler (✉)
Iwp Institute for Economic Psychology, Study Centre Stuttgart, FOM University of Applied Sciences for Economics and Management, Essen, Germany

Department of Addictive Behaviour and Addiction Medicine, Central Institute of Mental Health, Medical Faculty Mannheim, University of Heidelberg, Heidelberg, Germany
e-mail: mira.fauth-buehler@zi-mannheim.de

© Springer Nature Switzerland AG 2019
A. Heinz et al. (eds.), *Gambling Disorder*, https://doi.org/10.1007/978-3-030-03060-5_11

non-substance-related addictions are strikingly similar. Both are characterized by feelings of "tension or arousal before committing the act" and "pleasure, gratification or relief at the time of committing the act" [5]. The ego-syntonic nature of these behaviors may weaken over time, as the behavior (including substance taking) itself becomes less pleasurable and more of a habit or compulsion and is more motivated by negative reinforcement (e.g., relief of dysphoria or withdrawal) rather than by positive reinforcement (positive feelings, rewarding effects) [6].

For an informed decision, similarities and differences in several domains such as diagnostics, comorbidity, cognitive dysfunction and more importantly neurobiological processes need to be compared between gambling disorder and other potential behavioral addictions candidates. For more detailed information on the neurobiology of gambling disorder and substance use disorders, please refer to our relevant reviews (e.g., [7, 8]). In the following, we focus on excessive behaviors for which at least some scientific evidence exist for the relevant categories listed above. These are Internet gaming disorder, compulsive buying disorder and compulsive sexual disorder.

11.2 Similarities and Differences with Internet Gaming Disorder

A 22-year-old first-generation South Korean male with past psychiatric history of major depression with anxious features presented to the mental health clinic because his compulsive video game use had progressively interfered with his interpersonal relationships and motivation to work. He began playing video games at age 6 in the context of physically and verbally abusive parenting.

Within a week of going to college, he became engrossed with the Internet gaming culture and played online video games 10 h daily while maintaining minimal grades in order to pass his classes. He spent the subsequent 2½ years withdrawing from classes he could not complete as a result of his gaming habit. During his second year of college, he moved into an apartment with other gaming colleagues and was playing 14 h daily of online video games, such as first-person shooters and role-playing games (source: http://www.ncbi.nlm.nih.gov/pmc/articles/PMC4553653/).

11.2.1 Diagnostic Criteria and Clinical Characteristics

Users can show addiction-like behaviors when it comes to different forms or contents of the Internet such as gaming, use of social media, use of pornographic sites, gambling, etc. Internet gaming disorder is currently the best-studied domain and therefore the focus of this section. Internet gaming disorder is not yet a formal disorder in common diagnostic systems (*Diagnostic and Statistical Manual of Mental*

Disorders (DSM-5 [1]); International Classification of Diseases (ICD-10 [4])) due to limited available data. However, Internet gaming disorder is categorized as "condition for further study" in sect. III of the DSM-5 [1] highlighting the need for more scientific evidence before a decision regarding its classification can be made. In the latest revision of the ICD (ICD-11), gaming disorder has been added to the section on addictive disorders, initiating a discussion on the pros and cons of this potentially premature classification.

Diagnostic criteria for Internet gaming disorder share similarities with those outlined for gambling disorder, the first officially recognized behavioral addiction. These criteria include preoccupation or obsession with Internet games, withdrawal symptoms, tolerance, unsuccessful attempts to stop or control playing Internet games, loss of interest in other life activities, continued use despite negative consequences, lying about the extent of the problem and playing Internet games as a way to relieve anxiety or guilt.

Sociodemographic characteristics of addicted Internet users are male gender, younger age and higher family income [9].

Sociodemographic characteristics of Internet gaming disorder resemble those reported for individuals with disordered gambling. The majority of subjects with gambling disorder are male, and the disease onset is at a younger age [10].

11.2.2 Comorbidities and Family History

It is worth noting that comorbidities appear to be the norm, rather than the exception for individuals with excessive Internet use. Comorbid psychiatric disorders most frequently reported are depression, anxiety, attention deficit hyperactivity disorder and other substance use disorders [11]. Comorbid substance use disorders have also been found by other studies (e.g., [12, 13]). Black et al. [12] found that 38% of problematic computer users in their sample had a substance use disorder in addition to their behavioral problems/addiction. In a patient sample of 1826 individuals who were treated for substance addictions (mainly cannabis addiction), 4.1% were found to suffer from Internet addiction [13].

Thus, research findings indicate that individuals who suffer from Internet addiction have a higher likelihood to experience other addictions at the same time. This is in accordance with data from subjects with gambling disorder. Gambling disorder also shares commonalities with substance use disorders when looking into the prevalence of comorbid psychiatric conditions. Data from two large epidemiological surveys in the United States, the National Epidemiologic Survey on Alcohol and Related Conditions (NESARC [10]) and the National Comorbidity Survey Replication (NCS-R [14]), found the highest prevalence rates for substance use disorders, in particular nicotine dependence followed by alcohol use disorders. The second highest prevalence rates were observed for mood disorders. Own data in a large group of pathological gamblers in treatment support these findings: 88% of the gamblers had a comorbid diagnosis of substance dependence. We found the highest Axis I comorbidity rates for nicotine dependence (80%), followed by alcohol dependence (28%). First-degree family members of pathological gamblers were also more likely to suffer from substance dependence, in particular alcohol dependence, pathological gambling and suicide attempts [15].

11.2.3 Brain Functions

In order to come up with an informed decision, phenomenological similarity is appealing but not sufficient to classify two psychiatry conditions as addictive disorders. Similar underlying neurobiological mechanisms need to be present that indicate a neurobiological resemblance between diseases.

Therefore, the following section focuses in particular on relevant domains of addiction research, including impulsivity, and reward processing. We compare these findings to similar findings from research on gambling disorder and pathological gambling respectively. A more detailed overview of the research available on neurobiological correlates of Internet gaming disorder and similarities to pathological gambling can be found in a recent review [16].

11.2.3.1   Impulsivity

An early definition considers impulsivity as a behavior that is disinhibited to the degree that it is poorly conceived, premature, unduly risky and inappropriate to the context and likely has adverse consequences [17]. Different forms of impulsivity can be distinguished: While impulsive actions refer to the inability to inhibit inappropriate motor behavior, impulsive choice behavior is characterized by suboptimal decision-making, such as choosing immediate but less favourable rewards instead of more-favourable reward options in the long term. Alteration in fronto-striatal networks has been associated with impulsive behaviors [18].

Regarding impulsive actions, studies that assessed behavioral measures of response-inhibition abilities did not find any differences between Internet gaming disorder patients and controls (e.g., [19, 20]). These results are in line with findings for problem gamblers [21]. Neuroimaging studies suggest that altered functioning of a certain brain region, namely, the prefrontal cortex, may play a central role during response inhibition in both Internet gaming disorder patients and problem/pathological gamblers [19, 20, 21]. This brain region has previously been involved in behavioral-control-related actions, including motor-response inhibition [16].

Impairments to risk-evaluation capacity and elevated impulsive choice behavior have both been observed in both patient groups (see [16] for a summary). Both Internet gaming disorder patients and subjects with gambling disorder have been found to exhibit impairments in decision-making especially in situations when the evaluation of risk is involved. Further research is needed to investigate the reasons underlying the observed differences in brain-activity patterns between subjects with gambling disorder and Internet gaming disorder patients during decision-making in risky situations.

11.2.3.2   Reward

Reward sensitivity can be defined as increased physiological, emotional and cognitive reactivity to the prospect of obtaining tangible incentive objects as well as increased behavioral responsiveness to tangible incentive objects. Punishment sensitivity refers to the opposite: how strongly the individual reacts to aversive stimuli.

The brain structures grouped together under the term "mesocorticolimbic reward system" have been implicated in motivated behavior, processing of reward and punishment as well as reinforcement learning [22]. The striatum is considered a central node in a distributed network of highly interconnected subcortical and cortical brain structures, such as prefrontal cortex, amygdala, hippocampus and the ventral tegmental area of the midbrain [23].

Increased activity in the reward system of the brain can be observed in patients suffering from Internet gaming disorder when confronted with gaming-related stimuli. This finding suggests that increased incentive salience of gaming cues might underlie Internet gaming disorder patients' excessive gaming and urges to engage in online games. Comparable results have been reported for subjects with gambling disorder: the salience of stimuli associated with gambling is increased, and the functioning of the reward system is altered in gamblers compared to brain activation of healthy controls without gambling problems.

In addition, Internet gaming disorder is characterized by enhanced reward sensitivity and decreased loss sensitivity. Reward and punishment sensitivity have been demonstrated to be altered for monetary reward. It remains unclear whether this finding holds for other types of reward, such as primary rewards (e.g., food-related stimuli, sexual cues, etc.). Additionally, monetary reward processing has been shown to be altered in gambling disorder. Two neuroimaging studies found deactivation in the ventral striatum and ventral putamen during loss events in gamblers compared to controls, suggesting decreased loss sensitivity to also be a hallmark of gambling disorder. Due to heterogeneous findings, more research is needed to better understand reward sensitivity in both gamblers and gamers.

11.3 Similarities and Differences with Compulsive Buying Disorder

Ms. A says shopping is her primary social activity and entertainment. Though she works full time, she shops three or more times a week, cruising expensive department stores and discount outlets on evenings and weekends. She buys clothing, shoes, makeup, jewellery, antiques, household electronics and other items. She says her shopping is spontaneous and impulsive. Shopping gives her an emotional "rush" that is frequently followed by periods of guilt, and she often returns or gives away purchased items. She is disappointed at her inability to control her shopping behavior and ashamed of the financial crises she has caused (source: http://www.currentpsychiatry.com/home/article/ compulsive-shopping-when-spending-begins-to-consume-the-consumer/674 ab9a0d6ce256ffdb3f1ec6087d188.html).

11.3.1 Diagnostic Criteria and Clinical Characteristics

Key features of compulsive buying are repetitive, irresistible and overpowering urges to purchase goods. In general, the goods are inexpensive and useless [24]. For a diagnosis severe distress or interference in social, financial and occupational domains need to be present. Similarities between compulsive buying and gambling disorder exist in several diagnostic criteria. For example, an overpowering urge to buy, the repetitive loss of control over spending and the negative emotional state that emerges when not buying correspond to craving, drug-seeking behavior, loss of drug-taking behavior and withdrawal symptoms in gambling disorder. Accordingly, feeling "high" have been reported from both patients with compulsive buying while performing the buying act and subjects with gambling disorder while betting. As in gambling disorder positive reinforcement plays a role at the beginning of compulsive buying, while negative reinforcement is involved in the long-term maintenance of the behavior [25].

While most subjects with gambling disorder in treatment are male, the majority of compulsive buyers in treatment studies are female (~80%; [26]). Although some epidemiological data suggest somewhat lower numbers, subjects with gambling disorder and compulsive buyers differ in gender; namely, that subjects with gambling disorder are to their majority male.

11.3.2 Comorbidities and Family History

Patients suffering from compulsive buying often reveal other psychiatric comorbidities similar to gambling disorder [27]. Psychiatric comorbidities that are most frequently observed are anxiety disorders, substance use disorders, eating disorders and disorders of impulse control. Also commonly observed are Axis II disorders. This points to another similarity with gambling disorder [10, 14].

First-degree relatives of compulsive buyers were more likely to suffer from depression, alcoholism and drug use disorders than comparison relatives [26, 28]. A similar finding has been reported for pathological gambling [29]: Dannon and colleagues reported higher prevalence of alcohol, substance abuse, problematic gambling, depression and anxiety disorders in the pathological gamblers and their first-degree relatives than in the control group.

A direct relationship between compulsive buying and gambling disorder has been provided by the Iowa pathological gambling family study [30]. Results indicate that compulsive buying disorder were more frequent in the pathological gamblers and their first-degree relatives versus controls and their relatives.

11.3.3 Brain Function

Only a few studies exist so far that have focused on the neurobiological underpinnings of compulsive buying such as impulsivity as well as reward and punishment processing. In the following section, we will summarize research findings available on that topic.

11.3.3.1 Impulsivity
Neurocognitive assessment revealed deficits in response inhibition and risk adjustment in nontreatment-seeking compulsive buyers versus controls [31]. More research on different facets of impulsivity is needed for a clearer picture in compulsive buyers.

11.3.3.2 Reward and Punishment Sensitivity

The neural correlates of compulsive buying were studied using neuroimaging [32], and preliminary findings in a small group of compulsive buyers versus healthy controls revealed increased activity in the ventral striatum in compulsive buyers during the presentation of purchasable products. Decreased activation of the insula was found in the compulsive compared to normal buyers during the presentation of product and price. These results suggest that altered reward processing of the meso-limbic reward system may underlie compulsive buying. Future neuroimaging studies in larger samples are needed for a better insight in altered reward processes in compulsive buyers.

First results indicate that compulsive buyers show impairments in several cognitive domains similar to those found in subjects with gambling disorder supporting a likely neurobiological overlap between compulsive buying and gambling disorder. However, future neuroimaging studies in larger samples are needed for an informed decision.

11.4 Similarities and Differences with Compulsive Sexual Behavior

A 50-year-old married business executive neglected sales calls when out of town and visited massage parlors and prostitutes, despite knowledge that he was risking HIV infection. He was once an effective salesman, but his work performance suffered because of his sexual pursuits. He took alternative routes on trips in an effort to avoid massage parlors, but he was unable to control his urge to visit these establishments. His wife learned about his sexual activities when he was arrested for soliciting sex from an undercover policewoman posing as a prostitute. At that point, his marriage was in jeopardy, his children and friends shocked and his job future uncertain (source: http://www.jenniferschneider.com/articles/recognize.html).

11.4.1 Diagnostic Criteria and Clinical Characteristics

Compulsive sexual behavior is a relatively common disorder that has significant personal and public health ramifications. Compulsive sexual behavior can be found under various synonyms in the literature such as hypersexuality, sex addiction or excessive sexuality. The key characteristics are repetitive and intense preoccupations with sexual fantasies, urges and behaviors that are distressing to the individual and/or result in psychosocial impairment [33].

Two categories within compulsive sexual behaviors can be distinguished: paraphilic and nonparaphilic compulsive sexual behaviors [34]. Paraphilic behaviors refers to socially unacceptable sexual behavior involving nonhuman objects and suffering of one's self or a partner, children or a non-consenting person (e.g., fetishism, exhibitionism and paedophilia) [1]. Nonparaphilic behaviors relates to more socially accepted sexual behaviors that are conducted in excess. Behaviors subsumed under this category include compulsive sexual acts with multiple partners, constant fixation on a partner that may be considered unobtainable, compulsive masturbation, compulsive use of pornography and compulsive sex and sexual acts within a consensual relationship [35].

In the revision process of the DSM-5, diagnostic criteria have been proposed for nonparaphilic compulsive sexual behaviors. These criteria leaned on the existing criteria used for addictive disorders [36]. However, nonparaphilic compulsive sexual behaviors have been excluded from the DSM-5, and the issue of how to conceptualize compulsive sexual behaviors is still a matter of debate (e.g., [37]). In addition to the proposed diagnostic criteria, another similarity exists with respect to gambling disorder which is the gender distribution: The majority of patients with compulsive sexual behaviors seeking help are male as are subjects with gambling disorder [38].

11.4.2 Comorbidities and Family History

Comparing comorbidities reported in patients suffering from gambling disorder with those diagnosed with compulsive sexual behavior a significant overlap exist (see, e.g., review by [39]). High rates of affective disorders, in particular major depression (lifetime: 58%), anxiety disorders (lifetime: 96%) as well as substance use disorders have been found (lifetime: 71%) [40]. In addition, other behavioral addictions are more prominent among individuals suffering from compulsive sexual behaviors such as gambling disorder (4–11%) and compulsive buying (13–26%) [41].

In terms of family history, substance abuse is common in the relatives of individuals with compulsive sexual behavior. In a survey of 76 individuals in treatment, 40% of the patients reported at least one substance-dependent parent, 36% of the patients reported at least one sexually addicted parent, 30% had a parent with an eating disorder and 7% reported having at least one parent with excessive gambling [42]. Only 13% of individuals with compulsive sexual behavior had a family member without any addictions [43].

11.4.3 Brain Functions

Only a few neuroimaging studies have assessed the neurobiological underpinnings of compulsive sexual behavior. Of particular interest is the comparison of altered activation in brain networks of patients suffering from compulsive sexual behaviors with those involved in substance abuse and other behavioral addictions [35]. A cue-reactivity study that presented sexually explicit videos and nonsexual exciting videos found increased activation in the corticostriatal-limbic circuitry including ventral striatum, amygdala and dorsal anterior cingulate in individuals with compulsive sexual behavior relative to controls [44]. These regions overlap with those found to be activated in addictive disorders including gambling disorder [21, 45, 46].

In addition, an increased association between subjective sexual desire (wanting) and functional connectivity of the dorsal anterior cingulate-ventral striatum-amygdala network was found in participants with compulsive sexual behavior relative to those without (REF). Reward processing seems to be altered in compulsive sexual behavior comparable to gambling disorder. As in gambling disorder, later stages of the disorders are linked to increased wanting and decreased liking of the particular behavior consistent with theories of incentive motivation of drug addiction [47]. However, only limited evidence is available at present, and more studies are needed to support this conclusion.

11.5 Summary and Conclusion

Gambling disorder, also referred to as pathological gambling in ICD-10 [4], is the only behavioral addiction so far officially recognized in the new DSM-5 [1]. In recent years, research on gambling disorder including neurobiological characteristics has increased. When it comes to scientific studies that focus on other excessive behaviors that might show addictive characteristics such as compulsive Internet use, compulsive buying or sexual behaviors, the picture is different, with very few research studies on these psychiatric conditions. Most evidence is available for Internet gaming disorder. Yet not much is known whether other activities conducted using the Internet can also become addictive such as the use of social networks. In particular, more studies on the neurobiological basis of these activities are warranted for an informed decision regarding their classification as an addictive disorder. The identification of similar underlying neurobiological mechanisms would allow drawing the conclusion that those psychiatric diseases are related.

Research conducted so far suggest numerous similarities between gambling disorder and potential candidates such as Internet gaming disorder, compulsive buying disorder and compulsive sexual behavior (for a comparison see Table 11.1). What hinders a definite answer regarding the question which diagnostic category would be most appropriate for Internet gaming disorder, compulsive buying disorder and compulsive sexual behavior is not the lack of similarities but rather the scarceness of neurobiological studies in the field. More studies in larger samples are needed in order to replicate and extend existing findings. In particular, data from computational modeling and molecular studies in addition to neuroimaging work will help in the future to clear the picture. We might even get rid of the question: "Which category is most appropriate", following the ideas of the Research Domain Criteria (RDoC) launched by the National Institute of Mental Health (https://www.nimh.nih.gov/research-priorities/rdoc/index.shtml)? The central aim of this project is to transform diagnosis by incorporating genetics, imaging, cognitive science and biology to lay the foundation for a new classification system. Psychiatric conditions are characterized in a dimensional way by grouping them based on specific characteristics (i.e., domains) such as cognition, emotion or behavior. Sticking to the terminology of the research domain criteria, the central question would be whether compulsive buying, compulsive sexual behavior and Internet gaming disorders

Table 11.1 Comparison of different domains between gambling disorder and other potential behavioral addictions

	Gambling disorder	Internet gaming disorder	Compulsive buying disorder	Compulsive sexual behavior
Diagnostic criteria	Great overlap with criteria for substance use disorder	Great overlap with criteria for substance use disorder	Great overlap with criteria for substance use disorder	Great overlap with criteria for substance use disorder
Gender	More male	More male	More female	More male
Main comorbidities (Axis I)	Substance use disorders, depression, anxiety disorders	Substance use disorders, depression, anxiety disorders, attention deficit hyperactivity disorder	Anxiety disorders, substance use disorders, eating disorders, disorders of impulse control	Depression, anxiety disorders, substance use disorders, compulsive buying, gambling disorder
Main family history of psychiatric disorders	Substance use disorders, depression, anxiety disorders, gambling disorder, compulsive buying	Not known	Depression, substance use disorders, gambling disorder	Substance use disorders, compulsive sexual behavior, gambling disorder, eating disorder
Altered impulsivity	Yes	Yes	Yes	Yes
Altered reward processing	Yes	Yes	Yes	Yes

show similar alterations in certain neurobiological areas such as reward processing and impulse control.

Irrespective of the approach followed, be it diagnostic classification in line with the traditional classification systems or the proposed specification according to research domains criteria, it is inevitable to consider neurobiological characteristics (genetics, molecular, cellular and systems neuroscience including brain functions) in addition to clinical observations, diagnostics, comorbidities and family history and treatment response.

In summary, research on behavioral addictions remains scant and data are particularly sparse for compulsive buying disorder and compulsive sexual behaviors. However, available studies provide first evidence of similarities between gambling disorder and compulsive buying disorder, compulsive sexual behavior and Internet gaming disorder in different domains including diagnostics, comorbidities, family history, cognitive features and neurobiological mechanisms, in particular in relation to reward processing and impulse control.

References

1. American Psychiatric Association. Diagnostic and statistical manual of mental disorders. 5th ed. Washington, DC: American Psychiatric Association; 2013.
2. Grant JE, Potenza MN, Weinstein A, Gorelick DA. Introduction to behavioral addictions. Am J Drug Alcohol Abuse. 2010;36(5):233–41.
3. Holden C. 'Behavioral' addictions: do they exist? Science. 2001 Nov 2;294(5544):980–2.
4. World Health Organization. The ICD-10 classification of mental and behavioural disorders: clinical descriptions and diagnostic guidelines. Geneva: World Health Organization; 1992.
5. American Psychiatric Association. Diagnostic and statistical manual of mental disorders. 4th ed. Washington, DC: American Psychiatric Association; 2000. text revision (DSM-IV-TR)
6. Brewer JA, Potenza MN. The neurobiology and genetics of impulse control disorders: relationships to drug addictions. Biochem Pharmacol. 2008;75(1):63–75.
7. Fauth-Bühler M, Mann K, Potenza MN. Pathological gambling: a review of the neurobiological evidence relevant for its classification as an addictive disorder. Addict Biol. 2017;22(4):885–97.
8. Quester S, Romanczuk-Seiferth N. Brain imaging in gambling disorder. Curr Addict Rep. 2015;2:220–9.
9. Kuss DJ, Lopez-Fernandez O. Internet addiction and problematic internet use: a systematic review of clinical research. World J Psychiatry. 2016;6(1):143–76.
10. Petry NM, Stinson FS, Grant BF. Comorbidity of DSM-IV pathological gambling and other psychiatric disorders: results from the National Epidemiologic Survey on Alcohol and Related Conditions. J Clin Psychiatry. 2005;66(5):564–74.
11. Jorgenson AG, Hsiao RC, Yen CF. Internet addiction and other behavioral addictions. Child Adolesc Psychiatr Clin N Am. 2016;25(3):509–20.
12. Black DW, Belsare G, Schlosser S. Clinical features, psychiatric comorbidity, and health-related quality of life in persons reporting compulsive computer use behavior. J Clin Psychiatry. 1999;60:839–44.
13. Müller KW, Dickenhorst U, Medenwaldt J, Wölfling K, Koch A. Internet addiction as comorbid disorder in patients with a substance-related disorder: results from a survey in different inpatient clinics. Eur Psychiatry. 2011;26:1912.
14. Kessler RC, Hwang I, LaBrie R, Petukhova M, Sampson NA, Winters KC, Shaffer HJ. DSM-IV pathological gambling in the National Comorbidity Survey Replication. Psychol Med. 2008;38:1351–60.
15. Mann K, Lemenager T, Zois E, Hoffmann S, Beutel M, Vogelgesang M, Kiefer F, Fauth-Bühler M. Comorbidity, family history and personality traits in pathological gamblers compared with healthy controls. Eur Psychiatry. 2017;42:120–8.
16. Fauth-Bühler M, Mann K. Neurobiological correlates of internet gaming disorder: Similarities to pathological gambling. Addict Behav. 2017;64:349–56.
17. Daruma J, Barnes P. A neurodevelopmental view of impulsivity and its relationship to the superfactors of personality. In: McCown W, Johnson J, Shure M, editors. The impulsive client: theory, research and treatment. Washington, DC: American Psychological Association; 1993.
18. Fineberg NA, Chamberlain SR, Goudriaan AE, Stein DJ, Vanderschuren LJ, Gillan CM, Shekar S, Gorwood PA, Voon V, Morein-Zamir S, Denys D, Sahakian BJ, Moeller FG, Robbins TW, Potenza MN. New developments in human neurocognition: clinical, genetic, and brain imaging correlates of impulsivity and compulsivity. CNS Spectr. 2014;19:69–89.
19. Chen CY, Huang MF, Yen JY, Chen CS, Liu GC, Yen CF, Ko CH. Brain correlates of response inhibition in internet gaming disorder. Psychiatry Clin Neurosci. 2015;69(4):201–9.
20. Ding W, Sun J, Sun Y-W, Chen X, Zhou Y, Zhuang Z, et al. Trait impulsivity and impaired prefrontal impulse inhibition function in adolescents with internet gaming addiction revealed by a Go/No-Go fMRI study. Behav Brain Funct. 2014;10:20.
21. Van Holst RJ, van Holstein M, van den Brink W, Veltman DJ, Goudriaan AE. Response inhibition during cue reactivity in problem gamblers: an fMRI study. PLoS One. 2012;7:e30909.
22. Fiorillo CD, Tobler PN, Schultz W. Discrete coding of reward probability and uncertainty by dopamine neurons. Science. 2003;299:1898–902.

23. Volman SF, Lammel S, Margolis EB, Kim Y, Richard JM, Roitman MF, Lobo MK. New insights into the specificity and plasticity of reward and aversion encoding in the mesolimbic system. J Neurosci. 2013;33:17569–76.
24. Lejoyeux M, Weinstein A. Compulsive buying. Am J Drug Alcohol Abuse. 2010;36(5):248–53.
25. Müller A, Mitchell JE, de Zwaan M. Compulsive buying. Am J Addict. 2015;24:132–7.
26. Black DW. A review of compulsive buying disorder. World Psychiatry. 2007;6(1):14–8.
27. De Zwaan M. Psychiatric comorbidity and compulsive buying. In: Müller A, Mitchell JE, editors. Compulsive buying. Clinical foundations and treatment. New York: Routledge; 2011. p. 87–104.
28. Black DW, Repertinger S, Gaffney GR, Gabel J. Family history and psychiatric comorbidity in persons with compulsive buying: preliminary findings. Am J Psychiatry. 1998;155(7):960–3.
29. Dannon PN, Lowengrub K, Aizer A, Kotler M. Pathological gambling: comorbid psychiatric diagnoses in patients and their families. Isr J Psychiatry Relat Sci. 2006;43(2):88–92.
30. Black DW, Coryell W, Crowe R, Shaw M, McCormick B, Allen J. The relationship of DSM-IV pathological gambling to compulsive buying and other possible spectrum disorders: results from the Iowa PG family study. Psychiatry Res. 2015;226(1):273–6.
31. Derbyshire KL, Chamberlain SR, Odlaug BL, Schreiber LR, Grant JE. Neurocognitive functioning in compulsive buying disorder. Ann Clin Psychiatry. 2014;26(1):57–63.
32. Raab G, Elger CE, Neuner M, Weber B. A neurological study of compulsive buying behaviour. J Consum Policy. 2011;34:401–13.
33. Fong TW, Reid RC, Parhami I. Behavioral addictions: where to draw the lines? Psychiatr Clin North Am. 2012;35(2):279–96.
34. Coleman E, Raymond N, McBean A. Assessment and treatment of compulsive sexual behavior. Minn Med. 2003;86(7):42–7.
35. Fong TW. Understanding and managing compulsive sexual behaviors. Psychiatry (Edgmont). 2006;3(11):51–8.
36. Kafka MP. Hypersexual disorder: a proposed diagnosis for DSM-V. Arch Sex Behav. 2010;39:377–400.
37. Stein DJ, Black DW, Shapira NA, et al. Hypersexual disorder and preoccupation with internet pornography. Am J Psychiatry. 2001;158:1590–4.
38. Kaplan MS, Krüger RB. Diagnosis, assessment, and treatment of hypersexuality. J Sex Res. 2010;47:181–98.
39. Derbyshire KL, Grant JE. Compulsive sexual behavior: a review of the literature. J Behav Addict. 2015;4(2):37–43.
40. Raymond NC, Coleman E, Miner MH. Psychiatric comorbidity and compulsive/impulsive traits in compulsive sexual behavior. Compr Psychiatry. 2003;44(5):370–80.
41. Freimuth M, Waddell M, Stannard J, Kelley S, Kipper A, Richardson A, Szuromi I. Expanding the scope of dual diagnosis and co-addictions: behavioral addictions. J Groups Addict Recover. 2008;3(3–4):137–60.
42. Schneider JP, Schneider BH. Couple recovery from sexual addiction: research findings of a survey of 88 marriages. Sex Addict Compulsivity. 1996;3:111–26.
43. Carnes PJ. Out of the shadows: understanding sexual addiction. 3rd ed. Center City, MN: Hazelden; 2001.
44. Voon V, Mole TB, Banca P, Porter L, Morris L, Mitchell S, Lapa TR, Karr J, Harrison NA, Potenza MN, Irvine M. Neural correlates of sexual cue reactivity in individuals with and without compulsive sexual behaviours. PLoS One. 2014;9(7):e102419.
45. Crockford DN, Goodyear B, Edwards J, Quickfall J, el-Guebaly N. Cue-induced brain activity in pathological gamblers. Biol Psychiatry. 2005;58:787–95.
46. Goudriaan AE, de Ruiter MB, van den Brink W, Oosterlaan J, Veltman DJ. Brain activation patterns associated with cue reactivity and craving in abstinent problem gamblers, heavy smokers and healthy controls: an fMRI study. Addict Biol. 2010;15:491–503.
47. Everitt BJ, Robbins TW. From the ventral to the dorsal striatum: devolving views of their roles in drug addiction. Neurosci Biobehav Rev. 2013;37:1946–54.

Gambling Disorder and Substance-Related Disorders: Similarities and Differences

12

Anna E. Goudriaan, Wim van den Brink, and Ruth J. van Holst

12.1 Introduction

Since 2013, gambling disorder (GD) has been classified as the first behavioral addiction under the category of Substance-Related and Addictive Disorders in DSM-5 [1]. This is an important step because it implies that other so-called behavioural addictions such as Internet gaming disorder, which is currently included in an appendix in the DSM-5, could also be classified in this category. The reasons for the move of pathological gambling (PG) as one of the impulse control disorders in DSM-IV to GD as behavioral addiction in DSM-5 are based on the fact that GD is much more than just an impulse control disorder and the many similarities between GD- and substance-related addictions. These include similarities in symptom profile, in etiological factors like neurobiology, and similarities in the effectiveness of certain psychological and pharmacological treatments. In this chapter, similarities

A. E. Goudriaan (✉)
Department of Psychiatry, Amsterdam University Medical Center, Amsterdam Institute for Addiction Research, University of Amsterdam, Amsterdam, The Netherlands

Department of Research and Quality of Care, Arkin, Mental Health Care, Amsterdam, The Netherlands
e-mail: A.E.Goudriaan@amc.uva.nl

W. van den Brink
Department of Psychiatry, Amsterdam University Medical Center, Amsterdam Institute for Addiction Research, University of Amsterdam, Amsterdam, The Netherlands
e-mail: w.vandenbrink@amc.uva.nl

R. J. van Holst
Department of Psychiatry, Amsterdam University Medical Center, Amsterdam Institute for Addiction Research, University of Amsterdam, Amsterdam, The Netherlands

Donders Institute for Brain and Cognition, Radboud University Nijmegen, Nijmegen, The Netherlands
e-mail: r.j.vanholst@amc.uva.nl

© Springer Nature Switzerland AG 2019
A. Heinz et al. (eds.), *Gambling Disorder*, https://doi.org/10.1007/978-3-030-03060-5_12

and dissimilarities are discussed, and a framework for future interventions targeting working mechanisms is proposed.

First, we will discuss the symptoms of GD and the changes in the DSM classification of gambling disorder over time. This will be followed by a discussion on the etiological model for disordered gambling. A detailed account is given for underlying neurobiological and personality factors that predispose for and influence the development and course of disordered gambling. Differences in the characteristics of GD versus SUDs give rise to the question whether these differences play a role in specific vulnerabilities for disordered gambling and whether they affect the use of treatments currently applied in SUDs.

12.2   Symptoms in Gambling Disorders and Substance Use Disorders: Evolving Concepts

When we compare the symptoms of GD and SUDs, we can see a large overlap in the DSM criteria in both the current (DSM-5) and previous versions of the DSM, especially since the introduction of DSM-III-R (see Table 12.1). For the DSM-5, only the new SUD-criterion "craving" is not present as a criterion for GD. There are many studies in GD showing higher scores on self-reported craving and elevated responses in the reward circuitry in the brain of disordered gamblers, similar to processes in SUDs (see Sect. 12.4.2.1 on craving). However, there are also many unresolved issues, e.g., what are the physiological and psychological aspects that are relevant, is the urge related to the desire to engage in gambling or to the sensation of winning, what is the emotional character of craving, does it include craving for the positive emotional effects of gambling (reward craving) or is it related to the escape from negative feelings (relief craving), and finally is craving for gambling unique as an urge to perceive the experience of excitement when gambling? Furthermore, which stimuli elicit craving: visual stimuli when viewing gambling or gambling-related pictures, auditory stimuli when hearing the sounds that accompany certain forms of gambling such as the clicking of chips, or the sound of slot machines when in operation, or tactile stimuli like the handling of chips or gambling machines? These are questions that need to be addressed in order to answer the question which aspects of craving can be conceptualized as similar or dissimilar to craving in SUDs. On the other hand, in SUDs, craving is a multifaceted construct as well, and more research is needed in SUDs to characterize, for instance, the relation between self-reported craving and physiological responses to substance-related cues.

12.3   How Does Disordered Gambling Develop? Etiological Models

Just like in etiological models of SUDs, a multifactorial biopsychosocial model is used in GD to explain this complex behavioral disorder. Biological, psychological, and social factors interact in the development and course of gambling disorders.

Table 12.1 Classification criteria for the diagnostic and statistical manual over time

	DSM-III	DSM-III-R	DSM-IV-TR	DSM-5
Number of criteria needed for a pathological gambling diagnosis	One mandatory +3/6	4/10	5/10	4/9
A. *Criteria* (Persistent and recurrent maladaptive/problematic gambling behavior leading to clinically significant impairment or distress, as indicated by)				
– Unable to resist gambling urges	Mandatory			
– Arrests for illegal acts to obtain means for gambling (DSM-III-R)/Having committed illegal acts (e.g., theft, forgery, fraud) to finance gambling	×	×	×	
– Unable to release debts or financial difficulties	×			
– Relational or family problems due to gambling	×			
– Borrowing illegally to obtain money for gambling	×			
– Unable to account for money	×			
– Being absent from work due to gambling	×			
– Repeated unsuccesful efforts to stop or cut back gambling			×	×
– Relying on others to relieve a desperate financial situation		×	×	×
– Preoccupation with gambling or with ways to obtain money to gamble		×	×	×
– Gambling more or playing longer than intended		×		
– Needs to increase the amount or frequency of gambling to obtain the desired level of excitement (tolerance)		×	×	×
– Feeling restless or irritable when unable to gamble (withdrawal)		×	×	×
– Returning the next day to try to gain back losses (chasing losses)		×	×	×
– Gambling instead of doing what is expected regarding social or work obligations		×		
– Jeopardizing a job or social relations due to gambling activity		×	×	×
– Continuing gambling despite debts due to gambling		×		
– Gambling to relieve a negative mood or forget problems/gambling when feeling distressed			×	×
– Lying to relatives or others to hide gambling problems/concealing the extent of involvement with gambling			×	×
B. *The gambling cannot be better accounted for by a manic episode*	×	×	×	×

A well-known model for gambling disorder is the three-pathway model by Blaszczynski and Nower [2, 3]. In the three-pathway model, a first pathway is proposed for pathological gamblers who develop gambling problems through behavioral conditioning, and for whom no specific neurobiological vulnerability is present, but rather the availability and accessibility of gambling—and early engagement in gambling—play a major role in the development of their gambling problems. A second pathway is proposed for what Blaszczynski and Nower describe as the "emotionally vulnerable problem gambler," characterized by personality factors like risk-taking, depression and anxiety, a high level of sensation seeking, and substance use. This is coupled to underlying biological vulnerabilities. These vulnerabilities were specified in the model only at EEG and neurotransmitter levels, representing the state of the art of research in 2002, but now could include abnormalities in functional fronto-striatal abnormalities, underlying the proposed "emotional vulnerabilities" of risk-taking and substance use, for example. A third pathway is defined as the "antisocial impulsivist" pathway, and includes, on top of the factors included in the second pathway, impulsive traits, such as ADHD, impulsivity, antisocial behavior, and substance abuse, which influence the classical and operant conditioning. In all three pathways, the conditioning is influenced by arousal and excitement and related physiological factors, and by cognitive misperceptions, such as the illusion of control and biased evaluation. Although in terminology differences are present between this pathway model and dual processing models as present for SUDs, the major factors overlap: both behavioral factors related to conditioning and risk-taking/impulsivity and the influence of (psychophysiological) effects of rewards related to drugs and gambling are recognized; the biased evaluation in the pathway model can be viewed as equivalent to the abnormal reward processing or salience attribution as proposed in dual process models as in the I-RISA model (see also Sect. 12.4) [4].

For the social etiology of gambling disorders, the presence of games of chance and cultural embeddedness of gambling form a prerequisite for the development of gambling behavior or regular engagement in gambling [5]. Early wins in gambling can promote the development of regular gambling. Besides social factors, genetic vulnerability for the development of addictive behavior [6] in combination with a (neuro)biological vulnerability can result in certain neurobiological and psychological reactions to the experience of reward (winning money) in gambling. In gambling disorder, the development of craving is the result of changes in the brain's reward circuitry, which result in a stronger attention for stimuli related to gambling and a stronger drive or motivation (craving) to engage in gambling. All these interacting social, genetic, and (neuro)biological factors form the base for the development of a pathological form of gambling or gambling disorder [3]. For example, we know from recent research that deficits in frontal brain functions related to impulsivity, such as a diminished planning ability and a focus on immediate rewards (delay discounting), can promote the development of GD [7–9]. At the same time, these factors also pose a risk for relapse in GD after treatment [10, 11]. Impulsivity has been proposed as an important etiological factor for problem gambling, since it implies rash decision-making, lack of thinking about the negative consequences of gambling, and diminished control over gambling. In addition, patients with GD show diminished physiological responses (e.g., heart rate) preceding risky decisions, which could imply that this lack of physiological responses or "somatic markers" is a vulnerability for the development of a gambling disorder [12]. This lack of physiological responsiveness when facing negative consequences (losses) could also explain why people continue gambling despite frequent losses. Related, the anticipation of losses in PG, has been associated with stronger responses in the ventral striatum compared to alcohol-dependent patients and healthy controls [13], which indicates that there may be an impaired salience attribution to losses in PGs, which may promote the chasing of losses. On the other hand, in the same study, a diminished response to successful vs. unsuccessful loss avoidance was found in the right ventral and medial prefrontal cortex, correlating with PG severity. In GD patients, reduced neural responses after experiencing losses were present [14], which may also hamper the decision to stop gambling when facing losses. Taken together, although a mixed image appears regarding findings on reward responsiveness, depending on the different tasks employed in the studies, abnormal neural processing of loss anticipation and loss outcomes is present and may be related to the phenomenon of chasing losses and to the diminished attention paid to losses by disordered gamblers.

In etiological models of problem gambling, cognitive misperceptions on gambling are unique, and there is no comparable concept for this in SUD models. Cognitive misperceptions on gambling are, for instance, irrational thoughts about gambling, such as the "illusion of control": the impression that paying attention or trying hard will influence the chances of winning. Cognitive misperceptions are rooted in neural mechanisms, which have been investigated, for example, the phenomenon of near misses [15]; see Sect. 12.4.3.2. Another cognitive misperception is the higher attention payed to wins, and the downplaying of losses, which results in a perceptual filter resulting in better remembering wins than losses (for a discussion on the neurobiological mechanisms of reward and loss processing, see Sect. 12.4.3.1). In the following paragraphs, the etiological factors common for GD and SUD and the ones unique for GD are discussed, and findings in GD are compared to findings in SUDs.

12.4 Cognitive and Motivational Functions in Gambling Disorder Compared to Substance Use-Related Disorders

Recent reviews on SUDs give a consistent image of cognitive-motivational functions that are affected in persons with SUDs. These disorders have been associated with higher impulsivity and deficient executive functions (cognitive control) on the one hand and with changes in reward sensitivity as expressed in heightened attentional sensitivity to drug-related rewards and a diminished reward sensitivity to non-drug-related (natural) rewards. In SUD models these two factors result in dual process models, such as, for instance, in the Impaired Response Inhibition and Salience Attribution (I-RISA) model [4]. In this model, response inhibition refers to the cognitive component of SUDs, and salience attribution refers to the changes in the reward pathways and associated higher salience (i.e., attention) for addiction-related stimuli. The cognitive and motivational functions that are central in SUD models represent two interacting brain systems: (1) a dorsal prefrontal cortical brain circuit, including the dorsolateral prefrontal cortex and cingulate cortex, related to executive functions, impulsivity, and control over motivational functions, and (2) a motivational circuit consisting of subcortical limbic-orbitofrontal structures involving the striatum, amygdala, hippocampus, and orbitofrontal cortex.

12.4.1 Impulsivity in Gambling Disorder and SUDs

There is consensus in the literature that impulsivity is a multifaceted construct and that several relatively unrelated aspects can be discerned. One of the most frequently used ways to assess the personality aspects of impulsivity is by self-report measures (see below). However, these self-report questionnaires of impulsivity have a low correlation with behavioral measures of impulsivity, such as motor impulsivity, choice impulsivity, and cognitive impulsivity.

12.4.1.1 Self-Reported Impulsivity

Impulsivity can be studied with self-report measures, of which the Barratt Impulsiveness Scale, BIS-11 [16], is a well-known example, consisting of three related subscales: motor impulsivity, attentional impulsivity, and non-planning impulsivity. Although these terms suggest that they measure similar constructs as the behavioral measures of impulsivity outlined above (motor impulsivity, choice impulsivity, cognitive impulsivity), these subscales of the BIS-11 measure dissimilar constructs and in general do not correlate with performance on behavioral impulsivity tasks [17–19]. Another questionnaire is the UPPS [20], which was designed to measure impulsivity across dimensions of the five-factor model of personality (urgency, lack of premeditation, lack of perseverance, sensation seeking) [20]. In contrast to the BIS-11, for the UPPS, relationships have been established between the subdomains urgency and motor impulsivity on the stop signal task [21], whereas another study found that only a small part—12%—of motor inhibition tasks could be attributed by BIS trait impulsivity [22], indicating that trait impulsivity and behavioral measures of (motor) impulsivity tap largely into distinct constructs.

Several studies indicate that problem gamblers score higher on measures such as the BIS-11, see, for instance [23–27], as well as on the UPPS [28–32], and these scores tend to be related to symptom severity. A recent meta-analysis indicates that all aspects of the UPPS are associated with elevated scores in SUDs but that both positive and negative urgency had the largest effect sizes for SUDs [33]. As the UPPS has been developed more recently than the BIS-11, more studies on impulsivity scores as measured with the BIS-11 are present, which indicate that elevated BIS-11 levels in SUD populations [34, 35]. In prospective studies, personality measures of impulsivity in adolescence and childhood have been related to the development of problem gambling later in life [7–9]. In summary, these studies indicate that impulsivity traits as measured by self-report instruments are related to both GD, less severe levels of GD like problem gambling, and to SUDs and that these impulsivity traits form both a vulnerability for the development of SUDs and are related cross-sectionally to the presence of GD and SUDs.

12.4.1.2   Impulsivity: Motor Impulsivity/Response Inhibition

Response inhibition can be viewed as the most basic, motoric form of impulsivity. Theoretically, one can argue that people who are less able to inhibit their responses would have a tendency to use substances more or to gamble more often, because the control over their responses is lower, and therefore their ability to stop using substances or stop gambling is lower once they are gambling or using substances. Response inhibition has been investigated in substance use disordered populations quite frequently. In patient groups with a cocaine use disorder, a consistent image of diminished response inhibition emerges [36–40]. Also in patients with heroin dependence, diminished response inhibition has been observed [41–44], as well as in alcohol use disordered groups [45–47] and in MDMA users [48–50]. In (meth) amphetamine users, the evidence is mixed: some studies report on diminished response inhibition in this group [51, 52], whereas other research groups report no difficulties with response inhibition in (meth)amphetamine users [53]. Importantly, polydrug use is more often present than single SUDs. In these groups of poly-SUDs, for instance, with cocaine as primary drug of choice [36, 54], or heroin as the drug of choice [55, 56], diminished response inhibition has been found. An important question in SUDs is whether diminished response inhibition is a pre-existing problem or (partly) the consequence of drug use on the brain and, thus, whether response inhibition recovers after prolonged abstinence. In an overview, the effects of length of abstinence on neurocognitive functions were evaluated, and it was concluded that there was proof for short- (up to 1 month) and medium-long-term (1–6 months) effects of abstinence on improvement of response inhibition for cocaine, (meth) amphetamine, heroin, and alcohol [57]. However, longitudinal research is scarce, and specifically polydrug use and a higher number of detoxifications are associated with longer-term problems with neurocognitive functions such as response inhibition [58]. Compared to SUDs, the evidence for diminished response inhibition in gambling disorder is mixed. Some studies report that a diminished response inhibition is present in gambling disorder [46, 59], whereas in other studies, the diminished response inhibition in gambling disorder could be accounted for by high comorbidity, for instance, of ADHD in pathological gamblers, or by a diminished stimulus-response integration, a more basic cognitive function which can influence response inhibition [27, 60]. In a recent meta-analysis by Smith and colleagues, the conclusion was drawn that in both pathological gambling and SUDs like cocaine, MDMA, methamphetamine, tobacco, and alcohol dependence, diminished response inhibition was present; however, no consistent evidence was present for diminished response inhibition in opioid or cannabis dependence, nor for Internet addiction [61]. Given the findings of this meta-analysis, it can be concluded that in general GD is associated with diminished response inhibition. However, there are studies which do not report differences between GD and healthy controls—and also in SUD studies, heterogeneity is present. The heterogeneity in findings fits with the idea that several subtypes of problematic gamblers, requiring different treatments, are present [2]. The findings also are consistent with the renewed attention for personalized medicine, instigated by the findings of high variability in functions like response inhibition in SUDs, which also affect the clinical effects of certain (pharmacological) interventions in alcohol use disorders and problem gamblers [62, 63]. For instance, in an experimental study by Zack and Poulos, differential effects of the cognitive enhancer modafinil were found for high-impulsive versus low-impulsive pathological gamblers: in high-impulsive gamblers, modafinil decreased the desire to gamble and diminished disinhibition and risky decision-making, whereas in low-impulsive gamblers, modafinil had opposite effects [63]. This stresses the importance of investigating (neurobiological) factors in GD subgroups in order to find targets for personalized treatment. Regarding the underlying neurobiological mechanisms of deficient response inhibition in DG, a review of ERP and fMRI studies on response inhibition and error processing in SUDs and behavioral addictions indicates that both in SUDs as in pathological gambling, hypoactivation in the anterior cingulate cortex (ACC), inferior frontal gyrus, and dorsolateral prefrontal cortex is present, although these findings were less robust for pathological gambling and other behavioral addictions, given the small number of studies [64].

12.4.1.3 Impulsivity: Delay Discounting and Immediate Rewards

Sensitivity for reward can be measured—without a focus on potential negative long-term consequences as in so-called decision-making tasks—with delay discounting tasks. In this type of task, the discounting of delayed rewards is measured. When people engage in a delay discounting task, their tendency to choose for an immediate lower reward, compared to a delayed larger reward, is measured. For instance, when we have the choice for a monetary reward of 5 Euros now, or 10 Euros in a week from now, choice behavior will differ between persons. In this way, an indifference point can be calculated for which persons are indifferent in their choice for an immediate smaller versus a delayed larger reward. Several studies indicate that in patients with SUDs, there is a stronger tendency to choose for the immediate reward, instead of a larger delayed reward, thus indicating a discounting of delays. In a recent meta-analysis, a robust association was found between delayed reward discounting investigating the effects of severity compared to those studies which focused on quantity-frequency measures of use [65]. In this meta-analysis, no specific effects of addictive behavior were found, indicating similar delayed reward discounting across SUDs and GD.

There is an effect of immediate substance use on delay discounting. For instance, in persons with an alcohol use disorder, who are not abstinent, delay discounting is higher than in persons who have an alcohol use disorder, but are recently abstinent. However, both groups still have a higher delay discounting compared to persons without an alcohol use disorder [66]. In heroin and cocaine use disorder, still a stronger preference for immediate rewards has been found, compared to groups with alcohol use disorders and healthy controls [67, 68]. Comorbid disorders, e.g., the presence of antisocial personality disorder, only partly account for higher delay discounting in SUDs [69, 70]. When we look at the evidence in gambling disordered groups, several studies have also found higher delay discounting in comparison to control groups [71, 26], and see for a meta-analysis [65]. As a parallel to the effect of intoxication on delay discounting, also in problem gamblers, contextual factors can influence delay discounting. For example, problem gamblers who were confronted with high craving-eliciting gambling pictures showed steeper delay discounting curves than when confronted with low craving-eliciting gambling pictures [72].

12.4.1.4   Impulsivity: Decision-Making

Decision-making is a complex aspect of impulsivity, which is sometimes defined separately from impulsivity. In general, in the literature, it refers to the ability to make advantageous decisions, e.g., as in choosing for long-term rewards, instead of short-term rewards that are accompanied by long-term losses, as measured in the Iowa gambling task. Usually, decision-making tasks also involve learning reward contingencies and thus depend—at least partly—on the ability to learn which choice options are associated with advantageous or disadvantageous outcomes. In certain tasks, such as contingency learning tasks, a change in contingencies is presented at some point, and there, decision-making thus also assesses flexibility with regard to contingency learning. Decision-making tasks have been studied widely in SUDs. Diminished (disadvantageous) decision-making on the Iowa gambling task has been reported in groups with alcohol, cannabis, heroin, cocaine, and (met)amphetamine use disorders and in frequent tobacco smokers [41, 44, 73–79]. Like in the studies on delay discounting, comorbid personality disorders are associated with higher decision-making problems, but also in groups without comorbid personality problems, diminished decision-making is present [80, 81]. In addition, length of abstinence and comorbid factors do not influence decision-making in opiate-dependent groups [82], indicating that in opiate users, decision-making deficits are relatively stable. In pathological gamblers and problem gamblers, diminished decision-making has been reported, with disadvantageous decision-making strategies associated with long-term negative consequences, in comparison to control groups without pathological gambling [81, 83, 84]. Interestingly, pathological gamblers who engage in strategic games of chance (e.g., card games) have intact decision-making strategies [81], in contrast to pathological gamblers who engage in gambling activities solely determined by luck (e.g., slot machine players). Thus, both phenotypic and endophenotypic subtypes of pathological gamblers can be discerned, which may have relevance for treatment (see Sect. 12.5).

When reviewing all the evidence on personality measures of impulsivity and behavioral measures of impulsivity, consistent evidence is present regarding higher self-reported impulsivity in GD, as well as regarding increased delay discounting which is comparably present in GD and SUDs. Regarding response inhibition, diminished response inhibition and related diminished dorsolateral prefrontal and anterior cingulate reactivity have been reported in SUDs, but the number of studies in GD is lower, some inconsistencies are reported in the literature, and there are only a small number of studies investigating the evidence for neural abnormalities responsible for diminished response inhibition in GD. Therefore, more research into motor impulsivity/response inhibition is needed in GD. Diminished decision-making has been reported in both SUDs and GD frequently, although for GDs, strategic gamblers seem to be less affected. In some studies, comorbidity partially explains aspects of impulsivity in GD, pointing at the fact that besides GD, underlying comorbidity may result in higher levels of impulsivity.

12.4.2 Motivational Functions in Gambling Disorder and SUDs

12.4.2.1 Craving and Cue Reactivity

When talking about craving and cue reactivity, craving usually refers to the (self-reported) subjective experience of craving for substance use or gambling: the experience of a strong urge to use a substance or for gambling. The term cue reactivity is used in studies where the physiological or brain response to substance- or gambling-related cues is studied, for instance in psychophysiological studies on the cardiovascular, cortisol or skin conductance response to substance- or gambling-related cues, or in functional magnetic resonance imaging (fMRI) or electronic encephalogram (EEG) studies where the brain's responsivity to gambling or substance-related cues versus neutral cues is compared. Regarding studies on the subjective experience of craving in gambling, there is little consistency in the craving measures that have been used and that relatively little is known about their validity [85, 86]. One of the issues that has hampered the development of craving scales for gambling is that the concept of craving and its components in disordered gambling is still discussed [87]. In addition, although some craving questionnaires have been developed, including the Gambling Urge Scale [85] and the Gambling Craving Scale [86], the validation is mostly done in the general population, and it is not known whether these measures can be validly applied to patients with gambling disorder. These issues probably also resulted in not including craving as a criterion in the definition of DSM-5 gambling disorder. It is to be expected that when new research on the concept of craving in gambling emerges, that craving may also be included as a criterion in a future version of the DSM.

In SUDs, craving and its neurophysiological substrates have been studied extensively. Since 2013, for the first time, craving has been included as a criterion for DSM-5 substance use disorders. The common neural substrates behind subjective craving and cue reactivity include a higher responsivity in the (ventral) striatum, and functional-related areas such as the amygdala, pallidum, and anterior cingulate cortex, thus serving primary the motivational-emotional limbic circuit within the fronto-striatal brain circuit [88, 89]. In gambling disorder, the number of studies on craving and cue reactivity is limited, but they show involvement of a similar motivational-emotional brain circuit [90], including increased activation in frontal brain areas (dorsolateral prefrontal cortex, inferior frontal areas) and subcortical structures like limbic parahippocampal areas, the amygdala, and areas involved in the ventral visual attentional stream, such as the occipital lobe in disordered gamblers compared to healthy controls [91, 92]. Moreover, higher brain activation to gambling cues was associated with the subjective experience of higher craving in the pathological gamblers [92, 93]. It should be noted, however, that only a very limited number of cue reactivity studies are available and that this topic deserves more attention. Specifically, the experience of craving and its motivational mechanisms in the brain may also influence other factors relevant in pathological gambling, such as delay discounting. In an fMRI study, the presence of gambling cues increased delay discounting in problem gamblers [72], indicating the relatedness between cognitive and motivational processes in gambling. This is an example of research that stresses that cues have both emotional effects, like on subjective craving, but that they also influence our behavior and enhance the focus on immediate rewards, as in delay discounting. On the other hand, the presence of gambling cues in impulsivity tasks sometimes also enhances attention in problem gamblers [94]. Thus, more research on the interaction between motivational and the various aspects of impulsivity and reward processing is needed.

12.4.2.2 Attentional Bias

When people with a gambling disorder are confronted with cues related to gambling, this results in a higher attention toward these cues. This higher attention can be measured with neurocognitive tasks that assess this attentional bias toward cues related to the addictive behavior in question. One of these attentional bias tasks is the *dot-probe task*. In this task, one picture relevant to the addictive disorder in question and one picture not related to the addictive disorder are simultaneously presented on the left and the right side of a computer screen, and one has to watch a dot in the middle of the screen. Shortly after the presentation of the pictures, a "probe" or neutral sign appears at the place of one of the pictures, requiring a response. Faster responses to the probe that appears at the location of the previous addiction-related picture versus responses to the probe at the location of the neutral picture indicate attentional bias toward the addiction-related pictures. Several other tasks can measure attentional bias toward addiction-related stimuli, e.g., the addiction-relevant Stroop task. In this task, addiction-relevant words or neutral words are presented, and the color in which the words are printed needs to be named. Attentional bias is present when it takes longer, or more errors are made, for the words related to addiction versus neutral words. Attentional bias is present across SUDs, for several attentional bias tasks as, for instance, in alcohol use disorders, nicotine dependence, and heroin dependence [95–100]. Moreover, active use is associated with a higher attentional bias in heroin-dependent patients compared to abstinent heroin-dependent patients [101]. Related to this is the influence of whether persons with SUDs are in treatment or not. For instance, a negative attentional bias has been reported in patients with alcohol dependence currently in treatment [102, 103]. This can be interpreted as related to the changed motivation that is present in persons in treatment, for whom substance-related material has a lot of negative associations as well.

In disordered gamblers, several studies indicate that attentional bias is present for gambling-related stimuli. In an early study by McCusker and Gettings, attentional bias was present in a Stroop task study in members of gamblers anonymous compared to their non-gambling addicted spouses [104]. Another study employing a gambling-relevant Stroop task [105] indicated that in a group of persons who experienced loss of control over gambling, a higher attentional bias was present compared to gamblers with a high control over gambling. In a more recent set of studies, the specific components of attentional bias in problem gamblers and non-problem gamblers used a Posner attentional bias task, in which both initial orientation attentional bias and maintenance of attentional bias can be measured. In these studies, in active problem gamblers, a facilitation of attentional encoding was present [106], whereas in the abstinent problem gamblers, an avoidance bias was present [107]. This indicates that the status of problem gambling—in treatment, or actively gambling, differences in the presence or absence of motivation to change gambling behavior—can influence these attentional biases and needs to be taken into account when performing attentional bias research.

12.4.3 Unique Factors in Gambling Disorder

From the evidence reviewed above, there are important similarities between disordered gambling and SUDS, despite apparent differences in cognitive and motivational functions between several SUDS and some differences in severity of neurocognitive dysfunctions between GD and SUDs. Several aspects of gambling are however not present in SUDS. For instance, in gambling, one is never sure of the outcome of the gambling game, whereas for SUDs there is at least partly a security about the presence of a substance in the drug, differing dependent on the regulation of the substance. For instance, one can safely assume that a certain level of alcohol is present in a bottle of wine. For gambling on the other hand, with the placement of a bet, one is not sure of the outcome, either a win or a loss. Thus, when engaging in gambling, this is per se a risky activity, associated with uncertainty, and gambling can be subdivided in several stages: placing a bet or engaging in a certain gambling activity (and this engagement can differ from a high-risk bet to a low-risk bet and from a high stake to a low stake), waiting for the outcome (expectancy phase) and the experience of a win or loss (outcome phase). Several neurocognitive and neuroimaging studies have now focused on these different phases of gambling [108, 109], and also in SUDs there is a growing interest in the more theoretical process of reward expectancy and reward (outcome) experience and their neural mechanisms [110, 111].

Another aspect that differs between gambling and substance use is the role of expectancies and cognitions about the gambling game. Whereas the gamble in itself is uncertain and risky per definition, certain thoughts and ideas about the gambling game can influence how these risks are perceived and hence influence gambling behaviour. In disordered gambling, these abnormal cognitive processes are referred to as "cognitive misperceptions" and include, for instance, the overestimation of one's skill to influence the outcome of a gambling game, the overestimation of the chances of winning, or a bias in remembering wins versus losses, which could be related to attentional biases. Studies have shown that compared to non-gamblers, problem gamblers are more often overconfident in their own abilities—even in non-gambling-related abilities—and that this is related to less profitable betting behavior [112].

12.4.3.1 Reward Outcome and Expectancy of Reward

In the first fMRI studies focusing on reward processing in pathological gambling, the outcome phase of rewards was usually the focus. For instance, in a study on processing of monetary gains versus losses, disordered gamblers showed diminished activation in the ventral striatum and ventral prefrontal cortex when processing gains compared to losses [113]. In this study, because a direct comparison was made between reward and loss processing, the relative responsiveness of reward and loss processing could not be discerned. In a later study focusing on cognitive switching in which pathological gamblers could win money, lose money, or experience a neutral outcome, both brain responsiveness to wins and losses in the ventral prefrontal cortices were diminished in pathological gamblers compared to healthy controls [14]. On a psychophysiological level, responsiveness to wins in the Iowa gambling task also has been shown to be lower—heart rate decreased after wins in pathological gamblers compared to heart rate increases after wins in healthy controls [12], and diminished ventromedial prefrontal activity has been reported during performance of the IGT [114]. Thus, both a diminished responsiveness to rewards and to losses seem present in disordered gamblers. However, in a recent meta-analysis, SUD patients showed increased activation of the ventral striatum in reward outcome situations, whereas gambling addicts showed decreased activation of the dorsal striatum in reward outcome situations [115].

Regarding the anticipation to rewards and losses, or reward processing during the phase of gambling in which decisions regarding gambling are made, a different picture emerges. For instance, in an fMRI study focusing on poker players differing in the level of problematic playing and controls, higher activity in reward-related areas such as the ventral striatum, but lower activity in the cognitive control network (dorsolateral prefrontal activation), was present in poker players during deck selection on the IGT compared to healthy controls, and this activation correlated with levels of gambling problems [116]. In a study of problem gamblers, using a probabilistic choice game to model anticipatory processing, higher responsivity in the ventral striatum was present in pathological gamblers when anticipating larger wins compared to smaller wins [109]. Similarly, another fMRI study showed that both in pathological gamblers and cocaine-dependent patients, higher anticipatory activity was present in mesolimbic and ventrocortical regions, although in pathological gamblers higher activation was present in anticipation of a possible reward, whereas in cocaine-dependent patients, responsiveness to certain loss anticipation was higher [117]. In a study in which high-risk and low-risk gambles were presented, high-risk gambles led to a higher anticipatory response in reward-related areas, in problem gamblers, compared to controls [108, 118]. However, in two studies that used a more abstract modified monetary incentive delay (MID) task [110] in which subjects have to make speeded responses to acquire points/money or to prevent losing points/money, another picture emerges: pathological gamblers showed attenuated ventral striatal responses during reward anticipation as well as in response to monetary wins [119, 120]. Another MID study in GD and alcohol dependence found that activity in the right ventral striatum during loss anticipation was increased in GD patients compared with controls and alcohol-dependent patients. Moreover, PG patients showed decreased activation in the right ventral striatum and right medial prefrontal cortex during successful loss avoidance compared with controls, which was inversely associated with severity of gambling behavior [13]. Thus, it seems that in gambling-related contexts there is an increased anticipatory responsivity in reward-related brain circuitry in pathological gamblers, where higher activation is seen when higher risks or higher monetary rewards are involved, whereas a diminished responsivity is present when anticipating rewards outside of a gambling context and when experiencing the outcomes of wins and losses. With regard to the diminished responsivity to rewards and losses, however, context could also play a role: in an EEG study, hyper-reactivity in a higher medial frontal signaling after receiving monetary rewards was present in problem gamblers in high-risk bets [121], consistent with the fMRI study by Miedl et al. [108], in which higher responsivity to high-risk bets vs low-risk bets was found in reward-related brain circuitry. Thus, the evaluation of the height of the reward and the perception of the risk associated with the choice by problem gamblers versus healthy controls and discerning the evaluation of wins and losses both in the context of high-risk and low-risk situations are essential for the field to evaluate in which situations and how reward processes are affected in disordered gamblers.

In summary, abnormal reward and loss processing is present in both GD and SUDs, with diminished behavioral, psychophysiological, and neural responsiveness toward the experience of rewards and losses and in GD, whereas in SUDs, a higher neural responsiveness in striatal areas is present for reward outcomes. A similar diminished reward expectancy pattern is present in SUDs and GDs when a gambling-neutral context is present; however, when a gambling-relevant context is present, increased involvement of the striatal-limbic motivational circuit is seen in GD.

12.4.3.2 Cognitive Misperceptions and Near Misses

The existence of cognitive misperceptions is unique to disordered gambling and does not have its equivalent in SUDs. We refer to Chap. 4 on *Cognitive Distortions in Gambling Disorder* in this volume for a detailed review. Specifically, near misses have been associated with differences in its neurobiological mechanism in disordered gamblers versus non-problematic gamblers, and the presence of near misses affects gambling behavior of disordered gamblers differently than non-problematic gamblers.

Behavioral studies of near misses in gambling indicate that they are experienced as less pleasant than full wins but that they result in an increase in desire to gamble [15]. Importantly, in a study of gamblers differing in the level of problems they experienced, the propensity to continue gambling after near misses was predicted by skill-related cognitive misperceptions, indicating that there may be a link between the near misses (the experience that one is "almost there") and the development of cognitive misperceptions [122]. Psychophysiologically, more severe gambling problems are related to higher skin conductance responses and smaller interbeat interval changes in response to near misses compared to full losses or rewards [123]. In the brain, near-wins activate the same reward circuitry as is activated by real wins, but to a lesser extent. Studies indicate that the level of activation in the reward circuitry, elicited by near-wins, correlates with the urge to continue gambling, thus indicating that near-wins may play a role in the development of loss of control over gambling, due to the increase in gambling urges and activation of reward-related circuitry and thus may constitute a part of what makes gambling addictive [15]. Indeed, near misses elicit stronger responses in gamblers with a higher problem gambling severity [124, 125]. Finally, compared to controls, pathological gamblers show amplified striatal responses to near-miss outcomes, which was not influenced by dopamine antagonist (e.g., sulpiride [126]).

12.5 Novel Perspectives for Interventions in the Treatment of Gambling Disorders

Given the similarities between disordered gambling and SUDs, targeting novel intervention methods in disordered gambling that are being investigated in SUDS has high relevance. Recent reviews on SUDs and behavioral addictions discuss a potential development in addictive behaviors from impulsive behavior at the start of the disorder, toward compulsive-like behavior and underlying brain processes in the later stages of addictive behavior [127, 128]. When compulsivity in GD has similar neurobiological mechanisms to compulsive behaviors as present in obsessive-compulsive disorder, for instance, novel interventions could also be linked to novel developments in treatment for OCD, such as high dosage of SSRIs or clomipramine in GDs with high levels of compulsivity.

Besides cognitive behavioral and pharmacological interventions (see Chaps. 8 and 9 in this volume), recent developments in the treatment of SUDs concern neuromodulation interventions, ranging from cognitive training to repetitive transcranial neurostimulation rTMS), and maybe even deep brain stimulation for gambling disordered individuals who are highly compulsive. These novel interventions specifically target some of the neurobehavioral mechanisms that underlie both SUD and GD, for instance, by improving cognitive functions through improvement of dorsolateral prefrontal functioning, which may diminish impulsivity and craving. Alternatively, the presupplementary motor area may be a target for neuromodulation, as it has been related to diminished response inhibition in obsessive-compulsive disorder [129]. However, since there is a scarcity of studies investigating (underlying neural mechanisms of) response inhibition in GD, this topic needs to be further investigated before specific targets for neuromodulation in GD can be determined.

Neuromodulation may have broader effects than cognitive effects on the stimulated area of the dorsolateral prefrontal cortex. Indeed, a meta-analysis assessing the effect of neurostimulation such as repeated transcranial direct current stimulation (tDCS) and transcranial magnetic stimulation (rTMS) on the dorsolateral prefrontal cortex in reducing craving for substances or high-palatable food indicated a medium-effect size [130]. These neuromodulation interventions may also indirectly lead to improvement of treatment success, because of improvement in functions that are necessary for cognitive behavioral therapy. For instance, in developing skills to refuse gambling or developing a relapse prevention plan, planning and regulating of one's impulses is essential.

Cognitive training methods such as working memory training and attentional bias retraining have been investigated in SUDs. As for attentional bias retraining, which as the name indicates, focuses on diminishing the attentional bias for addiction relevant stimuli, mixed results are present: a recent meta-analysis indicates that cognitive bias modification has moderate effects on the presence of cognitive bias, but that effects on addiction outcomes are not present or limited to small-effect sizes for long-term effects [131]. Clearly, the field of cognitive training needs larger and more rigorous studies about the effects on cognitive bias and clinically relevant outcomes, including relapse and substance use. Related to the field of cognitive or attentional bias, retraining is the study on the effects of working memory training on craving. A recent study indicates that applying working memory training when experiencing craving reduces craving and relapse for substances [132]. For both neurostimulation and working memory training, studies in clinical groups that do not (only) focus on craving but on the effects on addictive behavior are scarce [133]. Regarding neurostimulation, some small studies have studied clinical effects of neurostimulation in SUDs. In a study with multiple sessions of rTMS, ten daily sessions of active rTMS over the DLPFC resulted in diminished cigarette use and levels of nicotine dependence compared to the placebo sham rTMS condition [134]. Although there is nascent evidence that rTMS could be effective in the reduction of craving and substance use in cocaine, nicotine, and alcohol use disorders, more adequately powered, rigorous, controlled efficacy studies are clearly needed. In summary, interventions with neurostimulation or cognitive training such as working memory training or attentional bias training in disordered gambling are also warranted given the similarities in vulnerability factors such as impulsivity, craving, and abnormalities in fronto-striatal brain functions in disordered gambling and SUDs (please also see Chap. 10 on *Innovative Treatment Approaches in Gambling Disorder*).

References

1. American Psychiatric Association. Diagnostic and statistical manual of mental disorders. 5th ed. Washington, DC: American Psychiatric Association; 2013.
2. Blaszczynski A, Nower L. A pathways model of problem and pathological gambling. Addiction. 2002;97(5):487–99.
3. Sharpe L. A reformulated cognitive-behavioral model of problem gambling. A biopsychosocial perspective. Clin Psychol Rev. 2002;22(1):1–25.
4. Goldstein RZ, Volkow ND. Drug addiction and its underlying neurobiological basis: neuroimaging evidence for the involvement of the frontal cortex. Am J Psychiatr. 2002;159(10):1642–52.
5. Raylu N, Oei TP. Role of culture in gambling and problem gambling. Clin Psychol Rev. 2004;23(8):1087–114.

6. Slutske WS, Eisen S, True WR, Lyons MJ, Goldberg J, Tsuang M. Common genetic vulnerability for pathological gambling and alcohol dependence in men. Arch Gen Psychiatry. 2000;57(7):666–73.
7. Slutske WS, Moffitt TE, Poulton R, Caspi A. Undercontrolled temperament at age 3 predicts disordered gambling at age 32: a longitudinal study of a complete birth cohort. Psychol Sci. 2012;23(5):510–6. 0956797611429708 [pii].
8. Vitaro F, Arseneault L, Tremblay RE. Dispositional predictors of problem gambling in male adolescents. Am J Psychiatr. 1997;154(12):1769–70.
9. Vitaro F, Arseneault L, Tremblay RE. Impulsivity predicts problem gambling in low SES adolescent males. Addiction. 1999;94(4):565–75.
10. Alvarez-Moya EM, Ochoa C, Jimenez-Murcia S, Aymami MN, Gomez-Pena M, Fernandez-Aranda F, et al. Effect of executive functioning, decision-making and self-reported impulsivity on the treatment outcome of pathologic gambling. J Psychiatry Neurosci. 2011;36(3):165–75.
11. Goudriaan AE, Oosterlaan J, de Beurs E, van den Brink W. The role of self-reported impulsivity and reward sensitivity versus neurocognitive measures of disinhibition and decision-making in the prediction of relapse in pathological gamblers. Psychol Med. 2008; 38(1):41–50.
12. Goudriaan AE, Oosterlaan J, de Beurs E, van den Brink W. Psychophysiological determinants and concomitants of deficient decision making in pathological gamblers. Drug Alcohol Depend. 2006;84(3):231–9.
13. Romanczuk-Seiferth N, Koehler S, Dreesen C, Wüstenberg T, Heinz A. Pathological gambling and alcohol dependence: neural disturbances in reward and loss avoidance processing. Addict Biol. 2015;20:557–69.
14. de Ruiter MB, Veltman DJ, Goudriaan AE, Oosterlaan J, Sjoerds Z, van den Brink W. Response perseveration and ventral prefrontal sensitivity to reward and punishment in male problem gamblers and smokers. Neuropsychopharmacology. 2009;34(4):1027–38. npp2008175 [pii].
15. Clark L, Lawrence AJ, Astley-Jones F, Gray N. Gambling near-misses enhance motivation to gamble and recruit win-related brain circuitry. Neuron. 2009;61(3):481–90. S0896-6273(09)00037-3 [pii]
16. Patton JH, Stanford MS, Barratt ES. Factor structure of the Barratt impulsiveness scale. J Clin Psychol. 1995;51(6):768–74.
17. Baumann AA, Odum AL. Impulsivity, risk taking, and timing. Behav Process. 2012;90(3):408–14.
18. Broos N, Schmaal L, Wiskerke J, Kostelijk L, Lam T, Stoop N, et al. The relationship between impulsive choice and impulsive action: a cross-species translational study. PLoS One. 2012;7(5):e36781.
19. Jentsch JD, Ashenhurst JR, Cervantes MC, Groman SM, James AS, Pennington ZT. Dissecting impulsivity and its relationships to drug addictions. Ann N Y Acad Sci. 2014;1327:1–26.
20. Whiteside SP, Lynam DR. Understanding the role of impulsivity and externalizing psychopathology in alcohol abuse: application of the UPPS impulsive behavior scale. Exp Clin Psychopharmacol. 2003;11(3):210–7.
21. Wilbertz T, Deserno L, Horstmann A, Neumann J, Villringer A, Heinze HJ, et al. Response inhibition and its relation to multidimensional impulsivity. Neuroimage. 2014;103:241–8.
22. Aichert DS, Wostmann NM, Costa A, Macare C, Wenig JR, Moller HJ, et al. Associations between trait impulsivity and prepotent response inhibition. J Clin Exp Neuropsychol. 2012;34(10):1016–32.
23. Fuentes D, Tavares H, Artes R, Gorenstein C. Self-reported and neuropsychological measures of impulsivity in pathological gambling. J Int Neuropsychol Soc. 2006;12(6):907–12. S1355617706061091 [pii].
24. Knezevic B, Ledgerwood DM. Gambling severity, impulsivity, and psychopathology: comparison of treatment- and community-recruited pathological gamblers. Am J Addict. 2012;21(6):508–15.

25. Kraplin A, Buhringer G, Oosterlaan J, van den Brink W, Goschke T, Goudriaan AE. Dimensions and disorder specificity of impulsivity in pathological gambling. Addict Behav. 2014;39(11):1646–51. S0306-4603(14)00170-1 [pii].

26. Petry NM. Substance abuse, pathological gambling, and impulsiveness. Drug Alcohol Depend. 2001;63(1):29–38.

27. Rodriguez-Jimenez R, Avila C, Jimenez-Arriero MA, Ponce G, Monasor R, Jimenez M, et al. Impulsivity and sustained attention in pathological gamblers: influence of childhood ADHD history. J Gambl Stud. 2006;22(4):451–61.

28. Albein-Urios N, Martinez-Gonzalez JM, Lozano O, Clark L, Verdejo-Garcia A. Comparison of impulsivity and working memory in cocaine addiction and pathological gambling: implications for cocaine-induced neurotoxicity. Drug Alcohol Depend. 2012;126(1–2):1–6.

29. Billieux J, Lagrange G, Van der Linden M, Lancon C, Adida M, Jeanningros R. Investigation of impulsivity in a sample of treatment-seeking pathological gamblers: a multidimensional perspective. Psychiatry Res. 2012;198(2):291–6.

30. Cyders MA, Smith GT. Clarifying the role of personality dispositions in risk for increased gambling behavior. Pers Individ Dif. 2008;45(6):503–8.

31. Grall-Bronnec M, Wainstein L, Feuillet F, Bouju G, Rocher B, Venisse JL, Sebille-Rivain V. Clinical profiles as a function of level and type of impulsivity in a sample group of at-risk and pathological gamblers seeking treatment. J Gambl Stud. 2012;28(2):239–52.

32. Michalczuk R, Bowden-Jones H, Verdejo-Garcia A, Clark L. Impulsivity and cognitive distortions in pathological gamblers attending the UK National Problem Gambling Clinic: a preliminary report. Psychol Med. 2011;41(12):2625–35. S003329171100095X [pii].

33. Berg JM, Latzman RD, Bliwise NG, Lilienfeld SO. Parsing the heterogeneity of impulsivity: a meta-analytic review of the behavioral implications of the UPPS for psychopathology. Psychol Assess. 2015;27(4):1129–46.

34. Littlefield AK, Stevens AK, Sher KJ. Impulsivity and alcohol involvement: multiple, distinct constructs and processes. Curr Addict Rep. 2014;1:33–40.

35. Stanford MS, Mathias CW, Dougherty DM, Lake SL, Anderson NE, Patton JH. Fifty years of the Barratt impulsiveness scale: an update and review. Personal Individ Differ. 2009;47:385–95.

36. Fillmore MT, Rush CR. Impaired inhibitory control of behavior in chronic cocaine users. Drug Alcohol Depend. 2002;66(3):265–73.

37. Hester R, Garavan H. Executive dysfunction in cocaine addiction: evidence for discordant frontal, cingulate, and cerebellar activity. J Neurosci. 2004;24(49):11017–22.

38. Kaufman JN, Ross TJ, Stein EA, Garavan H. Cingulate hypoactivity in cocaine users during a GO-NOGO task as revealed by event-related functional magnetic resonance imaging. J Neurosci. 2003;23(21):7839–43.

39. Moeller FG, Barratt ES, Fischer CJ, Dougherty DM, Reilly EL, Mathias CW, Swann AC. P300 event-related potential amplitude and impulsivity in cocaine-dependent subjects. Neuropsychobiology. 2004;50(2):167–73.

40. Verdejo-Garcia AJ, Perales JC, Perez-Garcia M. Cognitive impulsivity in cocaine and heroin polysubstance abusers. Addict Behav. 2007;32(5):950–66. S0306-4603(06)00216-4 [pii].

41. Clark L, Robbins TW, Ersche KD, Sahakian BJ. Reflection impulsivity in current and former substance users. Biol Psychiatry. 2006;60(5):515–22. S0006-3223(05)01397-1 [pii]

42. Ersche KD, Clark L, London M, Robbins TW, Sahakian BJ. Profile of executive and memory function associated with amphetamine and opiate dependence. Neuropsychopharmacology. 2006;31(5):1036–47. 1300889 [pii].

43. Gruber SA, Silveri MM, Yurgelun-Todd DA. Neuropsychological consequences of opiate use. Neuropsychol Rev. 2007;17(3):299–315.

44. Mintzer MZ, Stitzer ML. Cognitive impairment in methadone maintenance patients. Drug Alcohol Depend. 2002;67(1):41–51.

45. Bjork JM, Hommer DW, Grant SJ, Danube C. Impulsivity in abstinent alcohol-dependent patients: relation to control subjects and type 1-/type 2-like traits. Alcohol. 2004;34(2–3):133–50.

46. Goudriaan AE, Oosterlaan J, de Beurs E, van den Brink W. Neurocognitive functions in pathological gambling: a comparison with alcohol dependence, Tourette syndrome and normal controls. Addiction. 2006;101(4):534–47.
47. Kamarajan C, Porjesz B, Jones KA, Choi K, Chorlian DB, Padmanabhapillai A, et al. The role of brain oscillations as functional correlates of cognitive systems: a study of frontal inhibitory control in alcoholism. Int J Psychophysiol. 2004;51(2):155–80.
48. Morgan MJ. Recreational use of "ecstasy" (MDMA) is associated with elevated impulsivity. Neuropsychopharmacology. 1998;19(4):252–64. S0893-133X(98)00012-8 [pii].
49. Morgan MJ, Impallomeni LC, Pirona A, Rogers RD. Elevated impulsivity and impaired decision-making in abstinent ecstasy (MDMA) users compared to polydrug and drug-naive controls. Neuropsychopharmacology. 2006;31(7):1562–73. 1300953 [pii].
50. Quednow BB, Kuhn KU, Hoppe C, Westheide J, Maier W, Daum I, Wagner M. Elevated impulsivity and impaired decision-making cognition in heavy users of MDMA ("Ecstasy"). Psychopharmacology (Berl). 2007;189(4):517–30.
51. Monterosso JR, Aron AR, Cordova X, Xu J, London ED. Deficits in response inhibition associated with chronic methamphetamine abuse. Drug Alcohol Depend. 2005;79(2):273–7. S0376-8716(05)00060-8 [pii].
52. Salo R, Nordahl TE, Possin K, Leamon M, Gibson DR, Galloway GP, et al. Preliminary evidence of reduced cognitive inhibition in methamphetamine-dependent individuals. Psychiatry Res. 2002;111(1):65–74.
53. van der Plas EA, Crone EA, van den Wildenberg WP, Tranel D, Bechara A. Executive control deficits in substance-dependent individuals: a comparison of alcohol, cocaine, and methamphetamine and of men and women. J Clin Exp Neuropsychol. 2009;31(6):706–19. 906024863 [pii].
54. Colzato LS, van den Wildenberg WP, Hommel B. Impaired inhibitory control in recreational cocaine users. PLoS One. 2007;2(11):e1143.
55. Brand M, Roth-Bauer M, Driessen M, Markowitsch HJ. Executive functions and risky decision-making in patients with opiate dependence. Drug Alcohol Depend. 2008;97(1–2):64–72.
56. Pau CW, Lee TM, Chan SF. The impact of heroin on frontal executive functions. Arch Clin Neuropsychol. 2002;17(7):663–70.
57. Fernandez-Serrano MJ, Perez-Garcia M, Verdejo-Garcia A. What are the specific vs. generalized effects of drugs of abuse on neuropsychological performance? Neurosci Biobehav Rev. 2011;35(3):377–406. S0149-7634(10)00092-8 [pii].
58. Schulte MH, Cousijn J, den Uyl TE, Goudriaan AE, van den Brink W, Veltman DJ, et al. Recovery of neurocognitive functions following sustained abstinence after substance dependence and implications for treatment. Clin Psychol Rev. 2014;34(7):531–50. S0272-7358(14)00119-6 [pii].
59. Kertzman S, Lowengrub K, Aizer A, Vainder M, Kotler M, Dannon PN. Go-no-go performance in pathological gamblers. Psychiatry Res. 2008;161(1):1–10. S0165-1781(07)00210-7 [pii].
60. Kertzman S, Lowengrub K, Aizer A, Nahum ZB, Kotler M, Dannon PN. Stroop performance in pathological gamblers. Psychiatry Res. 2006;142(1):1–10. S0165-1781(05)00242-8 [pii].
61. Smith JL, Mattick RP, Jamadar SD, Iredale JM. Deficits in behavioural inhibition in substance abuse and addiction: a meta-analysis. Drug Alcohol Depend. 2014;145:1–33.
62. Joos L, Goudriaan AE, Schmaal L, Fransen E, van den Brink W, Sabbe BG, Dom G. Effect of modafinil on impulsivity and relapse in alcohol dependent patients: a randomized, placebo-controlled trial. Eur Neuropsychopharmacol. S0924-977X(12)00283-0 [pii]. 2012.
63. Zack M, Poulos CX. Effects of the atypical stimulant modafinil on a brief gambling episode in pathological gamblers with high vs. low impulsivity. J Psychopharmacol. 2009;23(6):660–71. 0269881108091072 [pii].
64. Luijten M, Machielsen MW, Veltman DJ, Hester R, de Haan L, Franken IH. Systematic review of ERP and fMRI studies investigating inhibitory control and error processing in people with substance dependence and behavioural addictions. J Psychiatry Neurosci. 2014;39(3):149–69.

65. Amlung M, Vedelago L, Acker J, Balodis I, MacKillop J. Steep delay discounting and addictive behavior: a meta-analysis of continuous associations. Addiction. 2017;112(1):51–62.

66. Petry NM. Delay discounting of money and alcohol in actively using alcoholics, currently abstinent alcoholics, and controls. Psychopharmacology. 2001;154(3):243–50.

67. Kirby KN, Petry NM, Bickel WK. Heroin addicts have higher discount rates for delayed rewards than nondrug-using controls. J Exp Psychol Gen. 1999;128:78–87.

68. Kirby KN, Petry NM. Heroin and cocaine abusers have higher discount rates for delayed rewards than alcoholics or non-drug-using controls. Addiction. 2004;99:461–71.

69. Dom G, De WB, Hulstijn W, van den Brink W, Sabbe B. Behavioural aspects of impulsivity in alcoholics with and without a cluster-B personality disorder. Alcohol Alcohol. 2006;41(4):412–20. agl030 [pii].

70. Petry NM. Discounting of delayed rewards in substance abusers: relationship to antisocial personality disorder. Psychopharmacology (Berl). 2002;162(4):425–32.

71. Dixon MR, Marley J, Jacobs EA. Delay discounting by pathological gamblers. J Appl Behav Anal. 2003;36(4):449–58.

72. Miedl SF, Buchel C, Peters J. Cue-induced craving increases impulsivity via changes in striatal value signals in problem gamblers. J Neurosci. 2014;34(13):4750–5.

73. Bechara A, Damasio H. Decision-making and addiction (part I): impaired activation of somatic states in substance dependent individuals when pondering decisions with negative future consequences. Neuropsychologia. 2002;40(10):1675–89.

74. Bechara A, Martin EM. Impaired decision making related to working memory deficits in individuals with substance addictions. Neuropsychology. 2004;18(1):152–62.

75. Dom G, De WB, Hulstijn W, van den Brink W, Sabbe B. Decision-making deficits in alcohol-dependent patients with and without comorbid personality disorder. Alcohol Clin Exp Res. 2006;30(10):1670–7. ACER202 [pii].

76. Ernst M, Grant SJ, London ED, Contoreggi CS, Kimes AS, Spurgeon L. Decision making in adolescents with behavior disorders and adults with substance abuse. Am J Psychiatr. 2003;160(1):33–40.

77. Ersche KD, Fletcher PC, Lewis SJ, Clark L, Stocks-Gee G, London M, et al. Abnormal frontal activations related to decision-making in current and former amphetamine and opiate dependent individuals. Psychopharmacology (Berl). 2005;180(4):612–23.

78. Rotherham-Fuller E, Shoptaw S, Berman SM, London ED. Impaired performance in a test of decision-making by opiate-dependent tobacco smokers. Drug Alcohol Depend. 2004;73(1):79–86.

79. Whitlow CT, Liguori A, Livengood LB, Hart SL, Mussat-Whitlow BJ, Lamborn CM, et al. Long-term heavy marijuana users make costly decisions on a gambling task. Drug Alcohol Depend. 2004;76(1):107–11.

80. Dom G, Sabbe B, Hulstijn W, van den BW. Substance use disorders and the orbitofrontal cortex: systematic review of behavioural decision-making and neuroimaging studies. Br J Psychiatry. 2005;187:209–20.

81. Goudriaan AE, Oosterlaan J, de Beurs E, van den Brink W. Decision making in pathological gambling: a comparison between pathological gamblers, alcohol dependents, persons with Tourette syndrome, and normal controls. Brain Res Cogn Brain Res. 2005;23(1):137–51.

82. Biernacki K, McLennan SN, Terrett G, Labuschagne I, Rendell PG. Decision-making ability in current and past users of opiates: a meta-analysis. Neurosci Biobehav Rev. 2016;71:342–51.

83. Brand M, Kalbe E, Labudda K, Fujiwara E, Kessler J, Markowitsch HJ. Decision-making impairments in patients with pathological gambling. Psychiatry Res. 2005;133(1):91–9.

84. Cavedini P, Riboldi G, Keller R, D'Annucci A, Bellodi L. Frontal lobe dysfunction in pathological gambling patients. Biol Psychiatry. 2002;51(4):334–41.

85. Ashrafioun L, Rosenberg H, Cross NA, Brian TJ. Further evaluation of the construct, convergent and criterion validity of the Gambling Urge Scale with university-student gamblers. Am J Drug Alcohol Abuse. 2013;39(5):326–31.

86. Young MM, Wohl MJ. The gambling craving scale: psychometric validation and behavioral outcomes. Psychol Addict Behav. 2009;23(3):512–22.

87. Ashrafioun L, Rosenberg H. Methods of assessing craving to gamble: a narrative review. Psychol Addict Behav. 2012;26(3):536–49.
88. Courtney KE, Schacht JP, Hutchison K, Roche DJ, Ray LA. Neural substrates of cue reactivity: association with treatment outcomes and relapse. Addict Biol. 2016;21(1):3–22.
89. Kuhn S, Gallinat J. Common biology of craving across legal and illegal drugs – a quantitative meta-analysis of cue-reactivity brain response. Eur J Neurosci. 2011;33(7):1318–26.
90. Noori HR, Cosa Linan A, Spanagel R. Largely overlapping neuronal substrates of reactivity to drug, gambling, food and sexual cues: a comprehensive meta-analysis. Eur Neuropsychopharmacol. 2016;26(9):1419–30.
91. Crockford DN, Goodyear B, Edwards J, Quickfall J, el-Guebaly N. Cue-induced brain activity in pathological gamblers. Biol Psychiatry. 2005;58(10):787–95.
92. Goudriaan AE, de Ruiter MB, van den Brink W, Oosterlaan J, Veltman DJ. Brain activation patterns associated with cue reactivity and craving in abstinent problem gamblers, heavy smokers, and healthy controls: an fMRI study. Addict Biol. 2010;15(4):491–503.
93. Limbrick-Oldfield EH, Mick I, Cocks RE, McGonigle J, Sharman SP, Goldstone AP, Stokes PR, Waldman A, Erritzoe D, Bowden-Jones H, Nutt D, Lingford-Hughes A, Clark L. Neural substrates of cue reactivity and craving in gambling disorder. Transl Psychiatry. 2017;7:e992.
94. van Holst RJ, van der Meer JN, McLaren DG, van den Brink W, Veltman DJ, Goudriaan AE. Interactions between affective and cognitive processing systems in problematic gamblers: a functional connectivity study. PLoS One. 2012;7(11):e49923.
95. Cox WM, Fadardi JS, Pothos EM. The addiction-stroop test: theoretical considerations and procedural recommendations. Psychol Bull. 2006;132(3):443–76. 2006-06233-005 [pii].
96. Loeber S, Vollstadt-Klein S, von der Goltz C, Flor H, Mann K, Kiefer F. Attentional bias in alcohol-dependent patients: the role of chronicity and executive functioning. Addict Biol. 2009;14(2):194–203. ADB146 [pii].
97. Lubman DI, Peters LA, Mogg K, Bradley BP, Deakin JF. Attentional bias for drug cues in opiate dependence. Psychol Med. 2000;30(1):169–75.
98. Sinclair JM, Nausheen B, Garner MJ, Baldwin DS. Attentional biases in clinical populations with alcohol use disorders: is co-morbidity ignored? Hum Psychopharmacol. 2010;25(7–8):515–24.
99. Townshend JM, Duka T. Attentional bias associated with alcohol cues: differences between heavy and occasional social drinkers. Psychopharmacology. 2001;157(1):67–74.
100. Weinstein A, Cox WM. Cognitive processing of drug-related stimuli: the role of memory and attention. J Psychopharmacol. 2006;20(6):850–9. 0269881106061116 [pii].
101. Constantinou N, Morgan CJ, Battistella S, O'Ryan D, Davis P, Curran HV. Attentional bias, inhibitory control and acute stress in current and former opiate addicts. Drug Alcohol Depend. 2010;109(1–3):220–5. S0376-8716(10)00040-2 [pii].
102. Townshend JM, Duka T. Avoidance of alcohol-related stimuli in alcohol-dependent inpatients. Alcohol Clin Exp Res. 2007;31(8):1349–57. ACER429 [pii].
103. Vollstadt-Klein S, Loeber S, von der Goltz C, Mann K, Kiefer F. Avoidance of alcohol-related stimuli increases during the early stage of abstinence in alcohol-dependent patients. Alcohol Alcohol. 2009;44(5):458–63. agp056 [pii].
104. McCusker CG, Gettings B. Automaticity of cognitive biases in addictive behaviours: further evidence with gamblers. Br J Clin Psychol. 1997;36(Pt 4):543–54.
105. Boyer M, Dickerson M. Attentional bias and addictive behaviour: automaticity in a gambling-specific modified Stroop task. Addiction. 2003;98(1):61–70.
106. Ciccarelli M, Nigro G, Griffiths MD, Cosenza M, D'Olimpio F. Attentional biases in problem and non-problem gamblers. J Affect Disord. 2016;198:135–41.
107. Ciccarelli M, Nigro G, Griffiths MD, Cosenza M, D'Olimpio F. Attentional bias in non-problem gamblers, problem gamblers, and abstinent pathological gamblers: an experimental study. J Affect Disord. 2016;206:9–16.
108. Miedl SF, Fehr T, Meyer G, Herrmann M. Neurobiological correlates of problem gambling in a quasi-realistic blackjack scenario as revealed by fMRI. Psychiatry Res. 2010;181(3):165–73. S0925-4927(09)00277-7 [pii].

109. van Holst RJ, Veltman DJ, Buchel C, van den Brink W, Goudriaan AE. Distorted expectancy coding in problem gambling: is the addictive in the anticipation? Biol Psychiatry. 2012;71(8):741–8. S0006-3223(12)00056-X [pii].

110. Knutson B, Adams CM, Fong GW, Hommer D. Anticipation of increasing monetary reward selectively recruits nucleus accumbens. J Neurosci. 2001;21(16):RC159.

111. Knutson B, Fong GW, Bennett SM, Adams CM, Hommer D. A region of mesial prefrontal cortex tracks monetarily rewarding outcomes: characterization with rapid event-related fMRI. NeuroImage. 2003;18(2):263–72.

112. Goodie AS. The role of perceived control and overconfidence in pathological gambling. J Gambl Stud. 2005;21:481–502.

113. Reuter J, Raedler T, Rose M, Hand I, Glascher J, Buchel C. Pathological gambling is linked to reduced activation of the mesolimbic reward system. Nat Neurosci. 2005;8(2):147–8.

114. Tanabe J, Thompson L, Claus E, Dalwani M, Hutchison K, Banich MT. Prefrontal cortex activity is reduced in gambling and nongambling substance users during decision-making. Hum Brain Mapp. 2007;28(12):1276–86.

115. Luijten M, Schellekens AF, Kuhn S, Machielse MW, Sescousse G. Disruption of reward processing in addiction : an image-based meta-analysis of functional magnetic resonance imaging studies. JAMA Psychiatry. 2017.

116. Brevers D, Noel X, He Q, Melrose JA, Bechara A. Increased ventral-striatal activity during monetary decision making is a marker of problem poker gambling severity. Addict Biol. 2016;21(3):688–99.

117. Worhunsky PD, Malison RT, Rogers RD, Potenza MN. Altered neural correlates of reward and loss processing during simulated slot-machine fMRI in pathological gambling and cocaine dependence. Drug Alcohol Depend. 2014;145:77–86.

118. Miedl SF, Fehr T, Herrmann M, Meyer G. Risk assessment and reward processing in problem gambling investigated by event-related potentials and fMRI-constrained source analysis. BMC Psychiatry. 2014;14:229.

119. Balodis IM, Kober H, Worhunsky PD, Stevens MC, Pearlson GD, Potenza MN. Diminished frontostriatal activity during processing of monetary rewards and losses in pathological gambling. Biol Psychiatry. 2012;71(8):749–57.

120. Choi JS, Shin YC, Jung WH, Jang JH, Kang DH, Choi CH, et al. Altered brain activity during reward anticipation in pathological gambling and obsessive-compulsive disorder. PLoS One. 2012;7(9):e45938.

121. Hewig J, Kretschmer N, Trippe RH, Hecht H, Coles MG, Holroyd CB, Miltner WH. Hypersensitivity to reward in problem gamblers. Biol Psychiatry. 2010;67(8):781–3. S0006-3223(09)01346-8 [pii].

122. Billieux J, Van der Linden M, Khazaal Y, Zullino D, Clark L. Trait gambling cognitions predict near-miss experiences and persistence in laboratory slot machine gambling. Br J Psychol. 2012;103(3):412–27.

123. Ulrich N, Ambach W, Hewig J. Severity of gambling problems modulates autonomic reactions to near outcomes in gambling. Biol Psychol. 2016;119:11–20.

124. Chase HW, Clark L. Gambling severity predicts midbrain response to near-miss outcomes. J Neurosci. 2010;30(18):6180–7.

125. van Holst RJ, Chase HW, Clark L. Striatal connectivity changes following gambling wins and near-misses: associations with gambling severity. Neuroimage Clin. 2014;5:232–9.

126. Sescousse G, Janssen LK, Hashemi MM, Timmer MH, Geurts DE, Ter Huurne NP, Clark L, Cools R. Amplified striatal responses to near-miss outcomes in pathological gamblers. Neuropsychopharmacology. 2016;41:2614–23.

127. Fauth-Buhler M, Mann K, Potenza MN. Pathological gambling: a review of the neurobiological evidence relevant for its classification as an addictive disorder. Addict Biol. 2016.

128. Figee M, Pattij T, Willuhn I, Luigjes J, van den Brink W, Goudriaan A, et al. Compulsivity in obsessive-compulsive disorder and addictions. Eur Neuropsychopharmacol. 2016;26(5):856–68.

129. de Wit SJ, de Vries FE, van der Werf YD, Cath DC, Heslenfeld DJ, Veltman EM, et al. Presupplementary motor area hyperactivity during response inhibition: a candidate endophenotype of obsessive-compulsive disorder. Am J Psychiatry. 2012;169(10):1100–8.
130. Jansen JM, Daams J, Koeter MW, Veltman DJ, van den Brink W, Goudriaan AE. Effects of non-invasive neuro-stimulation on craving: a meta-analysis. Neurosci Biobehav Rev. 2013;37(10):2472–80.
131. Cristea IA, Kok RN, Cuijpers P. The effectiveness of cognitive bias modification interventions for substance addictions: a meta-analysis. PLoS One. 2016;11(9):e0162226.
132. Skorka-Brown J, Andrade J, Whalley B, May J. Playing Tetris decreases drug and other cravings in real world settings. Addict Behav. 2015;51:165–70.
133. Salling MC, Martinez D. Brain stimulation in addiction. Neuropsychopharmacology. 2016;41(12):2798–809.
134. Amiaz R, Levy D, Vainiger D, Grunhaus L, Zangen A. Repeated high-frequency transcranial magnetic stimulation over the dorsolateral prefrontal cortex reduces cigarette craving and consumption. Addiction. 2009;104(4):653–60.

Roles of Culture in Gambling and Gambling Disorder

13

T. P. S. Oei, N. Raylu, and J. M. Y. Loo

13.1 Introduction

Gambling behaviour existed at the beginning of human civilisation and is widely engaged by individuals from different cultures and geographical locations worldwide. Furthermore, gambling acceptability and participation rates varies significantly among culturally and linguistically diverse (CALD) groups [1]. Problem gambling (PG) occurs when an individual's gambling is at a stage that it begins causing personal, interpersonal, legal and social difficulties [2]. The extent and nature of problematic gambling also appears to vary from one CALD group to the next [3, 4].

The heterogeneous nature of problem gamblers (PGs) in the development and maintenance of gambling depends on complex interactions between a number of variables (e.g. cognitive, personality, genetical, familial, psychological, biological, environmental and sociological factors), and these interactions vary from person to person [5, 6]. Individuals within a particular CALD group often have similarities in some of these factors (e.g. familial and environmental factors). For example, since

T. P. S. Oei (✉)
School of Psychology, The University of Queensland, St Lucia, QLD, Australia

CBT Unit, Toowong Private Hospital, Toowong, QLD, Australia

James Cook University, Singapore, Singapore
e-mail: oei@psy.uq.edu.au

N. Raylu
School of Psychology, The University of Queensland, St Lucia, QLD, Australia

J. M. Y. Loo
Jeffrey Cheah School of Medicine and Health Sciences, Monash University Malaysia, Bandar Sunway, Selangor Darul Ehsan, Malaysia

Research Department, The Salvation Army—Sydney Headquarters, Sydney, NSW, Australia
e-mail: jasmine.loo@monash.edu

© Springer Nature Switzerland AG 2019
A. Heinz et al. (eds.), *Gambling Disorder*, https://doi.org/10.1007/978-3-030-03060-5_13

social gambling is a common form of leisure activity among the Chinese [7], there is often high exposure to gambling for individuals in this group. Thus, differences in gambling and PG behaviour are not restricted to impacts of gambling accessibility and advertisements, but also to the milieu of a particular CALD group [1]. Some CALD groups are more likely to report lower social economic status and income levels and higher unemployment rates [8], all of which have been linked to increased risk of PG [9].

All of these above factors, however, cannot fully account for the differences in gambling and PG found among different CALD groups. This is supported by empirical studies that showed that high rates of PG among CALD individuals with a migration background could not be fully explained by demographic factors or preferred gambling form (e.g. [10]). Thus, there is a need to consider cultural specific variables to further examine these differences such as the meaning, role or purpose of gambling in different cultures that influence variations in gambling behaviours (i.e. forms of gambling chosen or gender distribution in gambling) and prevalence rates among different CALD groups [1, 4].

Due to factors such as immigration, the population in most Western countries are becoming more heterogeneous in nature [11, 12]. Inconsistencies are evident between PG rates and treatment-seeking rates among certain CALD groups, whereby certain groups including ethnic minority and indigenous gamblers were less likely to seek treatment for PG [13–15] and seek treatment as a last resort [16, 17]. An individual's cultural identity affects not only their gambling behaviours but also the likelihood they will seek treatment if their gambling gets out of control [1]. Better understanding of the prevalence of gambling and PG among various CALD groups as well as the cultural factors that may impact gambling could help provide adequate information on how to attract CALD PGs to treatment and improve future development of both prevention and intervention programmes.

We attempted to discuss the differences in prevalence rates among different CALD groups as well as the cultural variables that may play a role in the development and maintenance of gambling in our earlier paper [1]. At that stage very little was published in this area leading to inferences made from substance abuse literature to inform discussions on cultural variables that may impact gambling behaviour. As there is significant growth in research on cultural aspects of PG since then, the aim of this chapter is to expand and update our earlier review and (a) to discuss the gambling and PG rates among various CALD groups, (b) to provide an overview of the cultural variables that may play a role in the development and/or maintenance of PG, (c) to discuss implications of these findings in relation to the prevention and treatment of CALD PGs and (d) to take a critical look at the roles of culture in gambling.

A number of definitions have been used in the literature to indicate problematic gambling. For this chapter, the term "gambling disorder (GD)" will indicate excessive gambling behaviour that meet the diagnostic criteria in DSM-5. The term "problem gambling (PG)" will indicate subthreshold recurrent gambling behaviour with associated gambling-related problems, regardless of whether or not they meet any diagnostic criteria for GD. Culture will be defined as collective attitudes, practices, traditions, customs, laws and beliefs that are passed from one generation to the next via language, artefacts, rituals, myths, arts, texts and discourse modes of a group of individuals (i.e. [18]). A "culturally and linguistically diverse (CALD)" group is defined as a group of individuals who migrated from or had ancestors that migrated from a non-speaking English country or a group who may not have a migration history but are non-English multilinguists with different cultural norms and values. Thus, this includes aboriginal groups, which Breen and Gainsbury [4] identified as "first Nations, Indigenous or Aboriginal peoples who originate from or identify with a particular nation and who have deep abiding connections to their lands and ancestral culture" (p. 77). There are acknowledged challenges in defining these cultural terms comprehensively in an inclusive manner, and future improvements are imperative. Meanwhile, consistent with past research, these definitions will guide our discussions here.

In order to complete this article, relevant databases (e.g. PsycINFO, Social Science database, Humanities and Social Science collection, Health and Society database, Sociological Abstracts and Google Scholar) from 1975 to 2016 were searched using terms such as addiction, gambling, culture, ethnicity, race, prevalence and treatment. Online searches were also conducted using these words to access any other academically grounded published articles, government reports and conference papers.

13.2 Rates of Gambling and PG Among Different Cultural Groups

The studies published that explore the prevalence of gambling and PG among different CALD groups in Western countries are regarded as either aboriginal groups or ethnic minorities that have a migration background (in their own or ancestral background).

13.2.1 Aboriginal Groups

Studies on Native Americans (e.g. American Indians and Native Alaskans) have either reported no difference in lifetime [19] and past-year [20, 21] gambling rates or reported higher lifetime [22] and past-year [23] gambling rates between North American Aborigines compared to Caucasians or non-aboriginal samples. Although there is variation in GD rates, there is strong evidence that there is higher lifetime and current GD rates for this group using a range of measuring instruments and cut-offs compared to Caucasians or non-aboriginal groups (e.g. [24–26]). Williams et al. [27] reported that North American Aborigines tend to participate in more types of gambling than non-Aborigine groups. More recent studies suggest that Aborigines in North America are about 2–3 times more likely to develop gambling problems than Caucasians or non-aboriginal populations [20, 23, 27].

A number of studies with Native American adolescents have also supported high PG rates among this group compared to non-Native American adolescents

([28–31]). Studies have showed lifetime gambling among Native American adolescents to be 80–90% [32, 33]. Zitzow [30] reported that gambling among Native American adolescents not only commenced at an earlier age than Caucasians, they also had a greater participation in gambling.

Comparative studies of Native Americans with other CALD groups also exist. Westermeyer et al. [22] reported that the lifetime GD prevalence rate of Native American veterans (9.9%) was twice as high as Hispanic veterans (4.3%). Kong et al. [26] reported that Native Americans were less likely to admit to gambling five or less times per year in their lifetime (66.5%) compared to Caucasians (70.5%), African Americans (72.8%) and other racial/ethnic groups (72.3%) but more likely (30.1%) to score 0–2 on the DSM-IV criteria [34], compared to Caucasians (26.5%), African Americans (23.4%) and other racial/ethnic groups (24.7%). Although Native American GD rates were almost twice of Hispanics and Caucasians, they were similar to Asians and African Americans [35].

Research on indigenous groups from other countries (including Australia and New Zealand) are less in quantity. Nevertheless, they have presented similar findings as the North American studies where there are mixed findings in relation to gambling rates but higher GD rates compared to Caucasians or the general Western population. High rates of PG/GD have also being reported among Maoris in New Zealand [36, 37], where there is some evidence that although Maoris are less likely to gamble than the general population, they are more likely to experience gambling problems [4, 38, 39]. However, Volberg and Abbott [19] reported a non-significant difference in lifetime gambling rates but engagement in a higher number of gambling activities weekly and larger monthly amount spent on gambling among Maoris compared to Caucasians in New Zealand. They also reported that both the lifetime and past-year rates of GD were higher among Maoris (8.7% and 4.6%, respectively) compared to Caucasians (3% and 1.4%, respectively). Maoris also tend to engage in more types of gambling than the general population [39].

Indigenous Australians were more likely (80%) to engage in commercial gambling activities (especially gambling machines) compared to the general population, 64% [40, 41]. Stevens and Young [42] reported a GD rate of 13.5% among Aborigines in Australia based on one question on gambling in a health survey. Hing et al. [15] sampled Aborigines in Australia using PG Severity Index (PGSI [43]) to measure extent of GD and categorised 12.5% as low risk, 16.6% as moderate risk and 19.5% as PGs.

13.2.2 Ethnic Minorities with a Migration Background

Research from a number of countries including America, Canada, Australia, New Zealand and Sweden have reported higher rates of GD (lifetime or past year) among ethnic minorities with a migration background (i.e. those who themselves migrated or had ancestors that migrated from another country) [3, 21, 44–46]. Based on the US National Epidemiologic Survey on Alcohol and Related Conditions (NESARC) data, Alegria et al. [35] reported that the lifetime GD rates of groups with a migration history (Asians, 2.3%; African Americans, 2.2%) were twice that of Caucasians (1.2%) but similar to Native Americans (2.3%). Barry et al. [47] reported African Americans (0.96%) were more likely to report GD (5 or more on DSM-IV) than Caucasians (0.45%). Welte et al. [48] explored telephone survey data of individuals 14+ age and reported that Asians and African Americans were less likely to report gambling in the past year (66% and 67%, respectively) compared to Native Americans (83%), Caucasians (77%) and Hispanics (76%). However, all ethnic minority groups (African Americans, 5.5%; Hispanics, 4.6%; Asians, 5.3%), including Native Americans (5.4%), reported higher PG rates (using 3 or more past-year criteria threshold on DSM-IV) than Caucasians (1.9%).

Similar findings were reported for ethnic minority students/adolescents in a number of North American studies. Barnes et al. [49] conducted a phone survey of US residents aged 14–21 years using randomised sampling procedures and reported that African American youth were less likely to gamble in the past year (60%) compared to Hispanics (71%) and Caucasians (70%), but more likely to report having gambled 52 or more times in the past year (African Americans, 24%; Caucasians, 15%; and Hispanics, 21%). Welte et al. [50] explored past-year prevalence among the youth in a random phone study using the SOGS-RA [51] and found Asians (48%), mixed/unknown (45%) and African Americans (60%) were less likely to report having gambled than Caucasians (70%), Hispanics (71%) and Native Americans (83%). No significant difference in at-risk gambling (2 or more on SOGS-RA) or GD (4 or more on SOGS-RA) were found, but African Americans (18%) and Native Americans (28%) were more likely to report frequent gambling (on average two times or more per week) than other groups.

The above studies on adolescent and adult North American studies show that there are variations in which CALD group report higher rates. There are also variations in the results for certain CALD groups (e.g. the Hispanics/Latino). Alegria et al.'s [35] study showed no difference in lifetime GD prevalence rates between Latinos (1.0%) and Caucasians (1.2%). On the other hand, Barry et al. [52] evaluated the most recent NESARC data and reported that those that identified themselves as Hispanic (0.38%) reported lower rates of past-year GD compared to those that identified themselves as Caucasians (0.45%). In contrast to both of these findings, Welte et al. [21] reported past GD (5 or more on the SOGS-R [53]) rate was highest for Native Americans (5.3%), followed by Hispanics (4.2%), African Americans (3.7%), Caucasians (0.5%) and then Asians (0%). The limited studies that explored the GD rates among Hispanics/Latinos have produced varying results depending on the time frame used to assess problematic gambling (i.e. lifetime vs. past year) and sample characteristics [3, 52].

Studies in other countries have mirrored these findings in North America. A number of studies have reported higher GD rates among Pacific Islanders in New Zealand [37–39]. Some studies have reported that similar to Maoris in New Zealand, although Pacific Islanders in New Zealand are less likely to gamble, those that gamble are more likely to develop gambling problems [38, 39] with rates four times that of the general population for these two groups [4]. In another New Zealand study, Abbott and Volberg [54] reported that individuals that identified themselves as

Maori or Chinese were at high risk of developing gambling problems. In a lifestyle survey using the PGSI, GD rates among the CALD groups were found to be higher (Maori, 2.7%; Asians, 2.4%; Pacific Islanders, 0.6%) than Caucasians, 0.2% [55] in New Zealand. In an Australian study, the Victorian Casino and Gaming Authority [56] investigated gambling among those that spoke Chinese, Vietnamese, Arabic or Greek. They reported that although the gambling rates among the four groups were less than that of the general population, GD (SOGS score of 5 or more) rates for all four cultural groups were 5–7 times higher than the general community. Dickins and Thomas [57] review of gambling and PG among Australian CALD groups highlighted the lack of recent research in this area in Australia. They, however, stated that although CALD group may gamble less, they may be at greater risk of developing PG than Caucasians due to migration variables/stress, stigma/shame-related factors as well as variances in beliefs about luck and chance. A number of studies in Sweden also report being higher risk of PG among those who themselves migrated or had ancestors that migrated from another country [44, 58].

There has been significant research on Asian (especially Chinese) gambling and PG over the last decade [7, 59]. A number of studies conducted in Western countries using different measuring instruments have found higher rates of GD among Asians (research predominantly done on Chinese samples or by combining a number of CALD groups including Korean, Chinese, Cambodians, Vietnamese, Filipino, Japanese, Indian and/or Thai) compared to Caucasians or general population for both adults [7, 56, 60, 61] and student/youth samples [62–64]. Loo et al. [7] review of gambling and PG among the Chinese in a number of countries (including China, Macao, Australia, New Zealand, Canada and America) reported past-year GD prevalence rate of 2.5–4%. Some researchers have reported that although Asian youth are less likely to report gambling or have similar gambling rates compared to the general population or Caucasians, when they do gamble, they are more likely to report PG/GD [65–67].

Few studies have tried exploring rates for Asian groups other than Chinese. Petry et al. [68] assessed gambling prevalence among three South East Asian (Laos, Cambodia and Vietnam) refugees in America using a convenience sample and the SOGS and found that although lifetime rates were similar for the three countries, they were 10–25 times higher than the general population. Marshall et al. [69] reported a 10.4% and 3.5% lifetime GD prevalence rate among a probability sample (rather than a convenience one) of Cambodian refugees in America using a cut-off score of 5 or more and a score of 3–4 on the SOGS, respectively.

The GD rates reported in Asian countries show variability. Some studies from Hong Kong, Macao and Singapore have found adult GD rates higher than rates of Caucasians in Western countries [46, 70–72]. However, studies done in South Korea have shown very low lifetime [73] and past-year [74] rates of around 0.5–0.8%. Williams et al. [74] study also reported a low rate of past-year gambling of 41.8%. They stated this low rate of gambling and GD among South Koreans were probably due to low engagement in gambling by women in the country and overall negative viewpoint about gambling and limited access to gambling [74]. Liu et al. [75] reviewed studies in Asian countries assessing gambling and PG among the youth and reported there were significant differences in methodology between the studies from countries such as Singapore, Hong Kong, South Korea, Macau and Thailand. They stated that in these Asian countries, the youth gambling involvement rates varied between 32% and 60%, the PG problem rates varied between 1.5% and 5.0% and the GD rates varied between 0.07% and 2.66%. By highlighting the findings of Shaffer and Hall [76] meta-analyses study that showed that 10–15% of North American youth report at-risk gambling and 4–8% report GD, they stated that adolescent rates in Asian countries were less than rates found among North American adolescents.

13.2.3 Discussion and Summary of CALD Gambling and GD Prevalence Studies

Over the last decade although there have been significantly more published data on the prevalence of gambling and GD among various CALD groups, studies for various CALD populations are disproportionately represented. The above discussion also clearly shows there are significant methodological variations in these studies including variations in instruments, timeframe (lifetime vs. past-year gambling), cut-offs and data collection method (e.g. face-to-face vs. telephone administration, oversampling vs. randomised vs. survey, etc.) that influence reported rates [1, 46].

Besides these variations, there are a number of limitations in these studies. First, many assessment tools used are not normed for various CALD groups [77]. Second, measuring tools used are often translated and back translated, and there can be significant differences between the two versions. Third, a number of studies have categorised individuals into global categories (e.g. Caucasian vs. non-Caucasian or Hispanics, Asians, Pacific Islanders) without recognising that these global groups consist of many different subgroups [78]. Furthermore, there are also individuals from mixed cultural groups. Fourth, most of these studies do not distinguish origin of migrants [1]. Studies such as Blaszczynski et al. [60] have reported that those with a prior gambling history in the country they originated from are more likely to report PG. Finally, a large number of these studies used data based on self-reports, had small sample sizes and used non-random sampling procedures [79].

These methodological variations and limitations have led to variations in rates for same CALD groups from study to study. In spite of this, these studies generally show mixed findings in relation to the gambling rate but report higher GD rates among CALD populations compared to Caucasians or the general population. To better understand these cultural differences, it is important to evaluate specific cultural variables that could play a role in initiating and maintaining gambling, and this is discussed next.

13.3 Cultural Factors Implicated in the Development, Maintenance and Treatment of GD

Conceptualisations of cultural factors associated with GD can be examined through diverse viewpoints—personal, ethnic, societal, institutional and national cultures— that interact and co-exist together to impact cognitions and behavioural responses.

In the development and maintenance of GD behaviour, the individual is an active participant who executes a specific position within a cultural context, predetermined either by ethnic or societal norms, and national culture [80, 81]. These processes encompass a complex interaction of individual differences and mechanisms underlying gambling behaviour such as gambling urges, cognitions and psychological states [82–84], all of which are enacted within cultural norms. These perspectives will form the basis of discussions in subsequent sections in consideration of the impact of culture in an increasingly globalised environment.

13.3.1 Cultural Values and Beliefs in an Increasingly Globalised Environment

Although gambling activities are evident in most countries and cultural contexts, there are differential culturally mediated risks and protective factors that may increase or decrease GD propensity [3]. Cultural values and beliefs when passed on through familial means from one generation to another [1], through the mediation of cultural and sociodemographic contexts, can impact on decision-making processes and gambling behaviour. Research conducted on CALD populations residing in predominantly Western cultural contexts such as Iranians [45], Native Americans [20], Indigenous Australians [15, 40] and Asians [16, 85–88] have consistently reported differences in gambling motivations, cognitions, game preferences, presenting problems and help-seeking attitudes when compared between cultural groups. For instance, experimental investigations with a coin-toss task showed that Asian-Canadians were more susceptible to the gambler's fallacy (the belief that a win will follow after a series of losses), while Euro-Canadians are more susceptible to the "hot-hand fallacy" (belief that a winning streak will continue), which suggest cultural differences in gambling cognitions and decision-making processes [89]. These differences in the course of gambling development and personal antecedents were also evident among older adults [90]. Collectively, these findings have sparked an interest in further investigations to examine cross-cultural differences (or similarities) in the development of GD to continuously improve prevention and treatment efforts.

Meanwhile, findings reported in relation to CALD populations residing in ethnically matched cultural contexts or countries, though mainly Asian countries, suggested some similarities on top of common differences found in gambling-related cognitions, motivations and perceptions of risks [7, 91, 92]. For example, Chinese and American gamblers in Korean casinos were found to endorse similar superstitious beliefs, while games novelty and monetary gains were rated as highly important by Japanese and Korean gamblers, respectively [93]. It is clear that gambling serves different culturally mediated purposes and is understood or framed in a diverse manner according to an individual's cultural identity and the preference and game types played. Much work is needed in replicating or confirming some of these findings in other cultures, and consequently translating key findings to clinical or practical outcomes for policy or treatment reformations needs some caution.

The interaction effects between ethnic and national/geographical cultures on GD are complex mechanisms that are increasingly investigated through acculturation research [94, 95]. It is essential that our understanding of cultural differences is not constrained to defining cultures through concepts of ethnicity but encompasses the diversity of cultural values and beliefs in an increasingly globalised environment sparked by multi-generational migration. A match between ethnic cultures with permissive views of social gambling (e.g. Chinese and Korean cultures) and increased availability or accessibility of gambling venues in Western countries may further exacerbate risk of GD development [16]. Results from the US NESARC evidenced that second- and third-generation immigrants and nonimmigrants (native born Americans) were more likely to report PG, as compared to first-generation immigrants [96]. In other words, new migrants from CALD communities were least likely to report disordered gambling behaviour as compared to other groups. These patterns may be attributed to acculturation effects, where children of first-generation migrants may adjust their behavioural responses to match dominant culture and expectations [94]. These findings are interesting because the majority of past qualitative and quantitative studies on CALD populations have consistently reported higher GD prevalence rates among ethnic minorities (e.g. [97, 98]), in which significant cross-cultural differences in GD propensity may be partly attributed to statistically collapsing group effects of multi-generational immigrants.

On a familial level, cultural values and beliefs on social gambling and GD are passed on to younger generations through social learning and modelling of cognitive behavioural responses [1, 99]. Lower family functioning and social support are significantly associated with moderate risk and PG behaviour in a longitudinal-designed Canadian sample [100], highlighting the importance of family culture in GD propensity. Family members of treatment-seeking Chinese gamblers are constantly reported to have higher psychological distress and coping mechanisms that match Chinese cultural method of dealing with adverse circumstances [101]. Hence, ethnic cultural values and coping styles are evident in family systems and utilised similarly in GD behaviour. In a nationally representative sample, Italian adolescents who perceived higher parental knowledge of adolescent's life and whereabouts—indicative of higher parental involvement—were less likely to approve positive gambling beliefs, consequently contributing to lower gambling frequency [102]. Similarly, in a Macau sample, positive familial monitoring was a significant moderator of the relationship between lower risk-taking propensity and gambling cognitions [103]. Indeed, cultural values and beliefs transferred through family systems are important processes from which future investigations can expand on.

13.3.2 Culture, Motivations and Gambling Patterns

There are several ways in which cultural values and beliefs can influence gambling motivations and consequently patterns of gambling behaviour. Differentiated self-construal, construal of others and degree of interdependence between self and others [104] influence how individuals from varied cultures experience gambling, including gambling-related cognitions and motivations. It is traditionally viewed that in cultures that thrive on individuality and independence (e.g. Western cultures), gambling motivations will more likely include self-originated precipitant and maintenance factors such as sensation seeking, comorbidities with other addictions and gambling as means of remediating boredom or loneliness and means of escaping negative emotions [105, 106]. Meanwhile, individuals from cultures that thrive on community and interdependence (e.g. some Asian cultures) will most likely gamble for socialisation reasons within community norms, learnt through modelling of family or friends' behaviour [103] and for monetary gains [7, 107, 108]. These associations are not dichotomies but will vary in a continuum together with other contextual and psychosocial factors, especially in an increasingly globalised environment with merging of cultures and online access to gambling activities [109, 110].

Evidence suggests that gambling preferences and game types may vary between cultural groups. Results from Thailand's National Mental Health Survey indicated that 69.5% of the Thai population reported strongest preferences for lotteries [111]. Highest preferences for Lotto (New Zealand lotteries) were evident in all ethnic groups from the New Zealand National Gambling study on 6251 randomly selected households [112]. However, Maori and European adults reported highest frequency of participation in animal betting, Pacific Islanders in casino electronic gaming machines (EGMs) and Asians in casino table games and EGMs, as compared to other New Zealand cultural groups. Nevertheless, it has been argued that structural characteristics of gambling activities are stronger predictors of PG than generalised categorisations according to game types [113]. While game types and patterns are interesting avenues to identify at-risk cultural groups, it is worthwhile for future preventive efforts to expand our understanding of culture-mediated risks based on strategic versus non-strategic gambling activities [114], and specific game characteristics such as event and bet frequency, event duration and payout interval.

13.3.3 Culture, Gambling Recovery and Help-Seeking Behaviours

Numerous researchers have reported that certain CALD groups (e.g. Chinese, Korean, Arabic and Vietnamese) are less likely to seek PG treatment [1, 115, 116]. A number of factors have been suggested for this reduced treatment seeking among certain CALD groups including cultural mistrust, feelings of shame, stigma, language barriers, lack of recognition of problem severity and limited availability or awareness of culturally sensitive or cost-effective treatment facilities [14, 17, 117–119]. The process of recovery in CALD communities often times begins within the family and cultural community, as confidentiality, trust and rapport are important determinants of help-seeking behaviour and treatment retention. Some CALD populations (e.g. Chinese, Croatians and Indigenous Australians) demonstrated a tendency to rely on self, family and community to deal with PG [15, 115, 117, 119]. Thus, if family and community members have knowledge and awareness of PG and treatment options, they may effectively assist at risk and PGs [15].

Recovery, GD experiences and the rebuilding of self-construal and construal of others are reliant on culturally appropriate methods of prevention and treatment approaches [120]. The positive role family members play in professional help seeking has also been noted by researchers. For instance, Choong et al. [121] found that in a Malaysian sample, family members and loved ones are important catalysts in the initiation of help-seeking behaviour and the inclusion of family members (when appropriate) is beneficial to the recovery process. Recent evidence form a Spanish treatment evaluation found that the inclusion of a concerned significant other (CSO) into usual CBT treatment significantly improved attendance, adherence to recovery guidelines and retention rates, contributing to reduced relapse incidences, especially when including spousal CSO [122].

13.4   Implications in Relation to the Prevention and Treatment of PG

The above findings have important implications in relation to the prevention and treatment of gambling problems for CALD individuals.

13.4.1 Preventive Implications

A focus on prevention strategies would be a cost-effective approach to try to reduce gambling among at-risk CALD groups. Considering the barriers to treatment seeking such as low awareness or recognition of PG among certain CALD groups, one preventive measure is to provide information/psychoeducation to improve awareness and knowledge of PG, the negative consequences of gambling and the risk factors associated with gambling [4, 15, 123, 124]. Furthermore, there is also a need to increase knowledge of treatment options/services for CALD PGs as this may normalise help seeking and consequently encourage treatment seeking among these groups [1].

As many CALD gamblers seek assistance from family or community members [17, 123], these educational programmes need to widen target group beyond gamblers to include family and community members. An increase in concerned significant others (CSO) knowledge of gambling problems and possible treatment services may enable them to recognise if a distressed gambler or another CSO is suffering due to a PG. Being equipped with basic strategies to control or stop gambling especially at an earlier stage of gambling may further lead CSOs to encourage CALD PGs to seek treatment before the problems worsen. These programmes will assist CSOs to obtain support and guidance while supporting the gambler through recovery, even before the gambler is ready to seek professional treatment.

Strategies to persuade vulnerable CALD individuals to seek treatment are also important, especially given the aversion to help seeking among certain CALD groups. In order to encourage CALD PGs to access treatment services, information on PG and treatment services needs to be available and accessible to them in multiple languages and via several platforms. This would include making them available online on relevant ethnic websites as well as leaving information (e.g. pamphlets) in places they frequent (e.g. relevant community centres, various cultural celebrations/ festivals/gatherings/meetings, ethnic food stores/restaurants, senior citizens clubs as well as waiting area of health professionals they are likely to see) [1, 17]. Publication of articles on PG, its consequences as well as treatment (and places to obtain treatment) in relevant languages in cultural newspapers or publications, ethnic radios and TV would also be useful [1, 17]. Highlighting the availability of bi- or multilingual relevant ethnic community workers or treatment will help attract CALD PGs to treatment [1]. Having free help available via a telephone or Internet helpline [124] where users can access information about PG and treatment options or further access to clinicians who provide intervention in their preferred language [17] would be beneficial.

Early detection is a key to successful treatment outcome. Thus, it will be beneficial to educate targeted frontline workers who deal with vulnerable individuals from CALD groups on PG, recognition of early PG signs and guidance on appropriate treatment services. As high rates of gambling and PG are reported for some CALD youth, education and training to teachers, school psychologists or guidance counsellors can assist in enabling early intervention for at-risk youths. General practitioners (GP) training is especially important as many CALD groups (e.g. Asians) are more likely to consult with their GP for physical problems manifested from gambling-related behaviour [17] and are more willing to accept assistance from medical practitioners rather than psychologists due to social acceptability, expectations and preferences for medical remediation for health-related problems [119]. Such education and training can be provided to other health professionals (e.g. mental health and allied health professionals) who work with CALD individuals regularly. Other frontline workers include welfare groups, legal and debt agencies where gamblers may frequent when experiencing gambling-induced financial issues.

More acculturative assistance to vulnerable CALD groups can assist in adapting to host country through recreational and social opportunities as an explicit alternative to gambling [17]. Since migrants experience a number of deficiencies (e.g. language difficulties, or difficulties related to their qualifications not recognised in the host country) that can prevent them from accessing jobs that they may have been used to prior to migration, they may benefit from vocational training in language and job skills [1, 125].

Regardless of the type of prevention approach, all materials should be developed through consultations with community workers, leaders or experts from relevant communities to ensure programmes are culturally sensitive/appropriate [123]. These community leaders can effectively promote and distribute materials, as well as assist in promoting and implementing educational programmes among relevant at-risk community members.

13.4.2 Treatment Implications

There are a number of important treatment implications for CALD clients presenting to treatment. These relate to adequate assessment of CALD clients, design and implementation of culturally competent and effective treatment programmes to treat PG.

13.4.2.1   Adequate Assessment of CALD Clients

Assessment is crucial in accurate diagnosis, case formulation and treatment planning [126]. When a CALD client presents to treatment for PG, a number of assessment issues need to be considered. In the therapeutic setting, clinicians may need to assess and educate themselves about their client's cultural background, the relevance of gambling in that culture as well as any cultural ritual/practices or cultural beliefs that may be relevant to their gambling behaviours [1] to gain a better understanding of the role culture plays on the development and maintenance of their PG. It would also be beneficial for clinicians to learn about the CALD clients' culturally related beliefs about mental health problems as well as what may cause them [127]. Clinicians could utilise resources from the clients' cultural background to gather information such as community members/experts/leaders, cultural literature or consulting professionals with similar cultural backgrounds [12].

There will be variations in the exerted influence of family and community members on PGs of the same CALD group. A thorough assessment of the CALD clients needs to examine how gambling operates within their social-cultural context (i.e. their family and community) taking into account family and community behaviours, attitudes, perceptions and viewpoint towards gambling [77]. This is important as this will help establish impact of gambling on their family, the role of family members in maintenance or lapse/relapse of gambling behaviour [1] and subsequently chances of a successful treatment outcome within the context.

Assessment of cultural factors would not be complete without considering CALD PGs social environment. Richard et al. [79] highlighted important social and environmental risk factors for gambling and PG among CALD individuals including low socioeconomic status, lack of social/recreational activities and living close proximity to gambling opportunities. Thus, given the role environmental/social factors play in the development and maintenance of gambling, a thorough assessment of these factors is essential [79].

It would be useful for clinicians to examine family and social expectations/pressures (related to their own culture and the host culture) felt by CALD clients as well as how they are coping with these expectations/pressures [1, 77]. For migrants, it is also important to assess their migration history/journey and how the client and family members are adjusting to the new host culture in order to understand the role of migration in the development and maintenance of gambling, consequently identifying skills needed to facilitate adaption [77, 128].

There are several important issues related to gambling assessment tools and conceptualisation of gambling constructs among CALD clients. First, clinicians need to be careful in using assessment tools with CALD groups as most psychological measures to assess PG as well as gambling constructs (e.g. gambling cognitions, motivations or urges) were developed using predominantly Western populations and may not be normed/validated for use in other groups [77]. Second, in relation to assessing GD among CALD clients using measuring instruments, we need to start looking at alternative ways of obtaining more valid measure of GD. Traditionally, measuring instruments that assess GD symptoms have been used to assess at-risk clients. Since a scale that assesses symptoms is being used to measure symptoms, there is a possible confounding effect. An alternative approach would be to use measuring instruments that assess related variables that have been linked to increased risk of GD including impulsivity and gambling-related cognitions [6]. Thus, using validated measuring instruments to assess these variables (e.g. Gambling Related Cognitions Scale [1]) may be a more valid way to assess at-risk group for prevention work. Finally, any new instrument developed needs to be done in consultation with relevant community experts so that the cultural meanings of the concepts assessed are considered and culturally appropriate tools are developed [123].

13.4.2.2 Designing and Implementing Culturally Competent and Effective Treatment Programmes for CALD PGs

Researchers have considered various therapeutic styles that may suit CALD PGs. Pharmacological interventions may be provided to CALD communities with minimal cultural adaptations in treatment provision without compromising on retention rates due to the fact that CALD individuals prefer medical-based and physically tangible treatments over psychological therapy [59]. Treatment programmes that target both medical and psychological problems [129] may also help attract and maintain CALD PGs in treatment. The recurring effectiveness of integrating family coping strategies in gambling recovery among culturally diverse groups suggests that it is essential that we carefully integrate and support family members and CSOs while engaging with recovering PGs [101, 130]. It might be useful to work with clients' family members prior to seeing them in order to help decrease enabling and co-dependency behaviours, as well as reduce negativity felt for the gambler [119]. In some situations, family therapy may also be useful [1]. Richard et al. [79] stated that interventions such as motivational interviewing may be appropriate for CALD gamblers as it acknowledges each clients' values and autonomy. Furthermore, as it is brief in nature, it may be a cost-effective approach for those CALD clients with lower socioeconomic status [79]. Hettema et al.'s [131] meta-analytic study showed motivational interviewing was more effective for ethnic minorities compared to Caucasians. Cognitive behavioural treatment (CBT) has also shown to be successful in treating PG among the CALD groups [132–136]. Richard et al. [79] suggested using motivational interviewing to help CALD clients engage in treatment and gradually provide CBT strategies to treat their PG.

Treatment designers need to also consider treatment formats that best suit CALD PGs. Individuals that are not comfortable with seeking psychological intervention may be attracted to self-help approaches [15, 117, 119]. Unconventional self-help groups which are preferably facilitated by or in presence of a trusted community member (e.g. ethno-specific religions leader or respected community elder) and where there is more focus on encouragement, assistance, improving awareness and skill building rather than confrontation (similar to one suggested by Fong and Tsuang [119]) may be helpful. For those CALD PGs who do not easily share their difficulties due to stigma or shame, telephone counselling programme (e.g. one described by Parhami et al. [137]) may be appropriate [1, 17]. Accessing self-help treatment programmes via the Internet or through self-help treatment manuals/ books can be another alternative [79].

Regardless of treatment format or therapeutic style used, any treatment programme adapted for CALD PGs need to be culturally competent and sensitive. Griner and Smith [138] meta-analyses study reported that culturally adapted interventions were generally more effective, especially as treatments aimed at a particular CALD group were four times more effective than those that were delivered to mixed-CALD groups. To help modify treatment programmes to be more culturally competent/appropriate, a conference with leaders/experts from relevant communities would be essential [119]. A general sense of openness to investing in the development of cultural competencies among key stakeholders (policy developers, treatment providers, industry, etc.) is important in successfully reaching out to PGs and families.

There is only a handful of researchers who have reported on the effectiveness of culturally adapted treatment programmes for CALD PGs. Wong et al. [136] made a number of changes to a CBT programme including worksheet/discussion on culturally related gambling triggers (opportunities to test their luck, win money quickly or recoup losses) as well as culturally related cognitions (e.g. illusion of control, beliefs in luck) for Chinese PGs in Hong Kong. Those who received ten weekly sessions of individual counselling and group CBT (debt, supportive, grief and/or crisis intervention) reported greater reduction in gambling severity/frequency than the control group (only individual counselling). Okuda et al. [134] reported successfully treating a 51-year-old female afro-Caribbean immigrant with GD by modifying CBT techniques. Direct labelling of certain beliefs as irrational and challenging these beliefs may not be useful nor culturally appropriate for this client as it could be viewed as minimising the client's cultural beliefs [134]. They suggested instead subtly and gradually questioning the clients' beliefs. In relation to relapse prevention, they suggested teaching such clients to be assertive may not work if their family is a trigger. Thus, for such clients, discussing how they can set limits within their family and culture can assist the client to obtain more effective support from their family members.

A number of researchers have made suggestions in how to maintain CALD clients in treatment which can be relevant for treating CALD PGs. Therapeutic alliance can be improved by normalising CALD treatment experiences and reducing any stigma associated with mental health problems and their treatment via techniques such as education and empathy [127]. As therapy may be foreign to certain CALD clients, there needs to be a discussion on what therapy involves, roles and responsibilities of both clinician and clients in therapy and clients' treatment expectations in order to reduce treatment dropout [127]. Clinicians need to be mindful of the order and timing of treatment strategies used/implemented to help improve CALD clients' motivation to make changes (e.g. concentrating on problem-solving prior to commencing cognitive therapy) [127]. Given the collectivistic nature of some CALD groups, some CALD clients may not be comfortable to concentrate on individual goals, so clinicians need to ensure treatment goals are compatible with collectivistic goals/viewpoints [77]. Clinicians can combine cultural beliefs in treatment by using cultural metaphors, narratives, doctrines and teachings to help build rapport and help them understand concepts in intervention and thereby improving involvement in treatment [127]. For some CALD clients (e.g. Chinese) given their preference for goal- or solution-focussed tasks, in-session or homework exercises may need to be adapted accordingly [127, 139].

There are also a number of important interventions that treatment designers should consider including in treatment programmes for CALD PGs. Erroneous gambling-related cognitions (e.g. gambler's fallacies and superstitions that perpetuate betting behaviour) and motivations (e.g. gambling as means of earning quick money and increasing sense of belongingness) sparked by acculturative stress [95] should be addressed in prevention and treatment programmes, though these factors may not necessarily be presented clearly at initial intake. Treatments may need to focus on improving CALD clients' self-esteem and confidence so that they are better able to adapt to the host country rather than be attracted to gambling as means to improve their financial situation and standing [125]. Helping the family develop effective communication skills may help decrease intergenerational conflict [127]. Providing advice on coping with gambling-related debt or helping link such clients to organisations that help them deal with the debts and liaise with any debtors (especially those that have access to ethno-specific workers or translators) may be helpful for some CALD PGs.

A number of researchers have reported lower attrition rates for bicultural treatment programmes [140, 141]. Some researchers have also discussed increased utilisation of treatment services by ethnic minorities that had a bicultural programme [142]. Helping immigrants to become biculturally competent rather than adapt to the host country while giving up their cultural connections could help avoid acculturation problems and maintain useful cultural values [12, 127]. Fong and Tsuang [119] however highlighted that having multicultural programmes or providing clinicians with such cultural training can be difficult to achieve given lack of funding treatment services often usually encounter. In such situations, treatment providers may need to incorporate gambling assistant with already available treatment services [123], access already existing ethno-specific material using the Internet [119] or utilise existing services within the clients' community such as transport, financial, legal, language or other social services [12]. For treatment programmes that are not specific to CALD populations, other changes may need to be made to ensure CALD PGs are comfortable including using adequate signs for all programmes in different languages and having ethno-specific reading material in the waiting area [1].

Griner and Smith [138] meta-analyses study also reported that treatment delivered in CALD clients' non-English native language was twice as effective as those delivered in English. Some researchers have suggested that employing bi- or multilingual clinicians could help increase referral rates of CALD populations to treatment programmes [119, 142, 143]. This, however, may not always be practical. In these situations, clinicians could discuss with CALD clients their linguistic capabilities, emphasising their eagerness to assist despite these limitations and brainstorming with clients options such as bringing in significant others or other translators when discussing crucial subjects, using dictionaries or images to illustrate treatment concepts and/or speaking in a slower and clearer manner [144].

As important as it is for clinicians to be aware of the cultural background, beliefs, values and needs of CALD clients, it is also vital for them to be aware of their own personal and cultural values/biases as well as cultural stereotypes so that they do not interfere in working with different cultural groups [128]. Clinicians need to be careful about making stereotypical statements, generalisations and assumptions that can be offensive for some CALD clients [127]. Furthermore, even though considering clients' culture is essential in devising adequate treatment plans for CALD PGs, clinicians need to also acknowledge that there are individual differences between clients within a particular group so what may work with one individual from a particular CALD group may not for another in the same CALD group [144, 145]. Consequently, individualised assessment and treatment plan remains important [127, 128].

13.5   A Second Look at the Roles of Culture in Gambling

It is now generally accepted that culture plays important roles in the development, maintenance and treatment of many psychological and psychiatric disorders [1, 7, 59, 127, 130, 144]. The earlier sections of this review demonstrated there is enough evidence to support the importance of culture in our understanding and treatment of problem gambling. Although the positive and beneficial effects of culture and psychopathology and psychotherapy have been widely discussed, the negative or downside of the roles of culture in mental health and illness are seldom presented or discussed [130, 146]. Our intention of presenting the negative or the downside of culture in mental health and illness is not to decry the positive aspects of the progress already achieved but to alert readers that we need to watch out for the unintended negative aspects so that we can be more alert and ready to make sure that further progress can be made and that patients in the CALD would benefit more. Some of the major negative aspects in this context are outlined below:

1. A major downside is the lack of consensus in the definition of "culture". In the literature, the concepts of nation, ethnicity, race, religion, shared cognition, shared experiences, values, beliefs and behaviours are used interchangeably as culture. It is clear that nations, ethnicity and race can have some characteristics of culture, but they cannot be the same as culture [147].
2. There is a lack of a comprehensive theory outlining how "culture" operates and contributes to the psychopathology of mental illness and treatment outcome of psychotherapy. It is still unclear how the mechanisms of culture influence the existing theoretical constructs of known psychopathology of mental illness. For example, it is still unclear how culture interacts with Beck's cognitive triad in the psychopathology of mood disorders and also the treatment outcome of cognitive behaviour therapy. Similarly, evidence is sparse on how culture interacts with biochemical imbalance theory to impact mood disorders.
3. The psychological literature presents culture as if it is an "all "or "none" concept in a person. For example, a person is having an "individualistic" or a "collective"

cultural value. Also, it is assumed that once a person is determined as having a collective cultural value, that person holds the same value on most if not all of the issues. Research has shown that cultural value of a person is much more complex. A person can have a collective value for dealing with family issues but a capitalistic cultural value for dealing with financial matters. Similarly, a person can hold individualistic value at time 1 (e.g. young adult) but not at time 2 (e.g. old age).

4. It is now accepted that both individual and group psychotherapies are effective in the treatment of many psychological disorders. Equally, there is now plenty of literature showing the positive impact of culture in the conceptualisation and treatment outcome of individual psychotherapy. However, what roles do culture play in group psychotherapy treatment outcome, in particular group CBT, are still unclear as there is a lack of theoretical knowledge and empirical evidence in this area.

Current literature shows that culture plays an important role in our understanding and treatment of many psychological health and illness, including GD. However, there are unintended negative consequences that are seldom presented and openly discussed. It is hoped open discussions on these possible negative consequences will lead to further improvements and refinements on the positive roles on culture on psychopathology and psychotherapy. Perhaps one way of moving forward is to strengthen the contribution of culture further in the treatment of psychological problems but also be fully aware of the importance of individual differences in case formulations. In this way, both important cultural variables are assessed as unique individual differences for a client can be formulated using strong scientific methodology already existed in the literature. This, however, does not address the situation in group psychotherapy. Further, advances in this area are needed in the future.

13.6 Concluding Remarks

Despite some limitations in the studies, high rates of GD have been found for CALD individuals. Considering the role cultural variables in the development and maintenance of gambling, it is essential that treatment service providers are culturally competent and positively engage with key community and/or religious leaders to effectively reach out to multilingual and diverse groups, whereby online and hardcopy information sheets are made available in multiple languages. We acknowledge the fluidity of the concept of culture and our limited understanding of how culture specifically operates in psychopathology and psychotherapy. Thus, as a whole, cultural perspectives in GD require consistent evidence-based investigations and iterations, reflecting the fluidity of our concepts of culture and cultural norms in our increasingly globalised environments.

Acknowledgement Dr. Oei is now an Emeritus Professor of clinical psychology at the University of Queensland and a visiting professor of James Cook University, Singapore; Nanjing University, PR China; and Asia University, Taiwan.

References

1. Raylu N, Oei TPS. The gambling related cognitions scale (GRCS): development, confirmatory factor validation and psychometric properties. Addiction. 2004;99:757–69.
2. American Psychiatric Association. Diagnostic and statistical manual of mental disorders. 5th ed. Washington, DC: American Psychiatric Press; 2013.
3. Alegria M, Valentine A, Li H, Min G. Special population segments and the addiction syndrome. In: Shaffer H, LaPlante DA, Nelson SE, editors. APA addiction syndrome handbook: vol 2. Recovery, prevention, and other issues. Washington, DC: American Psychological Association; 2012. p. 297–331.
4. Breen H, Gainsbury S. Aboriginal gambling and problem gambling: a review. Int J Ment Health Addic. 2013;11:75–96.
5. Blaszczynski AP, Nower L. A pathways model of problem and pathological gambling. Addiction. 2002;97(5):487–99.
6. Raylu N, Oei TPS. A cognitive behavioural therapy program for problem gambling: therapists manual. UK: Routledge; 2010.
7. Loo JMY, Raylu N, Oei TPS. Gambling among the Chinese: a comprehensive review. Clin Psychol Rev. 2008;28(7):1152–66.
8. House J, Williams DR. Understanding and reducing socioeconomic and racial/ethnic disparities in health. In: Hofrichter R, editor. Health and social justice: politics, ideology, and inequity in the distribution of disease. San Francisco: Jossey-Bass; 2003. p. 89–131.
9. Johansson A, Grant JE, Kim SW, Odlaug BL, Götestam KG. Risk factors for problematic gambling: a critical literature review. J Gambl Stud. 2009;25(1):67–92.
10. Kastirke N, Rumpf H, John U, Bischof A, Meyer C. Demographic risk factors and gambling preference may not explain the high prevalence of gambling problems among the population with migration background: results from a German nationwide survey. J Gambl Stud. 2015;31:741–57.
11. Hochschild JL, Mollenkopf J. The complexities of immigration: why western countries struggle with immigration politics and policies. In: Stiftung B, editor. Delivering citizenship. Berlin, Germany: European Policy Centre, Migration Policy Institute; 2009.
12. Verney SP, Kipp BJ. Acculturation and alcohol treatment in ethnic minority populations: assessment issues and implications. Alcohol Treat Q. 2007;25(4):47–61.
13. Braun B, Ludwig M, Sleczka P, Bühringer G, Ludwig K. Gamblers seeking treatment: who does and who doesn't? J Behav Addict. 2014;3(3):189–98.
14. Gainsbury S, Hing N, Suhonen N. Professional help-seeking for gambling problems: awareness, barriers and motivators for treatment. J Gambl Stud. 2014;30(2):503–19.
15. Hing N, Breen H, Gordon A, Russell A. Gambling harms and gambling help-seeking amongst Indigenous Australians. J Gambl Stud. 2014a;30(3):737–55.
16. Kim W. Acculturation and gambling in Asian Americans: when culture meets availability. Int Gambl Stud. 2012;12(1):69–88.
17. Tse S, Wong J, Chan P. Needs and gaps analysis: problem gambling interventions among New Zealand Asian peoples. Int J Ment Health Addict. 2007;5:81–8.
18. Shweder RA. Thinking through cultures: expeditions in cultural psychology. Cambridge, MA: Harvard University Press; 1991.
19. Volberg RA, Abbott MW. Gambling and problem gambling among indigenous peoples. Subst Use Misuse. 1997;32(11):1525–38.
20. Patterson-Silver Wolf DA, Welte JW, Barnes GM, Tidwell MO, Spicer P. Sociocultural influences on gambling and alcohol use among Native Americans in the United States. J Gambl Stud. 2015;31(4):1387–404.
21. Welte JW, Barnes GM, Wieczorek W, Tidwell M, Parker J. Alcohol and gambling pathology among U.S. adults: prevalence, demographic patterns and comorbidity. J Stud Alcohol. 2001;62(5):706–12.
22. Westermeyer J, Canive J, Garrard J, Thuras P, Thompson J. Lifetime prevalence of pathological gambling Among American Indian and Hispanic American veterans. Am J Public Health. 2005;95(5):860–6.

23. Volberg RA, Bernhard B. The 2006 study of gambling and problem gambling in New Mexico. Albuquerque, NM: Responsible Gaming Association of New Mexico; 2006.
24. Belanger Y. Gambling with the future: the evolution of aboriginal gaming in Canada. Saskatoon: Purich Pubishing Ltd; 2006.
25. Belanger Y. Introduction. In: Belanger Y, editor. First nations gambling in Canada: current trends and issues. Winnipeg: University of Manitoba Press; 2011. p. 2–7.
26. Kong G, Smith PH, Pilver C, Hoff R, Potenza MN. Problem-gambling severity and psychiatric disorders among American-Indian/Alaska native adults. J Psychiatr Res. 2016;74:55–62.
27. Williams R, Stevens R, Nixon G. Gambling and problem gambling in North American aboriginal people. In: Belanger Y, editor. First nations gambling in Canada: current trends and issues. Winnipeg: University of Manitoba Press; 2011. p. 166–94.
28. Hewitt D, Auger D. Firewatch on aboriginal adolescent gambling. Edmonton, Alberta: Nechi Training, Research and Health Promotion Institute; 1995.
29. Stinchfield R. J Gambl Stud. 2000). Gambling and correlates of gambling among Minnesota public school students;16(2–3):153–73.
30. Zitzow D. Comparative study of problematic gambling behaviours between American Indian and non Indian adolescents within and near a northern plains reservation. Am Indian Alsk Native Ment Health Res. 1996;7(2):14–26.
31. Stinchfield R, Cassuto N, Winters K, Latimer W. Prevalence of gambling among Minnesota public school students in 1992 and 1995. J Gambl Stud. 1997;13:25–48.
32. Winters K, Stinchfield R, Fulkersen J. Adolescent survey of gambling behaviour in Minnesota. St. Paul, MN: Department of Human Services; 1990.
33. Peacock RB, Day PA, Peacock TD. Adolescent gambling on a Great Lakes Indian reservation. J Hum Behav Soc Environ. 1999;2(1–2):5–17.
34. American Psychiatric Association. Diagnostic and statistical manual of mental disorders. 4h ed. Washington, DC: American Psychiatric Press; 1994.
35. Alegria A, Petry NM, Hasin DS, Liu S, Grant BF, Blanco C. Disordered gambling among racial and ethnic groups in the US: Results from the National Epidemiologic Survey on Alcohol and Related Conditions. CNS Spectr. 2009;14(3):132–42.
36. Abbot MW, Volberg RA. The New Zealand national survey of problem and pathological gambling. J Gambl Stud. 1996;12(2):143–60.
37. Walker SE, Abbott MW, Gray RJ. Knowledge, views and experiences of gambling and gambling-related harms in different ethnic and socio-economic groups in New Zealand. Aust N Z J Public Health. 2012;36(2):153–9.
38. Abbott MW, Volberg RA. Taking the pulse on gambling and problem gambling in New Zealand: a report on phase one of the 1999 National Prevalence Survey. Report no. 3 of the New Zealand Gaming Survey. Wellington, New Zealand: New Zealand Department of Internal Affairs; 2000.
39. Gray R. New Zealanders' participation in gambling: results from the 2010 health and lifestyles survey. Wellington: Health Sponsorship Council; 2011.
40. Hing N, Breen H, Gordon A, Russell A. The gambling behavior of indigenous Australians. J Gambl Stud. 2014b;30(2):369–86.
41. Hing N, Gainsbury S, Blaszczynski A, Wood R, Lubman D, Russell A. Interactive gambling. Melbourne, Australia: Gambling Research Australia; 2014.
42. Stevens M, Young M. Reported gambling problems in the Indigenous and total Australian population. Melbourne: Gambling Research Australia; 2009.
43. Ferris J, Wynne H. The Canadian problem gambling index: final report. Submitted to Canadian Centre on Substance Abuse. 2001. http://www.ccgr.ca/en/projects/resources/CPGI-Final-Report-English.pdf
44. Abbott M, Romild U, Volberg R. Gambling and problem gambling in Sweden: Changes between 1998 and 2009. J Gambl Stud. 2014b;30(4):985–99.
45. Parhami I, Siani A, Campos MD, Rosenthal RJ, Fong TW. Gambling in the Iranian-American community and an assessment of motives: a case study. Int J Ment Health Addict. 2012b;10(5):710–21.

46. Williams RJ, Volberg RA, Stevens RMG. The population prevalence of problem gambling: methodological influences, standardized rates, jurisdictional differences, and worldwide trends. Report prepared for the Ontario Problem Gambling Research Centre and the Ontario Ministry of Health and Long Term Care. 2012.
47. Barry DT, Stefanovics EA, Desai RA, Potenza MN. Differences in the associations between gambling problem severity and psychiatric disorders among Black and White adults: findings from the National Epidemiologic Survey on Alcohol and Related Conditions. Am J Addict. 2010;20:69–77.
48. Welte JW, Barnes GM, Tidwell M, Hoffman JH. Gambling and problem gambling across the lifespan. J Gambl Stud. 2011;27(1):49–61.
49. Barnes GM, Welte JW, Hoffman JH, Tidwell MO. Gambling, alcohol, and other substance use among youth in the United States. J Stud Alcohol Drugs. 2009;70(1):134–42.
50. Welte JW, Barnes GM, Tidwell M, Hoffman JH. The prevalence of problem gambling among U.S. adolescents and young adults: results from a National survey. J Gambl Stud. 2008;24:119–33.
51. Winters KC, Stinchfield RD, Fulkerson J. Toward the development of an adolescent problem severity scale. J Gambl Stud. 1993;9:63–84.
52. Barry DT, Stefanovics EA, Desai RA, Potenza MN. Gambling problem severity and psychiatric disorders among Hispanic and White Adults: findings from a nationally representative sample. J Psychiatr Res. 2011;45(3):404–11.
53. Abbott MW, Volberg RA. Gambling and problem gambling in New Zealand: Report on phase one of the national survey of problem gambling. Research series no. 12. Wellington, New Zealand: New Zealand Department of Internal Affairs; 1991.
54. Abbott MW, Volberg RA. Gambling and pathological gambling: growth industry and growth pathology of the 1990s. Commun Ment Health New Zealand. 1994;9(2):22–31.
55. Devlin ME, Walton D. The prevalence of problem gambling in New Zealand as measured by the PGSI: adjusting prevalence estimates using meta-analysis. Int Gambl Stud. 2012;12(2):177–97.
56. Victorian Casino and Gambling Authority. The impact of gaming on specific cultural groups. Melbourne: Victorian Casino and Gaming Authority; 2000.
57. Dickins M, Thomas A. Gambling in culturally and linguistically diverse communities in Australia (AGRC discussion paper no. 7). Melbourne: Australian Gambling Research Centre, Australian Institute of Family Studies; 2016.
58. Volberg RA, Abbott MW, Rönnberg S, Munck IM. Prevalence and risks of pathological gambling in Sweden. Acta Psychiatr Scand. 2001;104(4):250–6.
59. Raylu N, Loo JMY, Oei TPS. Treatment of gambling problems in Asia: comprehensive review and implications for Asian problem gamblers. J Cogn Psychother. 2013;27(3):297–322.
60. Blaszczynski A, Huynh S, Dumlao VJ, Farrell E. Problem gambling within a Chinese speaking community. J Gambl Stud. 1998;14(4):359–80.
61. Chinese Family Service of Greater Montreal. Gambling and problem gambling among the Chinese in Quebec: an exploratory study. Quebec, Canada: Author; 1997.
62. Lesieur HR, Cross J, Frank M, Welch M, White CM, Rubenstein G, Moseley K, Mark M. Gambling and pathological gambling among university students. Addict Behav. 1991;16:517–27.
63. Luczak SE, Wall TL. Gambling problems and comorbidity with alcohol use disorders in Chinese-, Korean-, and White-American college students. Am J Addict. 2016;25:195–202.
64. Williams RJ, Connolly D, Wood RT, Nowatzki N. Gambling and problem gambling in a sample of university students. J Gambl Iss. 2006;16.
65. Chan AKK, Zane N, Wong GM, Song AV. Personal gambling expectancies among Asian American and White American college students. J Gambl Stud. 2015;31(1):33–57.
66. Kong G, Tsai J, Pilver CE, Tan HS, Hoff RA, Cavallo DA, Krishnan-Sarin S, Steinberg MA, Rugle L, Potenza MN. Differences in gambling problem severity and gambling and health/functioning characteristics among Asian-American and Caucasian high-school students. Psychiatry Res. 2013;210(3):1071–8.

67. Rinker DV, Rodriguez LM, Krieger H, Tackett JL, Neighbors C. Racial and ethnic differences in problem gambling among college students. J Gambl Stud. 2016;32(2):581–90.
68. Petry NM, Armentano C, Kuoch T, Norinth T, Smith L. Gambling participation and problems among the South East Asian refugees to the United States. Psychiatr Serv. 2003;54(8):1142–8.
69. Marshall GN, Elliott MN, Schell TL. Prevalence and correlates of lifetime disordered gambling in cambodian refugees residing in Long Beach, CA. J Immigr Minor Health. 2009;11(1):35–40.
70. Chen C, Wong J, Lee N, Chan-Ho M, Lau W, Fung JT-F. The Shatin community mental health survey in Hong Kong: II. Major findings. Arch Gen Psychiatry. 1993;50(2):125–33.
71. Fong D, Ozorio B. Gambling participation and prevalence estimates of pathological gambling in a far-east gambling city: Macao. UNLV Gaming Res Rev J. 2005;9(2). Retrieved from http://digitalscholarship.unlv.edu/grrj/vol9/iss2/2
72. Wong IL, So EM. Prevalence estimates of problem and pathological gambling in Hong Kong. Am J Psychiatr. 2003;160(7):1353–4.
73. Park S, Cho MJ, Jeon HJ, Lee HW, Bae JN, Park JI, Sohn JH, Lee YR, Lee JY, Hong JP. Prevalence, clinical correlations, comorbidities, and suicidal tendencies in pathological Korean gamblers: results from the Korean Epidemiologic Catchment Area Study. Soc Psychiatry Psychiatr Epidemiol. 2010;45(6):621–9.
74. Williams RJ, Lee C, Back KJ. The prevalence and nature of gambling and problem gambling in South Korea. Soc Psychiatry Psychiatr Epidemiol. 2013;48:821–34.
75. Liu L, Luo T, Hao W. Gambling problems in young people: experience from the Asian region. Curr Opin Psychiatry. 2013;26(4):310–31.
76. Shaffer H, Hall MN. Estimating the prevalence of adolescent gambling disorders: a quantitative synthesis and guide toward standard gambling nomenclature. J Gambl Stud. 1996;12:193–214.
77. Blume AW, Morera OF, de la Cruz BG. Assessment of addictive behaviors in ethnic-minority cultures. In: Donovan DM, Marlatt GA, editors. Assessment of addictive behaviors. 2nd ed. New York: Guilford Press; 2005. p. 49–70.
78. Bellringer M, Abbott M, Williams M, Gao W. Problem gambling: Pacific Island families longitudinal study. 2008. Retrieved from http://www.health.govt.nz/system/files/documents/pages/pif.pdf.
79. Richard K, Baghurst T, Faragher JM, Stotts E. Practical treatments considering the role of sociocultural factors on problem gambling. J Gambl Stud. 2016:1–17.
80. Egerer M. Problem drinking, gambling and eating-three problems, one understanding? A qualitative comparison between French and Finnish social workers. Nordic Stud Alcohol Drugs. 2013;30(1–2):67–86.
81. Venuleo C, Salvatore S, Mossi P. The role of cultural factors in differentiating pathological gamblers. J Gambl Stud. 2015;31(4):1353–76.
82. Loo JMY, Shi Y, Pu X. Gambling, drinking and quality of life: evidence from Macao and Australia. J Gambl Stud. 2016;32(2):391–407.
83. Oei TPS, Goh Z. Interactions between risks and protective factors on problem gambling in Asia. J Gambl Stud. 2015;31:557–72.
84. Raylu N, Oei TPS, Loo JMY, Tsai J-S. Testing the validity of a cognitive behavioral model for gambling behavior. J Gambl Stud. 2016;32(2):773–88.
85. Oei TPS, Lin J, Raylu N. The relationship between gambling cognitions, psychological states, and gambling: a cross-cultural study of Chinese and Caucasians in Australia. J Cross-Cult Psychol. 2008;39(2):147–61.
86. Oei TPS, Raylu N. The relationship between cultural variables and gambling behavior among Chinese residing in Australia. J Gambl Stud. 2009;25:433–45.
87. Oei TPS, Raylu N. Gambling behavior and motivation: a cross cultural study of Chinese and Caucasians in Australia. Int J Soc Psychiatry. 2010;56:23–34.
88. Zheng WY, Walker M, Blaszczynski A. Mahjong gambling and Chinese international students in Sydney: an exploratory study. J Psychol Chin Soc. 2008;9(2):241–62.
89. Ji L-J, McGeorge K, Li Y, Lee A, Zhang Z. Culture and gambling fallacies. Springerplus. 2015;4(1):510.

90. Medeiros GC, Leppink E, Yaemi A, Mariani M, Tavares H, Grant J. Gambling disorder in older adults: a cross-cultural perspective. Compr Psychiatry. 2015;58:116–21.
91. Lam D. Chopsticks and gambling. Piscataway, NJ: Transaction Publishers; 2014.
92. Loo JMY, Raylu N, Oei TPS. Testing the validity of an integrated cognitive behavioural model of gambling behaviour with a Chinese sample. In: Cavanna AE, editor. Psychology of gambling: new research. New York: Nova Publishers; 2012. p. 119–37.
93. Kim J, Ahlgren MB, Byun J-W, Malek K. Gambling motivations and superstitious beliefs: a cross-cultural study with casino customers. Int Gambl Stud. 2016;16:1–20.
94. Berry JW. Globalisation and acculturation. Int J Intercult Relat. 2008;32(4):328–36.
95. Jacoby N, von Lersner U, Schubert HJ, Loeffler G, Heinz A, Mörsen CP. The role of acculturative stress and cultural backgrounds in migrants with pathological gambling. Int Gambl Stud. 2013;13(2):240–54.
96. Wilson AN, Salas-Wright CP, Vaughn MG, Maynard BR. Gambling prevalence rates among immigrants: a multigenerational examination. Addict Behav. 2015;42:79–85.
97. Clarke D, Abbott M, Tse S, Townsend S, Kingi P, Manaia W. Gender, age, ethnic and occupational associations with pathological gambling in a New Zealand urban sample. N Z J Psychol. 2006;35(2):84–91.
98. Keen B, Pickering D, Wieczorek M, Blaszczynski A. Problem gambling and family violence in the Asian context: a review. Asian J Gambl Iss Public Health. 2015;5(1):1–16.
99. Oei TPS, Raylu N. Familial influence on offspring gambling: a cognitive mechanism for transmission of gambling behaviour in families. Psychol Med. 2004;34:1279–88.
100. Cowlishaw S, Suomi A, Rodgers B. Implications of gambling problems for family and interpersonal adjustment: results from the Quinte Longitudinal Study. Addiction. 2016;111(9):1628–36.
101. Chan EML, Dowling NA, Jackson AC, Shek D T-l. Gambling related family coping and the impact of problem gambling on families in Hong Kong. Asian J Gambl Iss Public Health. 2016;6(1):1–12.
102. Canale N, Vieno A, ter Bogt T, Pastore M, Siciliano V, Molinaro S. Adolescent gambling-oriented attitudes mediate the relationship between perceived parental knowledge and adolescent gambling: implications for prevention. Prev Sci. 2016;17(8):970–80.
103. Situ J, Mo Z. Risk propensity, gambling cognition and gambling behavior: the role of family and peer influences. J Educ Dev Psychol. 2016;6(1):77–94.
104. Markus HR, Kitayama S. Culture and the self: implications for cognition, emotion, and motivation. Psychol Rev. 1991;98(2):224–53.
105. Biback C, Zack M. The relationship between stress and motivation in pathological gambling: a focused review and analysis. Curr Addict Rep. 2015;2(3):230–9.
106. Sundqvist K, Jonsson J, Wennberg P. Gambling motives in a representative Swedish sample of risk gamblers. J Gambl Stud. 2016:1–11.
107. Lee C-K, Bernhard BJ, Kim J, Fong T, Lee TK. Differential gambling motivations and recreational activity preferences among casino gamblers. J Gambl Stud. 2015;31(4):1833–47.
108. Ma E, Lai IKW. Gambling motivation among tourists in Macau's casino resorts. Asia Pac J Tourism Res. 2016;21(11):1227–40.
109. Canale N, Santinello M, Griffiths MD. Validation of the reasons for gambling questionnaire (RGQ) in a British population survey. Addict Behav. 2015;45:276–80.
110. Henderson KV, Lyons B. The at-risk on-line gambler: a global issue with local implications. In: Spotts HE, Meadow HL, editors. Proceedings of the 2000 academy of marketing science (AMS) annual conference. Cham: Springer International Publishing; 2015. p. 151–7.
111. Assanangkornchai S, McNeil EB, Tantirangsee N, Kittirattanapaiboon P. Gambling disorders, gambling type preferences, and psychiatric comorbidity among the Thai general population: results of the 2013 National Mental Health Survey. J Behav Addict. 2016;5(3):410–8.
112. Abbott M, Bellringer M, Garrett N, Mundy-McPherson S. New Zealand 2012 National Gambling Study: overview and gambling participation. Wellington: Gambling and Addictions Research Centre & AUT; 2014a.
113. Griffiths MD, Auer M. The irrelevancy of game-type in the acquisition, development, and maintenance of problem gambling. Front Psychol. 2012;3:621.

114. Odlaug BL, Marsh PJ, Kim SW, Grant JE. Strategic vs nonstrategic gambling: characteristics of pathological gamblers based on gambling preference. Ann Clin Psychiatry. 2011;23(2):105–12.
115. GAMECS Project. Gambling among members of ethnic communities in Sydney: report on problem gambling and ethnic communities (part 3). Sydney: Ethnic Communities' Council of NSW; 1999.
116. Victorian Casino and Gambling Authority. Seventh survey of community gambling patterns and perceptions. Melbourne: Victorian Casino and Gaming Authority; 1999.
117. Breen HM, Hing N, Gordon A, Holdsworth L. Indigenous Australian gamblers and their help-seeking behavior. In: Baek Y, editor. Psychology of gaming. Hauppauge, NY: Nova Science Publishers; 2013. p. 93–120.
118. David EJR. Cultural mistrust, and mental health help-seeking attitudes among Filipino Americans. Asian Am J Psychol. 2010;1(1):57–66.
119. Fong TW, Tsuang J. Asian-Americans, addictions, and barriers to treatment. Psychiatry. 2007;4(11):51–9.
120. Reith G, Dobbie F. Lost in the game: narratives of addiction and identity in recovery from problem gambling. Addict Res Theory. 2012;20(6):511–21.
121. Choong LL, Loo JMY, Ng WS. The experience of recovering gamblers in Malaysia: a phenomenological study. Asian J Gambl Iss Public Health. 2014;4(1).
122. Jiménez-Murcia S, Tremblay J, Stinchfield R, Granero R, Fernández-Aranda F, Mestre-Bach G, Steward T, Del Pino-Gutiérrez A, Baño M, Moragas L, Aymamí N, Gómez-Peña M, Tárrega S, Valenciano-Mendoza E, Giroux I, Sancho M, Sánchez I, Mallorquí-Bagué N, González V, Martín-Romera V, Menchon JM. The involvement of a concerned significant other in gambling disorder treatment outcome. J Gambl Stud. 2016.
123. Hing N, Breen H. Indigenous Australians and gambling (AGRC discussion paper no. 2). Melbourne: Australian Gambling Research Centre; 2014.
124. Winslow M, Cheok C, Subramaniam M. Gambling in Singapore: an overview of history, research, treatment and policy. Addiction. 2015;110:1383–7.
125. Varma SC, Siris SG. Alcohol abuse in Asian Americans. Epidemiological and treatment issues. Am J Addict. 1996;5:136–43.
126. Raylu N, Oei TPS. Treatment planning for problem gamblers. Aust Clin Psychol. 2016;2(1):1–14. Retrieved from: file:///C:/Users/NRaylu/Downloads/acp_vol._2_issue_1_20110_raylu_n._oei_t._p._s.pdf
127. Hwang W. Culturally adapting evidence-based practices for ethnic minority and immigrant families. In: Zane N, Bernal G, Leong FTL, editors. Evidence-based psychological practice with ethnic minorities: culturally informed research and clinical strategies. Washington, DC: American Psychological Association; 2016. p. 289–308.
128. Díaz-Martínez AM. The case of Maria. Cultural approaches. Clin Case Stud. 2003;2(3):211–23.
129. Naegle MA, Ng A, Barron C, Lai TFM. Alcohol and substance abuse. West J Med. 2002;176(4):259–63.
130. Andrews T, Oei TPS. Development of Asian CBT research and network. Jpn J Behav Ther. 2016;42:21–33.
131. Hettema J, Steele J, Miller WR. Motivational interviewing. Annu Rev Clin Psychol. 2005;1(1):91–111.
132. Guo S, Manning V, Thane KK, Ng A, Abdin E, Wong KE. Predictors of treatment outcome among Asian pathological gamblers: clinical, behavioural, demographic, and treatment process factors. J Gambl Stud. 2014;30:89–103.
133. Manning V, Ng A, Koh PK, Guo S, Gomathinayagam K, Wong KW. Pathological gamblers in Singapore: treatment response at 3 months. J Addict Med. 2014;8:462–9.
134. Okuda M, Balán I, Petry NM, Oquendo M, Blanco C. Cognitive behavioural therapy for pathological gambling: cultural considerations. Am J Psychiatry. 2009;166:1325–30.
135. Pasche SC, Sinclair H, Collins P, Pretorius A, Grant JE, Stein DJ. The effectiveness of a cognitive-behavioral intervention for pathological gambling: a country-wide study. Ann Clin Psychiatry. 2013;25(4):250–6.

136. Wong DFK, Chung CLP, Wu J, Tang J, Lau P. A preliminary study of an integrated and culturally attuned cognitive behavioral group treatment for Chinese problem gamblers in Hong Kong. J Gambl Stud. 2015;31(3):1015–27.
137. Parhami I, Davtian M, Hanna K, Calix I, Fong TW. The implementation of a telephone-delivered intervention for Asian American disordered gamblers: a pilot study. Asian Am J Psychol. 2012a;3(3):145–59.
138. Griner D, Smith TB. Culturally adapted mental health intervention: a meta-analytic review. Psychother Theory Res Pract Train. 2006;43(4):531–48.
139. Hwang W, Wood JJ, Lin K, Cheung F. Cognitive-behavioral therapy with Chinese Americans: research, theory, and clinical practice. Cogn Behav Pract. 2006;13(4):293–303.
140. Sue S, McKinney H. Asian Americans in community mental health care system. Am J Orthopsychiatry. 1975;45:111–8.
141. True R. Mental health services in the Chinese American community. In: Ishikawa W, Hayashi N, editors. Service delivery in Pan Asian communities. CA: Pacific Asian Coalition; 1975.
142. Uba L. Meeting the mental health needs of Asian Americans: mainstream or segregated services. Prof Psychol. 1982;13:215–21.
143. Barrett L, Fraser S. The challenge of working with NESB communities experiencing gambling issues on the outskirts of Melbourne. Paper presented at the 9th National Association of Gambling Studies conference, Gold Coast, Australia, 1999.
144. Hwang W, Wood JJ. Being culturally sensitive is not the same as being culturally competent. Pragmat Case Stud Psychother. 2007;3(3):44–50.
145. Sue DW. Culture-Specific strategies in counselling: a conceptual framework. Prof Psychol Res Pr. 1990;21:424–33.
146. Oei TPS. The past, present and future of Asian CBT. Keynote presented at the 8th World Congress of behavioural and cognitive therapies, Melbourne, Australia. 2016.
147. Sawang S, Oei TPS, Goh YW. Are country and culture values interchangeable? A case example using occupational stress and coping. Int J Cross-cult Manag. 2006;6:205–19.

Preventing Adolescent Gambling Problems

14

Jeffrey L. Derevensky and Lynette Gilbeau

The landscape of gambling internationally has continued to evolve at an unprecedented rate. While traditional land-based gambling continues to flourish (e.g., casinos, racinos, card rooms, lotteries), technological advances have enabled more and more individuals to wager from the comfort of their own homes. Never before have there been such a multiplicity of different types of gambling activities that are easily accessible and readily available. Globally, gambling during the past decade has represented one of the fastest changing and growing industries in the world, with technological developments creating new innovative forms of gambling (e.g., fantasy and daily fantasy sports, skins gambling based upon skilled interactive games). While some jurisdictions (e.g., Atlantic City) have shown declines in gambling revenues, much of these revenues can be accounted for by increases in gambling opportunities in neighboring states. In other jurisdictions, for example, Macau, sociopolitical restrictions have limited the frequency of casino visits, ultimately curtailing revenues. In spite of these few blips, gambling continues to expand internationally. Gambling opportunities have become so prolific and widespread that it is difficult to find jurisdictions in which some form of gambling is not government controlled, regulated, organized, or owned, and even in jurisdictions without regulated forms of gambling, non-regulated gambling (e.g., among peers or online gambling) continues to flourish. Internationally, gambling continues to be viewed as a socially acceptable form of entertainment in spite of the acknowledged social, familial, and personal costs associated with excessive problematic gambling.

J. L. Derevensky (✉) · L. Gilbeau
International Centre for Youth Gambling Problems and High-Risk Behaviors,
McGill University, Montreal, QC, Canada
e-mail: jeffrey.derevensky@mcgill.ca; lynette.gilbeau@mcgill.ca

© Springer Nature Switzerland AG 2019
A. Heinz et al. (eds.), *Gambling Disorder*, https://doi.org/10.1007/978-3-030-03060-5_14

14.1   Adolescent Gambling

Most often considered an adult activity, there is a plethora of research suggesting gambling's popularity among adolescents (see [1–4]). This is likely a result of gambling's general social acceptability, governmental endorsements, advertisements, the allure associated with casinos, technological advances for easy accessibility, parental acquiescence, and the way in which gambling has been positively portrayed in the media. With television shows and movies depicting gambling's glamour and excitement (e.g., *21*, *Runner Runner*, *Casino Royale*, *The Gambler*, *CSI Las Vegas*, etc.) and televised world championship poker tournaments where young people win millions of dollars (recent World Series of Poker multimillion-dollar tournament winners have most often been in their 20s), gambling has become commonplace among youth. In spite of the fact that almost all jurisdictions have legislative statutes prohibiting children and adolescents from engaging in regulated forms of gambling (e.g., lottery, casinos, horse racing, machine gambling, online wagering), many young people continue to be actively engaged in both regulated and non-regulated (e.g., card games and sports wagering among peers, fantasy sports leagues, etc.) forms of gambling.

Prevalence findings examining youth gambling behavior have consistently revealed that adolescents (12–17 years of age) have managed to participate, to some degree, in practically all forms of social, government-sanctioned, and non-regulated gambling activities available in their homes and communities [1, 2, 4]. Typical forms of gambling among teens include card playing for money (poker, while waning, is still popular), sports wagering, dice, and board games with family and friends; betting with peers on games of personal skill (e.g., pool, bowling, basketball, and other sports); and arcade or video games for money and purchasing lottery tickets (especially scratch tickets). While a number of adolescents report engaging in other forms of gambling, including gambling in bingo halls and cardrooms and gambling on electronic gambling machines (slot machines, video poker machines, sports wagering through a bookmaker, wagering via Internet gambling sites), gambling on these types of activities are often age and accessibility dependent ([3–8].

In general, adolescents' gambling behavior has often been found to be dependent upon a number of factors including local availability/accessibility of games, the geographical proximity of gambling venues, the individual's gender (males gamble more frequently, wager larger amounts of money, and are typically more actively engaged in sports wagering, whereas female adolescents have been shown to prefer lottery ticket purchases and bingo), and age restrictions (age regulations in certain jurisdictions vary considerably and are often dependent on the type of gambling activity). For example, lotteries typically require a lower age than the age required to access a casino, with older teens and young adults preferring machine gambling, poker, and casino playing. There is also research suggesting one's cultural background and heritage, when controlling for accessibility, can influence adolescent gambling prevalence rates (see [4, 7, 9].

While there is ample research suggesting that adolescents typically have gambled for money sometime before reaching 18 years of age, most teens do so occasionally with few experiencing gambling-related problems. Youth gambling, similar to adult gambling, can be viewed on a continuum ranging from non-gambling to social/occasional/recreational gambling to problem/pathological/disordered gambling. Within the adolescent gambling literature, the terms *social/occasional/non-problematic/recreational gambling* have typically been used to denote occasional infrequent gambling. Adolescents deemed *at risk* for a gambling problem typically endorse a number of gambling-related problems on gambling diagnostic screens but fail to reach clinical criteria. Those individuals experiencing significant gambling-related problems, *disordered, problem, pathological*, or *compulsive gambling*, reach the clinical diagnostic criteria. Their gambling behaviors typically result in severe psychosocial, behavioral, economic, academic, interpersonal, mental health, and legal difficulties. It should be noted that youth exhibiting a gambling disorder often have a variety of concomitant mental health issues. For some, mental health issues drive these adolescents to gambling as a form of escape, while for others their gambling problems actually result in increased mental health disorders.

14.2 Adolescent Problem/Disordered Gambling

There is a large body of research suggesting that adolescents, as a developmental group, constitute a high-risk population for multiple risk-taking and addictive behaviors, including gambling problems ([1, 3, 4, 8–12]. Volberg et al. [4], while noting significant methodological differences in prevalence studies, concluded that between 60% and 80% of adolescents report having engaged in some form of gambling for money during the past year (age and accessibility dependent), with the vast majority of these adolescents being social, recreational, and occasional gamblers. However, reviews of prevalence studies of adolescent problem and disordered gambling have revealed that between 2% and 8% of adolescents report experiencing serious gambling problems with another 10–15% being at risk for the development of a gambling problem [4]. A recent analysis of international studies since 2000, with emphasis on European research, suggested that between 0.2% and 12.3% of youth meet the criteria for problem gambling [1]. These variability rates are often highly dependent upon different methodological approaches (e.g., instruments, different cut scores, use of different numbers of items, translations of instruments, timeframes) as well as accessibility and availability of gambling opportunities. There are also a number of recent longitudinal studies [13] that seem to suggest that disordered gambling may not be a stable construct over time for all individuals, with some individuals going from problem/disordered gambling to recreational/occasional gambling, while for others this can be a lifetime disorder. Examining the timeframe for disordered gambling remains quite important (e.g., past 6 months, past year, or lifetime gambling results in different prevalence rates). This also attests to the findings that lifetime disordered gambling rates are always higher than past year rates (some adolescent studies have looked at past 3 months).

Overall, given our current knowledge and reliance on existing screening instruments, there remains substantial evidence to suggest that adolescent prevalence rates of disordered gambling are considerably higher than that of adults. Yet, in spite of the increased diversity of gambling activities, increased technological advances, and increased availability and accessibility, the prevalence rates of disordered gambling among our youth have remained fairly constant during the past two decades. Nevertheless, two important facts are necessary to note: (a) the population of young people during the past two decades has increased, thus resulting in an increase in the absolute number of youth experiencing gambling problems in spite of relatively stable prevalence rates, and (b) the concomitant behavioral, familial, social, educational, mental health, economic, and legal problems associated with adolescent disordered gambling will have not only short-term but lifetime implications [3, 14–23]. It remains important to note that pathological/disordered gamblers do not constitute a homogeneous group (e.g., sports gamblers are often different from poker players who are different from casino gamblers) and that some forms of gambling, impacted by their structural or situational factors, may be more problematic and symptomatic of problem gamblers (e.g., slot machines and electronic gambling machines have been called the "crack cocaine" of gambling and are designed to result in repetitive play [24]).

14.3 Understanding Adolescent Problem/Disordered Gambling: A Precursor to Prevention

As previously noted, while a substantial proportion of youth engage in occasional gambling, it is only a relatively small percentage who go on to experience significant gambling and gambling-related problems. Yet, for these individuals and their families, the negative consequences are pervasive, with many experiencing a wide range of multiple disorders (e.g., alcohol and/or drug use disorder, nicotine dependence, mood disorders, anxiety disorder, personality disorders, impulsivity, depression, and delinquency) [21, 23, 25]. There is also evidence that these youth score more poorly on measures of resilience and coping in the face of adversity [26, 27]. Given the multiplicity of concomitant mental health issues, a more general mental health approach to prevention may be important.

Individuals with gambling problems typically report having a preoccupation with gambling; multiple attempts at recouping losses; increasing wagers; lying to family members and peers about their gambling; a perceived illusion of control; an inability to understand random events; and high levels of anxiety, impulsivity, and/or depression when trying to reduce their gambling. For many of these youth, gambling represents a coping strategy in order to escape daily problems (familial-, peer-, and school-related) [28]. The need for increased money often leads these youths to borrowing increasingly large sums of money from peers, family members, and loan sharks and/or criminal behaviors. Understanding the early warning signs of problem gambling can help deter youth from further gambling before their indebtedness becomes excessive.

There is little doubt that attention to the prevention of a gambling disorder as well as other mental health and behavioral disorders is important. A report from the National Research Council and Institute of Medicine concluded that there is emerging evidence for the cost-effectiveness of prevention initiatives for multiple mental, emotional, and behavioral disorders. We have long argued the potential value of prevention of gambling and other addictive disorders among youth but have stated that these programs should be evidence-based [3, 16].

14.4   The Correlates and Risk Factors Associated with Problem Gambling

Given youth problem or disordered gamblers are not a homogenous group, there is no single constellation of risk factors predictive of a gambling disorder. Nevertheless, considerable research during the last 25 years has focused on identifying those risk factors associated with excessive gambling problems and has identified possible protective factors as a way to minimize problems through early prevention strategies and clinical interventions [3, 23, 29–33].

Gupta et al. [34] and Derevensky [3] have suggested that adopting a bio-psycho-social-environmental framework may serve to promote a better understanding of the onset and developmental course of gambling problems. Addressing these correlates will likely enhance the robustness of prevention initiatives. Reviews by Derevensky [3] and Shead et al. [23] point to a wide range of empirical studies suggesting (a) gender differences (males tend to gamble more frequently, make larger wagers, have an earlier age of onset, engage in a wider variety of gambling behaviors, and report more pervasive gambling problems). Additionally, males report a preference for sports betting and wagering on games of skill, while females prefer gambling on the lottery and bingo; (b) youth with gambling problems frequently report having parents who gamble excessively, engage in other addictive behaviors, and/or have been involved in illegal activities; (c) for older adolescents, one's peer group plays an important role in endorsing or promoting gambling, and adolescent disordered gamblers report having friends with similar gambling interests; (d) youth with a gambling disorder report having positive attitudes toward gambling and perceive it to be a socially acceptable pastime; (e) while youth with gambling problems understand the negative consequences associated with excessive gambling, they don't view themselves as having a gambling problem; (f) risks associated with disordered gambling are viewed as a long-term consequence and not of immediate concern; (g) cultural, ethnic, and regional differences have been shown to impact disordered gamblers; and (h) problem gamblers who score higher on measures of excitability and extroversion tend to have difficulty conforming to societal norms, and experience difficulties with self-discipline, have been shown to exhibit higher state and trait anxiety scores, are more impulsive, are greater risk takers, and are more self-blaming and guilt prone. Adolescent disordered gamblers have multiple mental health issues, including being at heightened risk for suicide ideation, suicide attempts and risky behaviors.

14.4.1 Protective Factors

A limited number of studies have focused on identifying the protective and buffering factors thought to reduce and/or minimize the incidence of adolescent disordered gambling. While there exist some unique risk factors associated with problem gambling compared with other adolescent high-risk and addictive behaviors, Dickson-Gillespie et al. [16] in a comprehensive study concluded that family cohesion played a significant role as a protective factor. There is also evidence that familial and peer disapproval of gambling may be a reliable protective factor. In a number of studies, resilience has been shown to be a possible protective factor for youth gambling problems and other adolescent high-risk behaviors [27].

14.5 Prevention of Gambling Problems

Unlike prevention programs developed to help prevent substance abuse and dependency as well as a number of other mental health issues, prevention programs aimed to minimize disordered gambling have been hindered by a number of factors, myths, and common misconceptions including that (a) age restrictions on government-regulated gambling activities deter and prohibit adolescent participation, (b) disordered gambling is an adult disorder and as such underage individuals cannot have gambling problems, and (c) adolescents have little available discretionary funds for gambling. In spite of these misconceptions, the international prevalence research of youth disordered gamblers all point to addressing youth gambling within a social and public health policy framework. Historically, the focus in prevention research, in general, was initially to identify risk and vulnerability factors among at-risk populations. However, the identification of risk and vulnerability factors by themselves has been limited for prevention efforts since a large number of these factors are difficult to minimize (e.g., poverty) or identify (e.g., sexual abuse), as well as the fact that many high-risk youths never actually develop the anticipated negative behaviors. As a result, an attempt to identify variables and interactions between variables that might act as buffers or protective factors to counteract the risks associated with aberrant behavior has been postulated.

Predicated upon the belief that preventing mental health and substance use disorders and related problems in children, adolescents, and young adults remains critical to one's physical health and emotional well-being, early intervention is thought to have a better chance of reducing/minimizing the risks associated with mental health and substance use disorder. Thus, understanding the risk and protective factors of a specific disorder enables one to develop more effective prevention strategies. Williams et al. [35] argued that social scientists need to strive to develop *Best Practices* for programs and their implementation. Such policies could include (a) information dissemination, (b) education, (c) provisions for alternative activities, (d) strict regulatory and environmental policies and local community-based assistance, (e) the identification of high-risk individuals and activities, and (f) intervention for both high-risk individuals and those in need of treatment. While this sounds relatively simple, Ammerman et al. [36] suggest that potentially threatening public health challenges are indeed complex and that effective universal programs are difficult to develop.

14.5.1 Abstinence Versus Harm-Minimization Approaches

When addressing gambling prevention programs for youth, prevention approaches, in general, can be conceptualized as falling into two general categories: those emphasizing abstinence or those promoting harm minimization (sometimes referred to as harm reduction). While these two categories are not necessarily mutually exclusive, prevention programs for each of these approaches are predicated on different goals and processes. A harm-reduction framework incorporates policies, programs, or strategies that help individuals to reduce the harmful, negative consequences incurred through involvement in a risky behavior without requiring abstinence [30, 37]. In most jurisdictions, youths are typically (legally) prohibited access to government-regulated gambling venues, supporting an abstinence approach. However, the question remains as to whether abstinence is a realistic goal for youth when the research clearly suggests that the majority of adolescents report having gambled for money on one or more activities (some on regulated forms of gambling, while others report gambling among peers) and a growing body of research reveals that parents do not particularly view gambling among their underage children as being highly problematic [38]. This highlights both the paradox and the confusion as to which primary prevention approach to promote abstinence or harm reduction.

14.5.2 Harm-Minimization Programs

Universal adolescent harm-reduction programs are intended to modify inappropriate attitudes toward risky behaviors, enhance resilience and positive decision-making, as well as educate youth about the short- and long-term risks associated with a particular behavior [39]. Most youth gambling prevention programs promote a harm-minimization framework and emphasize "responsible gambling" [39]. The fact remains that there is universal acceptance that the age of onset of gambling is a significant factor associated with problem gambling (the earlier one begins gambling, the more likely they are to develop a gambling problem [4, 7, 11, 29, 30, 40]). As such, one salient approach, where feasible, is to delay the age of onset.

Most of the available gambling prevention programs designed for youth have typically incorporated a number of harm-minimization and educational objectives, including (1) highlighting the difference between games of chance and games of skill; (2) educating participants about erroneous cognitions, probability, and the independence of events; (3) dispelling the myth of the "illusion of control" regarding random events; (4) addressing issues of independence of events; (5) articulating the warning signs associated with problem gambling; and (6) providing resources to aid individuals either experiencing a gambling problem or who are at risk for a gambling problem [3, 41, 42]. Some more comprehensive prevention curricula seek to encourage the development of interpersonal skills, foster effective coping strategies, provide techniques to improve self-esteem, and offer ideas for resisting peer pressure [39].

Comprehensive and substantive elementary- and high school-based prevention programs for problem gambling are relatively rare but in fact do exist [35]. However, it should be noted that independent of the type of prevention program, for any program to be effective, it will require a sustained, multifaceted, and coordinated approach if it is to reach a wide range of youth. While this chapter is intended to discuss adolescent gambling prevention initiatives, it must be recognized that gambling problems represent only one type of high-risk behavior and that such programs should be generally thought of within a larger context of mental health programs.

While there exists a limited number of prevention initiatives for youth (see [43]; the International Centre for Youth Gambling and High-Risk Behavior's website www.youthgambling.com) (see Table 14.1), new forms of gambling, in particular online and mobile gambling, are making accessibility much easier. To compound this issue, we have online social casino games that simulate actual gambling activities with higher payout rates that may be encouraging individuals to gamble (see [44–46]). The similarities between gambling and gaming have been articulated by Griffiths et al. [47]. These types of games could be breeding a new generation of gamblers. The Morgan Stanley report [48], on social gambling, suggested that social gambling offers the potential to "teach young people to gamble." There is little doubt that such games actually normalize gambling among children and adolescents.

With the surge of online gambling, prevention experts have developed a number of online "responsible gambling tools" which include limit setting (both time and money), in-game informative messaging, self-appraisal quizzes, pop-up messaging reminding players of time and money wagered, enforced breaks in play, self-exclusion procedures, behavioral tracking tools, and personalized feedback. It should also be noted that there are a number of research studies suggesting more problem gamblers among individuals gambling over the Internet than in traditional land-based forms of gambling (e.g., [18, 43, 49]). In a recent study, early mobile gambling among adolescents was found to be predictive of gambling problems among adolescents [50]. These findings have led to the development, implementation, and evaluation of programs focused on providing personalized feedback to gamblers as a prevention strategy. Auer and Griffiths [51], in a series of studies, attempted to examine whether or not a personalized feedback and information system given to players in real time while gambling online could in fact impact future gambling behavior. Their results suggest that providing personalized feedback incorporating normative measures may be an effective tool in modifying gambling behavior. As more and

Table 14.1 Youth gambling prevention programs

Prevention program	School level	Developer	Website
Amazing Chateau	Grades 4–6	International Centre for Youth Gambling Problems and High-Risk Behaviors—McGill University	www.youthgambling.com
Clean Break	Grades 8–12	International Centre for Youth Gambling Problems and High-Risk Behaviors—McGill University	www.youthgambling.com
Don't Bet on It	Grades 10–12	Responsible Gambling Council	http://curriculum.org/resources/dont-bet-on-it-8211-a-youth-problem-gambling-prevention-program
Facing the Odds	Grades 5–8	Harvard Medical School—Division of Addictions	http://www.divisiononaddictions.org/curr/facing_the_odds.htm
Hooked City	Grades 6–8	International Centre for Youth Gambling Problems and High-Risk Behaviors—McGill University	www.youthgambling.com
Know Limits	Grades 7–12	International Centre for Youth Gambling Problems and High-Risk Behaviors—McGill University	www.youthgambling.com
Stacked Deck	Grades 9–12	Robert Williams and Robert Wood	http://www.uleth.ca/research/alberta-gambling-research-institute-agri
Wanna Bet?	Grades 3–8	Minnesota Council on Compulsive Gambling	http://www.nati.org/prevention_tools/youth.aspx
Youth Gambling: An Awareness and Prevention Workshop—Level I	Grades 4–6	International Centre for Youth Gambling Problems and High-Risk Behaviors—McGill University	www.youthgambling.com
Youth Gambling: An Awareness and Prevention Workshop—Level II	Grades 7–10	International Centre for Youth Gambling Problems and High-Risk Behaviors—McGill University	www.youthgambling.com

(continued)

Table 14.1 (continued)

Prevention program	School level	Developer	Website
Youth Making Choices: A Curriculum-Based Gambling Prevention Program	Grades 10–12	Centre for Addiction and Mental Health (CAMH)	http://www.problemgambling.ca/EN/ResourcesForProfessionals/Pages/CurriculumYouthMakingChoices.aspx
Youth Gambling Problems: Practical Information for Health Practitioners	Physicians	International Centre for Youth Gambling Problems and High-Risk Behaviors—McGill University	www.youthgambling.com
Youth Gambling Problems—Practical Information for Professional in the Criminal Justice System	Judges, Attorneys	International Centre for Youth Gambling Problems and High-Risk Behaviors—McGill University	www.youthgambling.com

more young people have smartphones, this represents a promising area for the development of prevention initiatives (for a comprehensive discussion see Marchica and Derevensky [52]).

A wide diversity of information/awareness campaigns have traditionally focused upon encouraging individuals to understand their gambling limits, provided warnings about the potentially addictive nature of gambling, enumerated the signs/symptoms/behaviors associated with problem gambling, provided information about where individuals can seek help for a gambling disorder, discussed the accurate mathematical odds associated with various gambling activities, dispelled common gambling fallacies and erroneous cognitions, and provided guidelines and suggestions for problem-free gambling [43]. A number of interactive, educational CD-ROM and DVD games as well as PowerPoint workshop presentations have been developed to help educate young people (see www.youthgambling.com/prevenmtion). As well, educational programs targeting professionals such as individuals in the legal system (judges, attorneys) and physicians have been developed. Such resources have been shown to result in improved knowledge of gambling and problem gambling while helping to dispel some of the erroneous myths and cognitions surrounding gambling.

14.6 The Importance of Developing Responsible Advertising Policies and Guidelines

Although there is only a limited amount of information available concerning the specific impact of gambling advertisements on gambling behavior, youth are continuously bombarded by advertisements enticing them to "live the dream" or visit a destination casino. Never in any of these advertisements promoting gambling is there an accurate balance between the benefits associated with gambling and the risks and the potential problems associated with gambling. Rather, adolescents frequently report that these advertisements depict individuals who are winning, happy, and excited. Youth report being bombarded through the Internet with pop-up messages enticing them to gamble and offers of sign-up bonuses with a growing number of online gaming operators using social media advertising to invite individuals to gamble money or to play on their free sites [53].

Young people, similar to adults, are resistant to enticing advertisements for all types of products. They see the newest trends, clothes, food products, and movies not to mention gambling advertisements (there is a reason cigarette and alcohol advertisements are prohibited). Adolescents report having a good knowledge and recall of popular gambling commercials, are familiar with the slogans of land-based casinos and lotteries, and easily remember the expressions of those who have won. In a study examining lottery playing among adolescents, while adolescents readily recall tickets being advertised, only problem gamblers were more likely enticed to purchase these tickets [54]. This further suggests that legislative policies concerning the minimum age to gamble must be strictly followed, monitored, and enforced. Few jurisdictions levy fines or remove licenses for selling lottery tickets to underage minors, although fines are more common for underage play among land-based casinos. St-Pierre et al. [55] found that only a moderate proportion of convenience store vendors (60%) were compliant with prohibiting underage youth from purchasing a lottery ticket in spite of legislative and regulatory statutes. Other strategies include prohibiting lottery products particularly attractive to youth. Currently, GamGard and ASTERIG, tools designed to assess lottery products for their appeal to vulnerable populations, are being used by a number of lottery vendors internationally.

While a number of prevention programs exist primarily for adults (e.g., self-exclusion, telephone "hotlines" and problem gambling call centers, limiting access to cash through ATMs, prohibition of credit, player card and behavioral tracking systems, forcing individuals to take a break in play, the incorporation of responsible gambling modifications to EGMs (electronic gambling machines), there is a real need for parental supervision and education both at home and in the classroom. In a series of studies, Derevensky and his colleagues found that among 13 potentially risky adolescent behaviors (e.g., drug and alcohol use, bullying, drinking and driving, etc.), gambling among teens was the least concerning activity as evaluated by parents, teachers, and even mental health professionals [38, 56–58] suggesting the need for further public awareness of the prevalence of youth gambling and the warning signs and consequences of adolescent problematic gambling.

14.6.1 Evaluating Prevention Programs

In the field of youth gambling prevention, there have been relatively few published evaluations of youth gambling prevention or intervention programs [59]. According to Ladouceur et al. [41] in their review of youth gambling prevention program, evaluations concluded that the majority of the evaluative studies did not include measures of gambling behaviors or long-term outcomes. Short-term benefits of these prevention programs point to improved knowledge and a reduction in misconceptions about gambling among youth [41, 60]. However, without follow-up evaluations and measurement of gambling behaviors, it is unclear whether gambling behavior is actually impacted in the long term [41].

14.7 Some Final Thoughts

The landscape of gambling is continually changing with technological advances, new forms of gambling, and increasing ease of access. This changing landscape, with an emphasis on technological advances and new gambling opportunities (online and mobile gambling, fantasy sports), the inclusion of social casino games, and the normalization and social acceptability of gambling and the growing popularity of e-sports wagering, represents a growing concern. Mental health specialists studying teens have long suggested that adolescence is a developmental stage marked by significant physical, social, cognitive, and emotional changes. The continued expansion of gambling, the glitz and glamour associated with gambling, and the social acceptance of the industry's expansion may result in more youth experimenting with gambling and ultimately more experiencing gambling-related problems. Whether these problems are short term or long term, the consequences can be quite severe. Researchers and clinicians have not yet realized *Best Practices* for treatment or prevention, and more longitudinal studies are needed.

Youth gambling, like many other adolescent risky behaviors, represents an important public health issue which needs to be addressed. Incorporating youth gambling into a public health framework [61, 62], using a multidimensional perspective recognizing the individual and social determinants, and simultaneously drawing upon health promotion principles, represent a plausible approach for addressing the issues of youth gambling and problem gambling. This issue is only beginning to gain attention.

References

1. Calado F, Alexandre J, Griffiths M. Prevalence of adolescent problem gambling: a systematic review of recent research. J Gambl Stud. 2017;33:397–424.
2. Delfabbro P, King D, Derevensky J. Adolescent gambling and problem gambling: prevalence, current issues and concerns. Curr Addict Rep. 2016;3(2):268–74.
3. Derevensky J. Teen gambling: understanding a growing epidemic. New York: Rowman & Littlefield Publishing; 2012.
4. Volberg R, Gupta R, Griffiths MD, Olason DT, Delfabbro P. An international perspective on youth gambling prevalence studies. In: Derevensky J, Shek D, Merrick J, editors. Youth gambling problems: the hidden addiction. Berlin: De Gruyter; 2010. p. 21–56.
5. Griffiths M, Parke J. Adolescent gambling on the internet: a review. Int J Adolesc Med Health. 2010;22(1):59–75.
6. Molinaro S, Canale N, Vieno A, Lenzi M, Siciliano V, Gori m, et al. Country and individual-level determinants of probable pathological gambling in adolescence: a multi-level cross-national comparison. Addiction. 2014;109:2089–97.
7. Productivity Commission. Gambling Productivity Commission Inquiry Report. Australian Government. 2010.
8. Welte J, Barnes G, Tidwell M, Hoffman J. The prevalence of problem gambling among US adolescents and young adults: results from a national survey. J Gambl Stud. 2008;24(2):119–33.
9. Abbott MW, Volberg RA, Bellringer M, Reith G. A review of research on aspects of problem gambling. Final report. Prepared for the Responsibility in Gambling Trust, London. 2004.
10. Jessor R, editor. New perspectives on adolescent risk behavior. Cambridge: Cambridge University Press; 1998.
11. National Research Council. Pathological gambling: a critical review. Washington, DC: National Academy Press; 1999.
12. Romer D, editor. Reducing adolescent risk: toward an integrated approach. CA: Sage Publications; 2003.
13. Williams R, Hann R, Schopflocher D, West B, McLaughlin P, White N, King K, Flexhaug T. Quinte longitudinal study of gambling and problem gambling. Report prepared for the Ontario Problem Gambling Research Centre and the Ontario Ministry of Health and Long Term Care. 2015.
14. Derevensky J, Gupta R. Adolescents with gambling problems: a synopsis of our current knowledge. eGambling. 2004. p. 10. Available at http://www.camh.net/egambling.
15. Derevensky J, Pratt L, Hardoon K, Gupta R. Gambling problems and features of attention deficit hyperactivity disorder among children and adolescents. J Addict Med. 2007;1(3):165–72.

16. Dickson-Gillespie L, Rugle L, Rosenthal R, Fong T. Preventing the incidence and harm of gambling problems. J Prim Prev. 2008;29(1):37–55.
17. Felsher J, Derevensky J, Gupta R. Young adults with gambling problems: the impact of childhood maltreatment. Int J Ment Heal Addict. 2010;8(4):545–56.
18. Griffiths M, King D, Delfabbro P. Adolescent gambling-like experiences: are they a cause for concern? Educ Health. 2009;27(2):27–30.
19. Hardoon K, Derevensky J, Gupta R. An examination of the influence of familial, emotional, conduct and cognitive problems, and hyperactivity upon youth risk-taking and adolescent gambling problems. Report prepared for the Ontario Problem Gambling Research Centre, Ontario. 2002.
20. Hardoon K, Gupta R, Derevensky J. Psychosocial variables associated with adolescent gambling: a model for problem gambling. Psychol Addict Behav. 2004;18(2):170–9.
21. Nower L, Blaszczynski A, Choi K, Glynn J. State of evidence: adverse effects of disordered gambling on individuals and families. Report prepared for Gambling Research Exchange Ontario. 2015.
22. Petry N. Pathological gambling: etiology, comorbidity, and treatment. Washington, DC: American Psychological Association Press; 2005.
23. Shead N, Derevensky J, Gupta R. Risk and protective factors associated with youth problem gambling. Int J Adolesc Med Health. 2010;22(1):39.
24. Schüll N. Addiction by design: machine gambling in Las Vegas. Princeton: Princeton University Press; 2012.
25. Barnes GM, Welte JW, Hoffman JH, Tidwell MCO. The co-occurrence of gambling with substance use and conduct disorder among youth in the United States. Am J Addict. 2011;20(2):166–73.
26. Lussier I, Derevensky JL, Gupta R, Bergevin T, Ellenbogen S. Youth gambling behaviors: an examination of the role of resilience. Psychol Addict Behav. 2007;21(2):165–73.
27. Lussier I, Derevensky J, Gupta R, Vitaro F. Risk, compensatory, protective, and vulnerability processes influencing youth gambling problems and other high-risk behaviours. Psychol Addict Behav. 2014;28:404–13.
28. Bergevin T, Gupta R, Derevensky J, Kaufman F. Adolescent gambling: understanding the role of stress and coping. J Gambl Stud. 2006;22(2):195–208.
29. Dickson L, Derevensky J, Gupta R. The prevention of youth gambling problems: a conceptual model. J Gambl Stud. 2002;18(2):97–159.
30. Dickson L, Derevensky J, Gupta R. Youth gambling problems: a harm reduction prevention model. Addict Res Theory. 2004;12(4):305–16.
31. St-Pierre R, Derevensky J. Youth gambling behavior: novel approaches to prevention and intervention. Curr Addict Rep. 2016;3(2):157–65.
32. St-Pierre R, Temcheff C, Derevensky J. Adolescent gambling and problem gambling: examination of an extended theory of planned behaviour. Int Gambl Stud. 2015;15:506–25.
33. St-Pierre R, Temcheff C, Derevensky J. Theory of planned behavior in school-based adolescent problem gambling prevention: a conceptual framework. J Prim Prev. 2015;36:361–85.
34. Gupta R, Nower L, Derevensky J, Blaszczynski A, Faregh N, Temcheff C. Problem gambling in adolescents: an examination of the pathways model. J Gambl Stud. 2013;29(3):575–88.
35. Williams R, West B, Simpson R. Prevention of problem gambling: a comprehensive review of the evidence, and identified best practices. Report prepared for the Ontario Problem Gambling Research Centre and the Ontario Ministry of Health and Long Term Care. 2012.
36. Ammerman A, Smith TW, Calancie L. Practice-based evidence in public health: improving reach, relevance, and results. Annu Rev Public Health. 2014;35:47–63.
37. Ariyabuddhiphongs V. Problem gambling prevention: before, during, and after measures. Int J Ment Heal Addict. 2013;11(5):568–82.
38. Campbell C, Derevensky J, Meerkamper E, Cutajar J. Parents' perceptions of adolescent gambling: a Canadian national study. J Gambl Iss. 2011;25:36–53.
39. Derevensky J, Gupta R. Youth gambling prevention initiatives: a decade of research. In: Derevensky J, Shek D, Merrick J, editors. Youth gambling problems: the hidden addiction. Berlin: De Gruyter; 2011. p. 213–30.

40. Jacobs D. Youth gambling in North America: an analysis of long term trends and future prospects. In: Derevensky J, Gupta R, editors. Gambling problems in youth: theoretical and applied perspectives. NY: Kluwer Academic/Plenum Publishers; 2004. p. 1–26.
41. Ladouceur R, Goulet A, Vitaro F. Prevention programmes for youth gambling: a review of the empirical evidence. Int Gambl Stud. 2013;13(2):141–59.
42. Turner N, Macdonald J, Somerset M. Life skills, mathematical reasoning and critical thinking: a curriculum for the prevention of problem gambling. J Gambl Stud. 2008;24(3):367–80.
43. Williams R, West B, Simpson R. Prevention of problem gambling: a comprehensive review of the evidence. Report prepared for the Ontario Problem Gambling Research Centre, Ontario, Canada. 2007.
44. Derevensky J, Gainsbury S. Social casino gaming and adolescents: should we be concerned and is regulation in sight? Int J Law Psychiatry. 2016;44:1–6.
45. Hollingshead S, Kim A, Wohl M, Derevensky J. The social casino gaming-gambling link: motivation for playing social casino games determines whether gambling increases or decreases. J Gambl Iss. 2016;33:52–67.
46. Kim A, Wohl M, Gupta R, Derevensky J. From the mouths of social media users: a focus group study exploring the social casino gaming-online gambling link. J Behav Addict. 2016;5(1):115–21.
47. Griffiths MD, King DL, Delfabbro PH. The technological convergence of gambling and gaming practices. In: Richard DCS, Blaszczynski A, Nower L, editors. The Wiley-Blackwell handbook of disordered gambling. Chichester: Wiley; 2014. p. 327–46.
48. Lewis V, Rollo J, Devitt S, Egbert J, Strawn M, Nagasaka M. Social gambling: click here to play. Morgan Stanley Research Report, Nov 14. 2012.
49. McBride J, Derevensky J. Internet gambling and risk-taking among students: an exploratory study. J Behav Addict. 2012;1:50–8.
50. Zhao Y, Marchica L, Derevensky J, Ivoska W. Mobile gambling among youth: a warning sign for problem gambling? Unpublished manuscript. McGill University. 2016.
51. Auer MM, Griffiths MD. The use of personalized behavioral feedback for online gamblers: an empirical study. Front Psychol. 2016;6:1406.
52. Marchica L, Derevensky J. Personalized normative feedback as an intervention method for gambling disorders: a systematic review. J Behav Addict. 2016;5(1):1–10.
53. Gainsbury SM, King D, Delfabbro P, Hing N, Russell A, Blaszczynski A, Derevensky J. The use of social media in gambling. Gambling Research Australia. 2015.
54. Felsher J, Derevensky J, Gupta R. Lottery participation by youth with gambling problems: are lottery tickets a gateway to other gambling venues? Int Gambl Stud. 2004;4(2):109–26.
55. St-Pierre R, Derevensky J, Gupta R, Martin I. Preventing lottery ticket sales to minors: factors influencing retailers' compliance behaviour. Int Gambl Stud. 2011;11:173–92.
56. Derevensky J, St-Pierre R, Temcheff C, Gupta R. Teacher awareness and attitudes regarding adolescent risky behaviors: is adolescent gambling perceived to be a problem? J Gambl Stud. 2014;30:435–51.
57. Hayer T, Griffiths M, Meyer G. Gambling. In: Handbook of adolescent behavioral problems. United States: Springer; 2005. p. 467–86.
58. Temcheff C, Derevensky J, St-Pierre R, Gupta R, Martin I. Beliefs and attitudes of mental health professionals with respect to gambling and other high risk behaviors in schools. Int J Ment Heal Addict. 2014;12:716–29.
59. Blinn-Pike L, Worthy SL, Jonkman J. Adolescent gambling: a review of an emerging field of research. J Adolesc Health. 2010;47(3):223–36.
60. Lupu IR, Lupu V. Gambling prevention program for teenagers. J Cogn Behav Psychother. 2013;13(2a):575–84.
61. Messerlian C, Derevensky J. Youth gambling: a public health perspective. J Gambl Iss. 2005;14.
62. Messerlian C, Derevensky J, Gupta R. Youth gambling problems: a public health framework. Health Promot Int. 2005;20:69–79.

Gambling Disorder: Future Perspectives in Research and Treatment

Nina Romanczuk-Seiferth, Marc N. Potenza, and Andreas Heinz

15.1   Gambling Disorder: Why It Needs More Attention

From a clinical viewpoint, the phenomenon of problem gambling is clearly a relevant public health concern. It is the first non-substance-use behavior formally recognized as a possible addiction by the American Psychiatric Association, appearing in the fifth edition of the organization's *Diagnostic and Statistical Manual of Mental Disorders* (DSM-5) in 2013. It similarly is recognized by the World Health Organization in the 11th edition of the International Classification of Diseases (ICD-11). However, its relevance to affected people and to society more broadly is relatively independent of the scientific debate on the appropriate diagnostic criteria and its categorization within diagnostic systems. Basic learning theory and research on habit formation in addictions suggest that engaging in specific behaviors with high frequency at the expense of other activities and in spite of negative consequences increases the probability of developing related health problems [1]. For gambling-related problems, very serious negative consequences, especially in social,

N. Romanczuk-Seiferth (✉) · A. Heinz
Department of Psychiatry and Psychotherapy, Charité—Universitätsmedizin Berlin,
Berlin, Germany
e-mail: nina.seiferth@charite.de; andreas.heinz@charite.de

M. N. Potenza
Yale Center of Excellence in Gambling Research, Yale University School of Medicine,
New Haven, CT, USA

Women and Addictions Core of Women's Health Research at Yale, Yale University School of
Medicine, New Haven, CT, USA

Yale University School of Medicine, New Haven, USA
e-mail: marc.potenza@yale.edu

© Springer Nature Switzerland AG 2019
A. Heinz et al. (eds.), *Gambling Disorder*, https://doi.org/10.1007/978-3-030-03060-5_15

psychological, and financial domains, are common. Gambling-related problems often include missing work and losing jobs, impaired relationships with spouses and other family members, and large debts that may lead to bankruptcy. Suicidal thoughts or behaviors may be prompted by gambling losses. Further, psychiatric comorbidity is the rule, not the exception. It is estimated from community data that 96% of individuals with gambling disorder have one or more psychiatric disorders and that 64% have three or more such conditions [2]. The prevalence of gambling disorder is approximately 0.5% [2, 3], slightly less than psychiatric disorders like bipolar disorder or schizophrenia. The impact of gambling disorder extends beyond those with the disorder as family, friends, employers, and others are affected. Thus, gambling disorder is a significant mental health issue that unfortunately receives relatively rather limited attention compared with other disorders [4]. Due to its relevance to society, gambling disorder should be of interest not only to physicians, psychologists, and other mental health care practitioners but also to government agencies, which typically pay too little attention to gambling-related problems. Although the possible harms related to problem gambling are well-documented, there is not a widespread public call for a strict regulation or even prohibition on gambling. Gambling is typically seen as a legitimate leisure-time pursuit, which most people can enjoy without problems. However, in order to protect the freedom of how individuals spend their time while at the same time promoting public health, it is important to understand how best to regulate gambling and prevent and treat gambling problems.

From a scientific perspective, gambling disorder deserves more attention. Albert Einstein once said, "Play is the highest form of research." More research is needed to understand why people play or gamble and how these common human behaviors may lead to harm in the case of gambling disorder and also gaming disorder. One of the most important scientific journals in the world, *Nature*, titled in its editorial in January 2018: "Science has a gambling problem." In this editorial, a criticism is raised that relatively few studies exist investigating the phenomenon of gambling and gambling problems in well-designed manners and which are conducted in real gambling environments [4, 5]. Such studies are needed to inform policymakers and clinicians as how best to handle the development of diverse online and offline gambling activities offered to people and potential gambling-related problems. Further, this approach should be applied to a broader range of behavioral addictions [6], particularly as gaming disorder will be included in ICD-11. Some countries have regulations to protect those who are most vulnerable to developing gambling problems – e.g., agreements with gambling establishments to ban people suffering from gambling disorder for fixed time periods. More empirical evidence is needed to show which strategies work best and to expand such approaches in order to better protect high-risk populations like adolescents. Ideally, this research should be independent from the related industry (e.g., funded by the government that is charged with protecting the public health).

In the above-mentioned Nature editorial, it is also argued that there may be some stereotypes associated with people spending money in the casino, at the racetrack, or elsewhere. Some portrayals of gambling in society may conjure images of glitter and luxury and of people seeming to take little responsibility for the consequences of their behaviors. Although the reality of most people affected by gambling disorder is typically far from this, such prejudices may decrease empathic reactions toward people suffering from significant gambling problems. Such stigmatizations share some similarities with historical views of people with substance-related disorders who may have been considered "weak-minded" or morally flawed in the past. Research on the development and maintenance of substance-use disorders has helped to mitigate such views by expanding the knowledge about these disorders. Thus, there is the need for governments to support research into gambling problems as is done for problematic alcohol and drug consumption.

15.2 Gambling Disorder: Future Directions

15.2.1 Rethinking Classification and Diagnostic Criteria

A significant change came with the publication of the DSM-5 in 2013. The condition "gambling disorder" was reclassified as a substance-related and addictive disorder, replacing pathological gambling that had been classified as an "impulse-control disorder not elsewhere classified" in earlier editions of the DSM. While the criteria remained nearly the same (with the removal of the illegal-acts criterion and changing of the diagnostic threshold from five of ten inclusion criteria to four of nine criteria), the reclassification of the disorder reflected evidence showing similarities with substance-use disorders in multiple domains including epidemiology, clinical phenomenology, genetics, neurobiology, prevention, and treatment [7, 8]. In an interview, Charles O'Brien, M.D., chair of the DSM-5 Work Group on Substance-Related and Addictive Disorders, stated: "The idea of a non-substance-related addiction may be new to some people, but those of us who are studying the mechanisms of addiction find strong evidence from animal and human research that addiction is a disorder of the brain reward system, and it doesn't matter whether the system is repeatedly activated by gambling or alcohol or another substance" [9]. Despite those clinical and neurobiological similarities which led to the changes in DSM-5 [10], future research should focus on both similarities and differences between gambling and substance-use disorders. For example, although tolerance development and withdrawal symptoms constitute core features of addictions in general [11], such symptoms in gambling disorder are usually milder than those in substance-use disorders. On the other hand, phenomena like craving and its influence on choice behavior as well as alterations in loss processing might be equally or even more relevant in non-substance-related problems due to the high generalizability of potentially triggering situations. Further, because non-substance-related addictions are not related to the use of specific substances, it may be possible to translate the concept of behavioral addictions to multiple aspects of human behavior. This comes with the potential danger and thus the responsibility for researchers as well as clinicians to consider the concept with caution in order to avoid stigmatization and to account adequately for variance in human behavior beyond mental illness (see also Chaps. 1 and 2).

Moreover, it is important to foster research that allows for a more complete view of the phenomena of gambling disorder. For example, different subtypes of gambling disorder have been proposed, like in the "pathways" model (see Chap. 3), and this model has gained empirical support. This and other models may be relevant in promoting advances in differential diagnosis and more targeted treatment options. It may also be helpful to include characteristics from cognitive research on gambling disorder, for example, gambling-related cognitive distortions may be assessed using psychometrically validated instruments in diagnosis and clinical practice (see Chap. 4).

Further, it is of interest for research in this field to move forward to a more continuous understanding of gambling behaviors and problems, with the understanding that gambling behaviors lie along a continuum of problem-gambling severity. From this viewpoint, there are many important reasons—including from a public health perspective [12]—to study continuous gambling phenotypes. This approach is also in line with efforts in understanding and treating psychiatric disorders from a dimensional perspective, including neurobiological approaches [13] and the research domain criteria (RDoC) initiative [14].

15.2.2 Understanding Neurobiological Mechanisms

From a neuroscientific perspective, gambling disorder may be of high interest to addiction research due to its non-substance-related nature. In contrast to substance-related addictive disorders, in gambling disorder there are not necessarily substance-related effects on the brain, e.g., neurotoxic effects of alcohol consumption on neurons in alcohol-use disorder. Thus, behavioral addictions such as gambling disorder may serve as an important model disease for studying the mechanisms underlying addiction. Therefore, it might also be of importance to better understand the neurobiological similarities as well as the differences between gambling disorder and substance-use disorders. Other behavioral addictions also warrant consideration. Research on other potentially relevant behavioral addictions, like compulsive buying, compulsive sexual behavior, and internet gaming disorder, appears rather scant to date (see Chap. 11), especially with regard to neurobiological studies.

As mentioned, neuroscientific research that identified neurobiological similarities between gambling and substance-use disorders contributed to a recategorization of gambling disorder in DSM-5. In comparison to the similarities, potential differences between substance-use disorders and gambling disorder have arguably received less attention. In order to deepen the understanding of differences (see Chap. 12), also specifically on a neural level (see Chap. 7), it is of high interest to further study gambling disorder in comparison to other conditions in domains like loss processing. The clinical phenomenon of loss chasing is a diagnostic criterion for gambling disorder that is not shared with substance-use disorders, although the concept of "chasing" (e.g., chasing drug highs or going on drug runs) may also apply more broadly to substance-use disorders. Alterations in loss processing as well as in the processing of near-misses on behavioral and neural levels may motivate loss chasing [15–20], but further research is needed to get a more complete picture. More research should also investigate relevant learning mechanisms at behavioral and neural levels that may lead to the development and maintenance of gambling disorder. While recent research exploring alterations in learning mechanisms in substance-use disorders may help to explain key features of these disorders [21–23], the role of similar mechanisms is relatively unexplored in gambling disorder. To this end, it may also be helpful to consider gambling disorder from a transdiagnostic dimensional perspective, as proposed by the RDoC initiative mentioned above [14]. Further, the specific alterations in relevant neurotransmitter systems in addiction in general [24] and also in gambling disorder [25, 26] are an ongoing debate; thus new insights can be expected in the future.

Commonly used neuroimaging methods may be extended by using alternate analytic strategies or adding other approaches. For example, using connectivity-based approaches like independent component analysis may provide additional insight over standard general linear model-based approaches [20, 27]. Additionally, as both genetic and environmental factors have been linked to the development of gambling disorder (see Chap. 5), it will also be helpful in the future to more intensively study the interplay of genetic variations and alterations in neurocircuitry in gambling disorder by using an imaging genetics approach, as it has been done in some studies of gambling disorder [28, 29] and more extensively for other psychiatric disorders like depression [30].

In addition, animal models for gambling disorder may permit additional insight into the condition as has been the case for substance-use disorders. A more comprehensive understanding of subtypes of individuals with gambling disorder or an identification of the most relevant functional mechanisms may lead to delineating a conceptual framework for animal research in this field. This can in turn lead to refinement of animal models with high translational validity, including rodent gambling and slot-machine tasks, that may be employed in studies using procedures and manipulations that are not permissible in humans (see Chap. 6).

Further, as an addition to the more classical approaches in neurobiological research, using computational models often allows for an improved mapping of neural substrate functions to clinically relevant behaviors. Thus, strengthening the use of computational modeling in the research on gambling disorder is likely to further increase our knowledge of the neurobiological basis of disordered gambling (see Chap. 7), as is the case in substance-use disorders [23, 31]. Decisively, computational approaches may provide generative models describing the key steps processed in the brain when adapting to a changing environment [1, 32]. Thus, by helping to understand alterations of neuronal processing in gambling disorder, these approaches may also allow for the development of new treatment options targeting core features of gambling disorder in a more direct way.

15.2.3 Advancing Prevention and Treatment

Fortunately, increasing effort is spent on the development of specific treatment programs as well as prevention strategies. With a focus on psychotherapy, studies have shown that the studied treatment programs yield benefits in reducing gambling problems, particularly cognitive-behavioral therapy in individual as well as in group settings. Since many interventions for gambling disorder suffer from low engagement and completion rates, it is important to foster the development of brief interventions and to find alternative ways of supplying help to affected people (see Chap. 9). Therefore, self-directed, computer-facilitated, web-based, and virtual reality interventions all warrant investigation and may extend the reach of existing treatments in the future. Moreover, the development of innovative approaches for the treatment of gambling disorder includes the evaluation of different cognitive and mindfulness trainings (see Chap. 10).

Despite the public health impact of gambling disorder and unlike in other psychiatric disorders, there are no medications formally approved for treatment of gambling disorder. Further, the above-described evidence shows that gambling disorder does not present with a homogeneous clinical picture, but different subtypes may exist [33]. This situation makes it important to understand the effects of medications on different symptoms of disordered gambling and, therefore, which medications may be best for specific subgroups of patients (see Chap. 8). Further insights are needed in order to develop customized pharmacological treatment strategies for the most severely affected. Moreover, there is a need for larger clinical trials, giving the opportunity of studying medication effects in different subtypes, doses, and treatment durations and/or with the focus on shorter-term and longer-term outcomes. To improve available treatment options, it is crucial to further elucidate how pharmacotherapy and other agents (e.g., nutraceuticals) may interact with psychotherapy [34, 35].

Further psychological and neurobiological insights may increase effectiveness and suitability of interventions by translating scientific results into clinical solutions. For example, some studies aim at the development of new pharmacological strategies based on the knowledge about neurobiological dysfunctions in addictions, like using a fast-working nasal spray containing naloxone that may potentially be used in high-craving situations [36].

Altogether, gambling disorder is associated with negative consequences in different domains of everyday life. Thus, developing more efficient prevention programs is essential for the general population and for specific groups like adolescents (see Chap. 14). Given elevated rates of gambling disorder in some populations (e.g., in immigrant groups), it is important to develop specific prevention strategies in high-risk populations and to ensure that such treatments reach affected people in a sufficient way by including multilingual material and cross-cultural skills into prevention and treatment (see Chap. 13). In general, it is necessary to incorporate the prevention of gambling disorder into our understanding of public health in order to draw public attention to this topic and to foster the development of new strategies for dealing with a changing landscape of gambling including new phenomena like mobile gambling and gambling elements in gaming.

References

1. Heinz A. A new understanding of mental disorders. Computational models for dimensional psychiatry. Cambridge, MA: MIT Press; 2017.
2. Kessler RC, et al. DSM-IV pathological gambling in the national comorbidity survey replication. Psychol Med. 2008;38:1351–60.

3. Petry NM, Stinson FS, Grant BF. Comorbidity of DSM-IV pathological gambling and other psychiatric disorders: results from the national epidemiologic survey on alcohol and related conditions. J Clin Psychiatry. 2005;66:564–74.
4. Nature. Science has a gambling problem. Nature. 2018;553:379. http://www.nature.com/doifinder/10.1038/d41586-018-01051-z. Retrieved 6 Oct 2018.
5. Ladouceur R, Shaffer P, Blaszczynski A, Shaffer HJ. Responsible gambling: a synthesis of the empirical evidence. Addict Res Theory. 2017;25:225–35.
6. Potenza MN, Higuchi S, Brand M. Call for research into a wider range of behavioural addictions. Nature. 2018;555:30.
7. Petry NM. Should the scope of addictive behaviors be broadened to include pathological gambling? Addiction. 2006;101:152–60.
8. Potenza MN. Should addictive disorders include non-substance-related conditions? Addiction. 2006;101:142–51.
9. Psychiatry Online. Gambling disorder to be included in addictions chapter. Psychiatr News 2013;48:5. http://psychiatryonline.org/doi/abs/10.1176/appi.pn.2013.4b14. Retrieved 6 Oct 2018.
10. Romanczuk-Seiferth N, van den Brink W, Goudriaan AE. From symptoms to neurobiology: pathological gambling in the light of the new classification in DSM-5. Neuropsychobiology. 2014;70:95–102.
11. Edwards G. Withdrawal symptoms and alcohol dependence: fruitful mysteries. Br J Addict. 1990;85:447–61.
12. Korn DA, Shaffer HJ. Gambling and the health of the public: adopting a public health perspective. J Gambl Stud. 1999;15:289–365.
13. Heinz A. Dopaminergic dysfunction in alcoholism and schizophrenia – psychopathological and behavioral correlates. Eur Psychiatry. 2002;17:9–16.
14. Insel T, et al. Research domain criteria (RDoC): toward a new classification framework for research on mental disorders. Am J Psychiatry. 2010;167:748–51. http://psychiatryonline.org/doi/abs/10.1176/appi.ajp.2010.09091379. Retrieved 30 July 2018
15. Balodis IM, et al. Diminished frontostriatal activity during processing of monetary rewards and losses in pathological gambling. Biol Psychiatry. 2012;71:749–57.
16. Chase HW, Clark L. Gambling severity predicts midbrain response to near-miss outcomes. J Neurosci. 2010;30:6180–7.
17. Genauck A, et al. Reduced loss aversion in pathological gambling and alcohol dependence is associated with differential alterations in amygdala and prefrontal functioning. Sci Rep. 2017;7:16306.
18. Romanczuk-Seiferth N, Koehler S, Dreesen C, Wüstenberg T, Heinz A. Pathological gambling and alcohol dependence: neural disturbances in reward and loss avoidance processing. Addict Biol. 2015;20:557–69.
19. Worhunsky PD, Malison RT, Rogers RD, Potenza MN. Altered neural correlates of reward and loss processing during simulated slot-machine fMRI in pathological gambling and cocaine dependence. Drug Alcohol Depend. 2014;145:77–86.
20. Worhunsky PD, Potenza MN, Rogers RD. Alterations in functional brain networks associated with loss-chasing in gambling disorder and cocaine-use disorder. Drug Alcohol Depend. 2017;178:363–71.
21. Deserno L, et al. Chonic alcohol intake abolishes the relationship between dopamine synthesis capacity and learning signals in the ventral striatum. Eur J Neurosci. 2015;41:477–86.
22. Garbusow M, et al. Pavlovian-to-instrumental transfer effects in the nucleus accumbens relate to relapse in alcohol dependence. Addict Biol. 2016;21:719–31.
23. Heinz A, et al. Targeted intervention: computational approaches to elucidate and predict relapse in alcoholism. Neuroimage. 2017;151:33–44.
24. Nutt DJ, Lingford-Hughes A, Erritzoe D, Stokes PRA. The dopamine theory of addiction: 40 years of highs and lows. Nat Rev Neurosci. 2015;16:305–12.
25. Potenza MN. How central is dopamine to pathological gambling or gambling disorder? Front Behav Neurosci. 2013;7:206.

26. Potenza MN. Searching for replicable dopamine-related findings in gambling disorder. Biol Psychiatry. 2018;83:984–6.
27. Xu J, et al. Large-scale functional network overlap is a general property of brain functional organization: reconciling inconsistent FMRI findings from general-linear-model-based analyses. Neurosci Biobehav Rev. 2016;71:83–100.
28. Grant JE, et al. A proof of concept study of tolcapone for pathological gambling: relationships with COMT genotype and brain activation. Eur Neuropsychopharmacol. 2013;23:1587–96.
29. Yang B-Z, Balodis IM, Lacadie CM, Xu J, Potenza MN. A preliminary study of DBH (encoding dopamine beta-hydroxylase) genetic variation and neural correlates of emotional and motivational processing in individuals with and without pathological gambling. J Behav Addict. 2016;5:282–92.
30. Pereira LP, et al. Imaging genetics paradigms in depression research: systematic review and meta-analysis. Prog Neuropsychopharmacol Biol Psychiatry. 2018;86:102–13.
31. Yip SW, Scheinhost D, Nich C, Potenza MN, Carroll KM. Connectome-based prediction of future cocaine abstinence. Am J Psychiatry. In press.
32. Friston KJ, Stephan KE, Montague R, Dolan RJ. Computational psychiatry: the brain as a phantastic organ. Lancet Psychiatry. 2014;1:148–58.
33. Blaszczynski A, Nower L. A pathways model of problem and pathological gambling. Addiction. 2002;97:487–99.
34. de Brito AMC, et al. Topiramate combined with cognitive restructuring for the treatment of gambling disorder: a two-center, randomized, double-blind clinical trial. J Gambl Stud. 2017;33:249–63.
35. Grant JE, et al. A randomized, placebo-controlled trial of n-acetylcysteine plus imaginal desensitization for nicotine-dependent pathological gamblers. J Clin Psychiatry. 2014;75:39–45.
36. The Guardian. Nasal spray aimed at tackling gambling addiction to be trialled in Finland | Science | The Guardian. 2018. https://www.theguardian.com/science/2018/jan/08/finnish-researchers-gambling-addiction-nasal-spray. Retrieved 6 Oct 2018.